INDIRECT HANDBOOK FOR ADVANCED NURSING ROLES

BEYOND THE BEDSIDE

PATTI RAGER ZUZELO, EdD, RN, ACNS-BC, ANP-BC, CRNP, FAAN

Clinical Professor, Nursing
Drexel University
College of Nursing & Health Professions
Advanced Nursing Practice Department/Doctor of Nursing Practice Program
Philadelphia, Pennsylvania
Associate Editor, *Holistic Nursing Practice*
Past President, *National Association of Clinical Nurse Specialists*

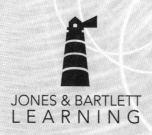

JONES & BARTLETT
LEARNING

World Headquarters
Jones & Bartlett Learning
5 Wall Street
Burlington, MA 01803
978-443-5000
info@jblearning.com
www.jblearning.com

Jones & Bartlett Learning books and products are available through most bookstores and online booksellers. To contact Jones & Bartlett Learning directly, call 800-832-0034, fax 978-443-8000, or visit our website, www.jblearning.com.

Production Credits

VP, Product Management: David D. Cella
Director of Product Management: Amanda Martin
Product Manager: Rebecca Stephenson
Product Assistant: Christina Freitas
Production Manager: Carolyn Rogers Pershouse
Vendor Manager: Molly Hogue
Senior Marketing Manager: Jennifer Scherzay
Product Fulfillment Manager: Wendy Kilborn
Composition: S4Carlisle Publishing Services
Project Management: S4Carlisle Publishing Services
Cover Design: Kristin E. Parker

Rights & Media Specialist: John Rusk
Media Development Editor: Troy Liston
Cover Image: © Mehau Kulyk/Science Photo Library/ Getty Images (Abstract pattern, Computer artwork), © Magurova/iStock/Getty Images (Abstract border- Illustration); Chapter Opener: © Mehau Kulyk/Science Photo Library/Getty Images (Abstract pattern, Computer artwork)
Printing and Binding: McNaughton & Gunn
Cover Printing: McNaughton & Gunn

Library of Congress Cataloging-in-Publication Data
Names: Zuzelo, Patti Rager, author.
Title: Indirect care handbook for advanced nursing roles : beyond the bedside
  / Patti Rager Zuzelo.
Description: 1st edition. | Burlington, MA: Jones & Bartlett Learning,
  [2020] | Includes bibliographical references and index.
Identifiers: LCCN 2018016318 | ISBN 9781284144109 (paperback)
Subjects: | MESH: Nurse Clinicians--organization & administration | Nurse's
  Role | Nursing Care--organization & administration
Classification: LCC RT89 | NLM WY 128 | DDC 362.17/3068--dc23 LC record available at https://lccn.loc.
  gov/2018016318

6048

Printed in the United States of America
22 21 20 19 18   10 9 8 7 6 5 4 3 2 1

Contents

Chapter 10 Recognizing and
                Responding to
                Risk, Harm, and
                Liability 343

*Patti Rager Zuzelo, EdD, RN, ACNS-BC, ANP-BC,
CRNP, FAAN and Joanne Farley Serembus,
EdD, MSN, RN, CCRN (Alumnus), CNE*

Acknowledgments

Drexel University's College of Nursing and Health Professions' Graduate Nursing Program provided tangible support during manuscript development under the leadership of Dr. Al Rundio, Associate Dean for Nursing & Continuing Nursing Education, Chief Academic Nursing Officer, Clinical Professor of Nursing; Dr. Kymberlee Montgomery, Associate Clinical Professor, Chair, Department of Advanced Practice Nursing, Nurse Practitioner and Doctor of Nursing Practice Programs; and Dr. Brenda Douglass, Assistant Clinical Professor, DNP Program Director. I am privileged to work with this talented administrative team and am appreciative of their enthusiastic support and collegiality.

Preface

This book builds on the approach used in *The Clinical Nurse Specialist Handbook* (2007, 2010), a book designed to offer a resource that was highly readable, usable, and helpful to students, educators, and practitioners. Over the decade or so of these two editions, I occasionally heard from nurse educators who were using the book for graduate students enrolled in non-CNS programs. Faculty members would share with me that the book provided students with practical information about responsibilities that were often inherent in advanced roles but were rarely explored in depth during clinical residencies or during didactic learning experiences. Educators and students emphasized the value of the coaching style of the book and its relevance to practice.

These conversations occurred simultaneous to the early years of interprofessional education (IPE) with its emphasis on teamwork, collegiality, and shared problem solving. The Patient Protection and Affordable Care Act (ACA) was the overlay to IPE and, during some of this time, the Advanced Practice Registered Nurse Consensus Model was also in its final development and implementation stages. These conversations made it evident to me that nurses continue to struggle with understanding and appreciating the unique and shared expertise of *intra*-professional colleagues. We persist in struggling with role confusion among nurse practitioners, CNSs, clinical nurse leaders, staff development experts, and other important roles that require advanced education and practice expertise. Although nurses are doing a good job of learning how to effectively work with other disciplines via interprofessional collaboration, there is still a need to appreciate the shared responsibilities and expertise that nurses have with other nurses, including those with master's or practice doctorate degrees.

Many conversations with new or established colleagues led to a recognized need for a book that offers guidance around shared goals and work responsibilities that cross formal role boundaries. A resource was needed to encourage advanced nurses of all types to recognize the value and power in collaboration *within* nursing—recognizing that there is plenty of work that needs to be done and interprofessional plus intraprofessional may be the route to success. Educators and advanced nurses shared with me that they enjoyed the original handbook because they used it across programs; the topics were relevant to a wide range of advanced nursing roles. The ACA has encouraged healthcare professionals to view work differently and while tensions continue to persist between different types of providers, at the sharp point of care, healthcare professionals are increasingly working together to improve outcomes measurement and care delivery processes, reduce harm risk, minimize threats of workplace violence, and develop the professionalism of self and peers, all while reducing consumption and encouraging sustainability!

The intended purpose of this book is to provide nursing graduate and doctoral study students and their faculties with the resources needed to address simple and wicked challenges in health care regardless of specific academic tracks or selected roles. Whether an advanced practice registered nurse, clinical nurse leader, manager, informatics department administrator, or staff educator is writing a self-evaluation, providing a peer review, or appraising a subordinate, the information needed and skills required are shared. When nurses have an interest in reducing the environmental impact of the healthcare agency by designing sustainability projects or establishing resource utilization guidelines, a collective group of advanced nurses coming to the table with unique and shared perspectives is likely the most effective way to maximize the impact of the ecofriendly plan. Of course, adding interprofessional colleagues to the mix is important as well.

We practice in a tumultuous period of time. There are threats and opportunities, recognized weaknesses and strengths across all systems of care. This handbook is crafted to maximize the *esprit de corps* that is needed to ensure a safe workplace and to improve all sorts of important outcomes. This book is novel in its approach and in its content. I hope that it provides opportunities for new learning around topics that trigger interesting projects and possibilities.

Please feel free to reach out and share your ideas, experiences, and critiques.

Thank you, colleagues.

About the Author

Patti Rager Zuzelo, EdD, RN, ACNS-BC, ANP-BC, CRNP, FAAN
Dr. Zuzelo is a Clinical Professor of Nursing in the Doctor of Nursing Practice Program of Drexel University in Philadelphia, Pennsylvania. She serves as Associate Editor of *Holistic Nursing Practice* and is a Past President (2010) of the National Association of Clinical Nurse Specialists. Dr. Zuzelo is nationally certified as an Adult Nurse Practitioner and an Adult Health Clinical Nurse Specialist and is a Fellow of the American Academy of Nursing. She is the author of *The Clinical Nurse Specialist Handbook* (2007, 2010), the 2007 *American Journal of Nursing*'s Book of the Year in the Advanced Nursing Practice Category. Dr. Zuzelo has been recognized with the Christian R. and Mary F. Lindback Award for Distinguished Teaching while teaching at La Salle University as a tenured Professor of Nursing. For 10 years, Dr. Zuzelo held a faculty-practice research appointment with Einstein Healthcare Network in the capacity of Associate Director of Nursing for Research.

Dr. Zuzelo earned an EdD in Higher Education Leadership from Widener University; a master's degree from the University of Pennsylvania in Nursing Administration; and a BSN from The Pennsylvania State University. She has a post-master's certificate from La Salle University in the Adult Nurse Practitioner program.

Contributors

Mary Beth Kingston, RN, MSN, NEA-BC
Executive Vice President and Chief
  Nursing Officer
Aurora Health Care
Milwaukee, WI
2018 President-Elect, American
  Organization of Nurse Executives

**Joanne Farley Serembus, EdD, RN, CCRN
  (Alumnus), CNE**
Associate Clinical Professor
Drexel University, College of Nursing
  and Health Professions
Philadelphia, PA

Reviewers

Jill Beavers-Kirby, DNP, MS, ACNP-BC, ANP-BC
Program Coordinator and Associate
  Professor
Mount Carmel College of Nursing
Columbus, OH

Eva M. Bell, DNP, APRN, FNP-BC, PMH CNS, PMHNP-BC
Assistant Professor
Texas A&M University,
Corpus Christi, TX

Karen Camargo, PhD, RN
Assistant Professor
MCPHS University
Boston, MA
UHV University
Victoria, TX

Jan Foecke, PhD, MS, RN, ONC
Director of Continuing Nursing
  Education/Education Assistant
  Professor
University of Kansas School of
  Nursing
Lawrence, KS

Peggy Jenkins, PhD, RN
Assistant Professor/Specialty Director
  iLEAD
University of Colorado College of
  Nursing
Aurora, CO

Deirdre Krause, PhD, ARNP, FNP-BC
Associate Professor
NOVA Southeastern University
  College of Nursing
Fort Lauderdale, FL

Shirley Levenson, FNP-BC
Professor
Texas State University, School of
  Nursing
Round Rock, TX

Amelia Malcolm, APRN, DNP, FNP-BC
FNP Program Coordinator
Brenau University
Gainesville, GA

Tammy McGarity, DNP, MSN, RN, NEA-BC
President/CEO, Clinical Advisory Team
University Health System
San Antonio, TX

Judy Phillips, DNP, FNP-BC, AOCN
Assistant Professor
Cancer Center of Western N.C.
Lenoir-Rhyne University
Asheville, NC

Beverly Reynolds, RN, EdD, CNE
Professor, Graduate Nursing Program
Saint Francis Medical Center College
  of Nursing
Peoria, IL

Terri Shumway, DNP, APRN, FNP-BC
Lead Faculty FNP Program, Assistant
  Professor
Saint Francis Medical Center College
  of Nursing
Peoria, IL

Julie G. Stewart, DNP, MPH, FNP-BC, FAANP
Associate Professor and Director of
  FNP and DNP Programs
Sacred Heart University
Fairfield, CT

Ruth Stoltzfus, PhD, CPNP-PC
Professor of Nursing, Director of
  Graduate Program in Nursing
Goshen College
Goshen, IN

Rhonda K. Tower-Siddens, PhD, MSN, APRN, FNP-C, CNE
Assistant Clinical Professor
Sacred Heart University
Fairfield, CT
Family Nurse Practitioner
Winnsboro Internal Medicine
Winnsboro, TX

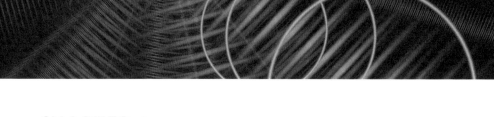

CHAPTER 1

Strategic Career Planning: Professional and Personal Development

Patti Rager Zuzelo, EdD, RN, ACNS-BC, ANP-BC, CRNP, FAAN

Nurses have access to a wide variety of career paths and a masters or a doctoral degree provide entrance to any number of advanced roles. Some roles are considered advanced *practice*, including clinical nurse specialists (CNSs), nurse practitioners (NPs), nurse anesthetists (NAs), and nurse midwives (NMs). These advanced practice roles require national certifications and state-specific credentialing. The educational programs that provide the degrees needed for advanced practice credentialing examinations are periodically evaluated by recognized accrediting bodies that have verified the quality of the program and its adherence to established curricular requirements.

In addition to these advanced practice registered nurse (APRN) roles, nurses have options to prepare for advanced roles that do not fall under the *practice* designation. These roles directly or indirectly influence health care in some sort of clear or tangential way; but, a nurse with a graduate degree from an educational program exclusive of the four APRN roles is likely not directly engaging with patients as would nurses in advanced practice. Nonetheless, although these nurses are not titled as APRNs, their contributions to informatics, administration, education, quality assurance/improvement, risk management, and other key health care system components are important and valuable.

Given the many diverse role opportunities available to nurses, it is not uncommon for nurses to lack full understanding of the work performed by those who practice in unrelated advanced roles, including APRN roles. One such example is the lack of familiarity that many nurses express regarding knowledge of the roles and responsibilities of the CNS. The specialization of the CNS and the organizing framework of CNS practice, known as the CNS spheres of influence (National CNS Competency Task Force, 2010), are sometimes difficult to articulate when comparing them to the role and responsibilities of the clinical nurse leader (CNL) who may have many years of clinical practice within a particular specialty plus a graduate degree as a "nurse generalist." Some nurses are confused by the responsibilities of a certified registered nurse anesthetist (CRNA). Nurse informatics specialists are often called on to explain their unique specialization. The nurse practitioner title is highly recognizable and is usually appreciated as an APRN role; however, many members of the health care team continue to be misinformed as to the role's uniqueness as compared to physician assistants or physicians.

The takeaway message is that role diversity in nursing is one of the profession's strengths while simultaneously contributing to role confusion and, at times, role antagonisms within and outside of nursing practice. Advanced nurses, those in APRN roles and those practicing in other roles that require advanced education, specialization, and expertise, share common job tasks and professional performance expectations. Getting to know each other and working together to meet common goals are important outcomes that require acknowledgment and attention. A good starting point is to consider how nurses can strategically bloom in their respective roles while supporting other advanced nurse colleagues, working with nonnursing health care team members, and improving health care processes and health outcomes. This book is written to encourage knowledge within nursing about various roles and their unique contributions to health care outcomes while also sowing a sense of appreciation for and recognition of the tremendous contributions of all types of advanced nurses to improved individual and public health.

This chapter focuses on both professional and personal development. Professional development is considered from two vantage points: advanced expertise and professional or scholarly development. Personal development is approached as a requisite component of professional practice, in other words, a call for advanced nurses, APRNs and others, to attend to the self and to role model the health-promoting behaviors that nurses advocate as important for clients, colleagues, and family members.

▶ Reflection and Self-Appraisal: Know Yourself

Prior to beginning the activities of this chapter, it is important to reflect on individual accomplishments, learning needs, challenges, expectations, talents, and experiences. Honest appraisal requires self-knowledge. For example, if an advanced nurse is beginning a search for a new expanded opportunity, it is important to proactively consider aspects of potential employment prospects that are most appealing and least appealing, to distinguish opportunities that may be a good fit from those that are likely a poor match.

If routinized work patterns are not appealing, contributing to diverse projects, taking risks and addressing systems issues that require rapid change improvements may sound intriguing. An advanced role, in this case, with a focus on short-term projects, data-driven systems changes, or Lean Six Sigma project implementation may be an ideal match. On the other hand, if careful attention to detail, stability, and an interest in patient education, staff development, and continuous quality improvement activities are of interest, a position as a unit or program-based advanced nurse with shared responsibilities for outcomes management or staff education may be very suitable.

For the nurse who feels accomplishment when "watching things grow" and appreciates opportunities to tend to the needs of developing nurses when facilitating professional growth, a position that includes teaching, evidence-based practice coaching, or shared governance activities might be best. Advanced nurses who prefer working with professionally diverse colleagues and shepherding new initiatives via interprofessional teams may be well served by looking for opportunities that focus on improving systems efficiencies by using nursing science and analytical sciences. Knowing what is personally appealing versus unappealing about work environments, job tasks, and role responsibilities is an important preliminary step for effective career building.

Contemplate Self-Care Practices

Reflecting on the personal self is a valuable activity and may be useful to do in partnership with professional reflection activities. Professional nurses frequently advise patients, families, and colleagues to take time out for self-care. Nurses recognize that there is value in leisure, exercise, and physical fitness and that these behaviors are critical for long-term physical and mental health. Yet, many nurses have poor diets with resulting excess body weight or obesity (Miller, Alpert, & Cross, 2008). Many nurses use tobacco products, do not exercise, and internalize stress. The *Healthy Nurse, Healthy Nation* movement is a nationwide effort in which nurses participate to improve their personal health and that of their families and their patients (American Nurses Association [ANA], 2018). This initiative provides an opportunity to register at no cost and complete a health behaviors survey that assesses health strengths, risks, and possibilities for improvement. Respondents are encouraged to commit to individualized improvement goals and, if desired, communicate with others for support and networking via an active discussion board that is organized around topics of interest.

Tobacco Cessation

One particularly concerning health behavior that warrants serious reflection is tobacco use. Conversations about cigarette smoking can be difficult to initiate with colleagues because striking a balance between actively and energetically promoting nicotine cessation versus berating and chastising smokers is challenging (Zuzelo, 2017). Self-appraisal is associated with its own set of challenges because nurses who smoke often experience guilt, self-blame, and remorse. They may conceal the extent of their smoking habits. While a majority of health care professionals has not smoked, a significant number are smokers (Sarna, Bialous, Nandy, Antonio, & Yang, 2014). The good news is that the number of registered nurse (RN) smokers has dramatically decreased since 2003 with one-third fewer nurses smoking by 2011 (Sarna et al., 2014). A review of literature did not reveal RN smoking rates organized by differing types of roles; but, it is likely that the RN smoker group includes nurses practicing in advanced capacities.

The experiences of nurses who smoke are influenced by their status as health care professionals. One research study used focus groups to describe issues related to nurses' attitudes toward smoking and quitting while also examining nurses' preferences for smoking cessation strategies (Bialous, Sama, Wewers, Froelicher, & Danao, 2004). Thematic analysis revealed that nurses' experiences with smoking addiction and cessation were consistent with those experienced by the general public, including feelings of shame and guilt. These emotional experiences were particularly applicable to nurses since family and friends believed that nurses were in a position to make better choices (Bialous et al., 2004).

Advanced nurses need to consider smoking cessation as a critical intervention for self-health and also as a necessary contribution to workplace health, particularly professional role modeling. Utilizing cessation opportunities and supports, both pharmacological and nonpharmacological, may enable the advanced nurse to successfully quit tobacco usage and promote the cessation efforts of others. Tobacco Free Nurses (2017) is an initiative that works to build capacity among nurses to equip them to assist patients with tobacco dependence and to become more involved in tobacco control efforts. Its website (https://tobaccofreenurses.org/) provides links to smoking cessation programs that advanced nurses may use or recommend to staff colleagues. Cessation programs may also be available in workplace settings and, if so, they are often accessible through employee assistance or employee health programs.

Stress Management

Nurses, including those in advanced roles, are challenged by work stress, shift schedules, and other circumstances that thwart healthy well-being. Many nurses are overweight due to job stress, snacking, inadequate exercise, and a work environment that encourages junk food, end-of-shift desserts, pizza, and pastries (Jackson, Smith, Adams, Frank, & Mateo, 1999). Nurses often do not engage in regular physical activity and live with irregular eating patterns (Nahm, Warren, Zhu, An, & Brown, 2012). Obese people are generally stigmatized in society (Zuzelo & Seminara, 2006) and these negative attitudes may be particularly pronounced in the health care setting.

Diet and Physical Activity Challenges

Nutritional deficiencies, caloric excess, and the need for self-care may be awkward conversation topics for nurses to have with their providers or colleagues but they are concerns that require contemplation and action. Approximately 20 years ago, Jackson et al. (1999) called for nurses to engage in and promote healthy lifestyles and confront the mixed message that patients receive when interacting with obese health care professionals. These concerns persist and are likely just as significant when it is the advanced nurse who is overweight with poor physical stamina given that nurses in leadership roles are perceived as role models and often expected to serve as examples for staff and care recipients.

Nurses tend to inconsistently address body mass index measurement with patients and avoid dietary counseling. They worry about hurting patients' feelings. As a result, many nurses avoid difficult conversations with patients about the need to diet, exercise, and lose weight (Zuzelo & Seminara, 2006). It is likely that conversation topics around nutritional challenges are equally challenging for nurses to initiate with colleagues.

Physical activity is a key determinant of health condition. Midlife women are particularly at risk for inactivity and although the percentage of men in nursing has increased by 12.5% between the years 2000 and 2010, the nursing workforce is predominately female at 91% (ANA, 2014). Compiled nurse demographics reveal that most nurses are in their fifth decade and female. Over 53 percent of working nurses are over 50 years of age (ANA, 2014). Midlife women tend to experience physiological and psychological transitions that decrease the amount of personal time available for physical activity (Dearden & Sheahan, 2002). Lack of physical activity contributes to weight gain, heart disease, and colon cancer, whereas exercise benefits physical health and mood while reducing distressing signs and symptoms of menopause (Dearden & Sheahan, 2002).

Postmenopausal women are at risk for obesity as well as osteoporosis and reduced joint flexibility. These factors contribute to musculoskeletal compromise as do many of the features inherent in nurse work, including prolonged walking and standing. Technologies such as standing computer stations or computerized medication administration carts increase musculoskeletal risks by reducing opportunities to sit, contributing to problems with feet and lower legs (Zuzelo, Gettis, Hansell, & Thomas, 2008). Advanced nurses need to carefully consider these concerns and develop strategies to reduce employee health risks and enhance well-being, particularly since the health care system needs aging nurses to stay in the workforce and contribute as productive and highly skilled professionals.

Advanced nurses must evaluate their personal health profiles and encourage staff and colleagues to do the same (**TABLE 1-1**). They should think about exercise, smoking cessation, sleep patterns, stress management, habits of health promotion, and weight. Advanced roles are incredibly challenging. Whether responding to project deadlines, orchestrating work assignments across disciplines, addressing health outcomes, responding to staffing challenges, or dealing with financial ramifications associated with reimbursement penalties, nurses in advanced roles certainly work within complicated and stressful practice environments.

Prioritize Self-Care Needs

While these challenges are onerous in their own right, compounding the unhealthy effects is the nurse's tendency to place role demands ahead of self-care activities. It is easy to justify a lack of exercise when the physical work of nursing is so demanding; however, a long day at work is not equal to a 20-minute brisk walk or aerobic exercise with weights. Jackson et al. (1999) suggest that nurses must begin "walking the walk of a healthy life style" (p. 1) and this directive certainly includes advanced nurses.

Keep Up with Personal Primary Care Needs

One excellent tool to assist advanced nurses in their quest for good health is the *electronic Preventive Services Selector* (ePSS) (https://epss.ahrq.gov/PDA/index.jsp) developed by the Agency for Healthcare Research and Quality (AHRQ, n.d.) and available to download at no charge. Designed to assist primary care practitioners to offer evidence-based recommendations to patients, the ePSS tool offers U.S. Preventive Services Task Force (USPSTF) recommendations and provides them in rank order based on appraised evidence. Interventions range from *recommended* to

TABLE 1-1 Queries to Guide a Personal Health Improvement Plan

Psychological/Social Queries	Physical Health Queries
Do I have quiet, reflective time for rejuvenating? Is there an opportunity for me to lead efforts to improve the practice environment so that a healthy milieu is created and maintained? How might I increase my opportunity for calm and solace? Is there an opportunity for incorporating meditation in my daily work routine? How do I increase my mindfulness? Alcohol intake inventory: Does my intake suggest a pattern of misuse? Depression screening Relationship health check: What is the status of my relationships? How do I want them to change and what do I need to do to achieve these goals? Am I safe from interpersonal violence?	Physical screenings. What is my current status? ■ Blood pressure ■ Blood glucose ■ Colonoscopy ■ Mammography ■ Lipid panel ■ Dental examination and cleaning ■ Vision examination ■ Sex-specific screenings: gynecologic or prostate ■ Hepatitis C virus testing ■ Bone health evaluation, including osteoporosis assessment if needed ■ Peripheral vascular health Sexual health, if sexually active: ■ Gonorrhea and chlamydia screening ■ Human immunodeficiency virus status ■ Am I a candidate for preexposure prophylaxis (PrEP)? Body mass index: ■ What is my height/weight/body mass? ■ How has my weight and body composition changed? Is this pattern cause for concern? Nutritional intake: ■ Meal patterns ■ Diet composition Tobacco-related behaviors Sleep patterns Exercise and physical activity routines

selectively recommended to *not recommended* and culminate in *uncertain* (AHRQ, n.d.). Specific USPSTF recommendations are provided with rationales, assessments, clinical considerations, burden of disease descriptions, and links to tools, including those for screening purposes. The ePSS provides an excellent guide not only for coordinating patient care but also for self-care planning. Many nurses work outside of primary care and keeping up with changes in primary care can be challenging for nurses who already struggle to maintain specialty expertise. The ePSS can be accessed via the web or downloaded onto a variety of electronic devices. It also has an application (app) available for smartphones.

The low rates of influenza vaccination among health care providers (HCPs) when compared to the 90% Healthy People 2020 target (Centers for Disease Control and Prevention [CDC], 2014) provides an excellent example of the need for advanced nurses to act on primary care and CDC health recommendations—not only to protect patients but also to protect themselves and their loved ones. Advanced nurses should serve as role models to colleagues and to the public. The CDC analyzed data that were retrieved from an internet panel survey conducted on HCPs. Findings revealed that early 2014–2015 season flu immunization rates among HCPs were 64.3%. Vaccination coverage in descending rank order by occupation reveals that pharmacists had the highest coverage followed by nurse practitioners and physician assistants, physicians, nurses, and other clinical professionals (CDC, 2014).

Advanced nurses have a role to play in improving these rates, not only by personally contributing to successful immunization campaigns via self-immunization but also by (1) exploring policies mandating immunizations; (2) developing systems to track rates while identifying and responding to barriers; and (3) educating employees about the evidence that underlies the push to immunize for flu. Survey findings exposed learning needs of health care professionals by revealing that the most common justification for nonimmunization status was an inaccurate belief that flu vaccines do not work (CDC, 2014). The CDC recommends that flu vaccination should be conveniently accessible to health care works at no cost. While many health care systems do provide free and convenient vaccination, there is room for improvement and, in particular, more attention is required to long-term care employee immunization rates. This is only one example of where advanced nurses may contribute to improving the healthiness of work environments.

It may be difficult for advanced nurses to prioritize personal health needs. Many organizational cultures are more inclined to implicitly reward the sacrificing, busy, tired advanced nurse rather than the nurse who insists on time for exercise, healthy lunches, bathroom breaks, personal time, and adequate hydration. However, it is empowering and necessary to promote self-health. Leading staff toward positive health practices may improve the quality of health-promotion activities in which nurses engage with patients.

Most nurses recognize the importance of teaching patients about health promotion and disease prevention. They may be neglectful of promoting these behaviors among colleagues and within their advanced practice peer group. Self-care is a worthwhile endeavor, but it must be a deliberately planned activity or it will be unaddressed. Advanced nurses should take the lead and promote smoking cessation, regular exercise, normal weight maintenance, snacking avoidance, routine healthy breakfast intake, regular sleep patterns with 7–8 hours nightly, and moderate alcohol intake. They can demonstrate this commitment to health as they strategically plan their professional *and* personal lives. They must proactively address both of these areas, never one at the consistent expense of the other. Professional success is enhanced by a state of personal well-being, and certainly longevity is improved when positive health practices become a routine way of life.

Advanced nurses influence through example. Those involved and engaged in professional activities tend to have more opportunities to share with interested staff. They have an increased ability to mentor because their repertoire of activities and experiences is greater than that of nurses who are less engaged. This premise applies to self-care practices as well. Advanced nurses cannot be haphazard in their approach to professional practice and must be equally disciplined in their approach to self-care. Leaders who manage their time and activities to benefit their health also benefit their families, colleagues, patients, and the organization (**EXEMPLAR 1-1**).

EXEMPLAR 1-1 The *Too Much to Do* Snare: Risking It All by Avoiding Self-Care

Judy Moore, DNP, RN, NEA-BC, is a busy administrator responsible for directing a cardiopulmonary program at a hectic university teaching hospital. Her partner, Tanya Johnson, MSN, RN, ANP-BC, is also very busy providing advanced care services in a primary care practice. Both Judy and Tanya are passionate about nursing practice and they work hard to satisfy the many professional demands of their respective roles. Their workdays begin early, typically arising by 0530 and ending late with a home arrival time that is usually around 1830. They have a teenage daughter living at home and an older son in college. Their financial status is secure although they both worry about paying for their son's college expenses while saving for their daughter's upcoming tuition following high school graduation. Judy's mother lives with them and she is helpful but does require some assistance managing her type 2 diabetes.

Judy does not provide direct care but is quite engaged with her team and values the close relationship that she has with managers and staff. Tanya practices in a stressful work environment that is understaffed and underresourced. Although she enjoys her job and is dedicated to the population that she serves, Tanya is conflicted about the toll that work is having on her personal health status and worries that she and Judy are failing to realistically address their personal health needs. Both women are 50 years old and experiencing menopause. Both are committed to service and teaching and they are actively involved in running health fairs and blood pressure screening events at their place of worship. They recently participated in a community blood glucose screening event. Neither is current in their age-appropriate screenings and immunizations. Judy has not had time for a mammogram for 2 years, and Tanya needs a vision screening given her family history of glaucoma and increased intraocular pressure findings revealed during her last appointment, approximately 2 years ago. Neither woman has had cervical cancer screening for the past 4 years.

During a particularly busy workday, Judy dropped in on the employee health fair with the sole intention of receiving the required influenza immunization. The fair booth had a variety of informational pamphlets and recommended Web resources. A Healthy Nurse, Healthy Nation™ (HNHN; http://www.healthynursehealthynation.org/) flyer caught her eye and she began to chat with a clinical nurse specialist (CNS) who had familiarity with the program and expertise in women's health. Judy shared with the CNS that both she and her partner were approximately 20–30 pounds overweight. They often purchased prepared meals and enjoyed ice cream and "treats" with a glass of wine or two in the evening before bed. Insomnia was a commonly experienced symptom for the both of them, and Judy had also noticed that she was waking in the morning with a cough, sore throat, and unpleasant taste in her mouth. She suspected that she had gastroesophageal reflux disease but was self-treating it with over-the-counter, intermittently administered medications.

The CNS enthusiastically encouraged Judy to consider exploring the HNHN website at home. Judy was intrigued enough to agree to do so with a tentative plan to speak with the CNS at some point over the following week. Later that evening, Judy and Tanya completed the HNHN survey and each responded to the queries related to nutrition, quality of life, physical activity, rest, and safety. Both were distressed to find that their survey results demonstrated high to moderate risk in every category. Tanya then suggested that they quickly take a look at the Agency for Health Care Research and Quality (AHRQ) Electronic Preventive Services Selector and conduct a candid evaluation of their current state of screenings and compile these results in combination with the HNHN survey results. Their daughter became involved in the conversation as well and

EXEMPLAR 1-1 The *Too Much to Do* Snare: Risking It All by Avoiding Self-Care *(continued)*

pointed out that both parents were overweight, highly stressed, and poor sleepers. She followed this observation with questions about their family history. Judy and Tanya began to earnestly consider their genograms and were compelled to recognize that Judy's familial risk for cardiovascular disease and diabetes was well established; while Tanya had a clear pattern of cardiovascular disease, glaucoma, and breast cancer.

Later that evening, Judy and Tanya developed a prioritized list of the U.S. Preventive Services Task Force recommendations that were relevant to their circumstances. They created a checklist that included mammography, colonoscopy, cervical cancer screening, and eye examinations. Tanya noted that her practice was emphasizing the importance of hepatitis screening, particularly hepatitis C. Additionally, both noted that they had not been tested for human immunodeficiency virus (HIV). They shared their disappointment in their lack of attention to their personal health, particularly given the influence that these behaviors may have on their children's prioritization of health screenings and health-promotion activities. They reflected on evidence supporting that nurses are less healthy than the average American (ANA, 2018) and are more likely to be overweight and highly stressed. The nurses also agreed that feelings of sleeplessness and sleepiness were more typical than feeling rested and that they often lamented these concerns during conversations at the dinner table that extolled their fatigue, stress, and workload anxiety.

The couple developed a plan that included their daughter so as to demonstrate the importance of self-care and to role-model behaviors that they recognized as essential to healthy aging and quality of life. This plan included biweekly engagement on the HNHN website to explore suggestions, strategies, and peer support in partnership with other nurses. Other self-care management goals included:

Judy and Tanya committed to contacting their primary care nurse practitioner to arrange for:

☐ complete physical examinations
☐ lipid panels
☐ cervical cancer screening
☐ blood glucose screening/glycosylated hemoglobin
☐ hepatitis screening
☐ total body skin checks
☐ blood pressure screening
☐ referrals for mammography and colorectal cancer screening

Age-appropriate immunizations (please refer to https://www.cdc.gov/vaccines/schedules/hcp/imz/adult.html):

☐ tetanus/diphtheria/pertussis
☐ influenza
☐ pneumococcal conjugate immunization (see Centers for Disease Control and Prevention recommendations)
☐ pneumococcal saccharide immunization
☐ hepatitis A
☐ hepatitis B
☐ Shingrix (herpes zoster protection; https://www.cdc.gov/vaccines/vpd/shingles/public/shingrix/index.html)

(continues)

EXEMPLAR 1-1 The *Too Much to Do* Snare: Risking It All by Avoiding Self-Care *(continued)*

Health promotion plan:

- ☐ routine exercise program including flexibility, strengthening, and stamina activities
- ☐ weekly shopping plan to include healthy foods and routine meal preparation
- ☐ reduced alcohol consumption
- ☐ reduced simple carbohydrates, including avoidance of white sugar and flour in meal planning
- ☐ a sleep program that includes restful downtime 1 hour before bed, herbal tea, and no electronic devices with a scheduled time frame that allowed for 7.5 hours nightly
- ☐ Scheduled eye examination

Judy and Tanya were pleased with their plan. They recognized the challenges but also appreciated the risks associated with a continued pattern of *too much to do and not enough time to do it!* They reflected on the piece written by Kreider (2012) and attached a small sign to their refrigerator, reading "Avoid the busy trap!"

The excited nurses brought their story to their colleagues at work and encouraged their nursing friends and coworkers to consider joining the HNHN™ Grand Challenge. They discussed the HNHN™ program with the nursing administration team and established an ad hoc committee to explore a partnership relationship with the program in hopes that the promotional materials and other resources might encourage participation (http://www.healthynursehealthynation.org/globalassets/all-images-view-with-media/partners/hnhn-gc-toolkit-final.pdf).

Judy and Tanya printed their primary care and health-promotion plan checklist and shared it as well. A few colleagues contributed additional items to the checklist. Many of the nurses shared their own personal health pitfalls and they collectively decided to support one another and celebrate those who came to work sharing stories about feeling rested and happy in their lives. They vowed to bring in healthy snacks to share rather than chips, pretzels, and soda. Caffeine consumption was discussed without resolution but there was firm resolve to cut back on caffeinated beverages during the second half of each shift. The nurses working with Tanya resolved to devote 15 minutes of each weekly staff meeting sharing health-promoting tips and exploring ideas for enhancing the healthfulness of the work environment.

Advanced nurses are encouraged to build on this health-promotion plan and consider the checklist created by Judy and Tanya. While doing so, advanced nurses should reflect on the following questions:

- How might an advanced nurse begin the process of learning to prioritize self-care, if this is an area of care requiring improvement?
- What barriers to self-care are often experienced by advanced nurses? How are some nurses able to manage these challenges? What may be learned from these "positive deviants"? (Refer to Chapter 9 for information about positive deviants.)
- What sorts of workplace changes could be designed to maximize the health care setting's positive impact on nurses' and other employees' health status?
- Is there a need for interprofessional opportunities for self-care support?
- What does the published literature reveal about workplace opportunities to improve employee health, including weight management, exercise, and stress reduction programs or self-care education?

Relationships Matter: Nurture Connections

In addition to attending to physical self-care needs, nurses usually recognize that relationships are important and need to be attentively tended to be healthy and resilient. Relationships require effort and engagement. However, nurses in all sorts of roles, including advanced nurses, may neglect to set aside deliberate time for nurturing relationships that are important to them. Despite advising others to attend to these needs, many times nurses are neglectful of their own personal priorities.

For example, it is not uncommon for advanced nurses to become involved in local, regional, and, in some cases, national organizations. These activities are rewarding but time consuming. The needs can be great, and nurses are accustomed to taking obligations very seriously. As a result, these committed nurses may experience personal burnout as they juggle family, clinical work, scholarship, and organizational activities.

It is imperative for nurses to carefully determine the time that is available for professional work within the context of the priorities of particular periods in life while consciously deciding to recognize and celebrate the events of life. "Living each moment" or "Live life to the fullest" are phrases that may be rather overdone, but they are important to keep in mind when working to effectively meet the demands of advanced nursing roles.

▶ Reflective Practice: Developing the Professional Self

Reflective practice is advocated in the United Kingdom (UK) as a learning process that encourages self-evaluation with subsequent professional development planning. UK practitioners are expected to meet a continuing professional development (CPD) standard, and reflection is a strategy that facilitates meeting this standard for revalidation (Royal College of Nursing [RCN], 2018). Registered nurses and midwives are required to develop a minimum of five written reflections related to selected activities. A template is provided to guide these written reflections and nurses are expected to reflect in and on action—defined as reflecting on an activity while in the midst of carrying it out or considering the practice event post hoc and creating knowledge from this consideration (RCN, 2018).

Tools are offered as resources to improve reflection, including a template to guide the written reflection, a list of tips to prepare reflections, a video that explores how to reflect as a component of revalidation, and RCN advice on reflection and reflective discussion (RCN, 2018). Several reflective models are provided to assist those nurses interested in a structured approach to reflections. Selected models highlighted by RCN (2018) include the reflective cycle by Gibbs, Johns's Model of Structured Reflection that connects reflective cues to Carper's (1978) patterns of knowing (specifically aesthetics, personal, ethics, and empirics), and Driscoll's (2007) cycle. Each model is linked to supplementary resource materials. The revalidation resources provide solid descriptive information and are rich with practical information, exemplars, and strategies (https://www.rcn.org.uk/professional-development /revalidation/reflection-and-reflective-discussion). Much of the work describing reflective practice as a strategy for facilitating continued, lifelong learning and for promoting professional competence has been published in UK journals.

In the United States, the term *reflective practice* is increasingly visible in the nursing literature, particularly in education-focused publications. Reflective activities are popular in baccalaureate and graduate nursing programs because the activities are valued as self-discerning. Students learn to question their practice and analyze situations to consider alternative behaviors and develop plans for future action. Journal-keeping is one particular learning strategy that encourages self-reflection and promotes critical analysis. This useful tool is now available as a feature on many popular distance or Web-based teaching platforms.

Reflection is a useful strategy for advanced nurses. It facilitates critical self-query and encourages movement toward the personal ideal of one's best nursing self. It is important to differentiate between thinking about daily work and reflecting on an experience, which requires intentionality and skill (Driscoll & Teh, 2001). Johns (2013) notes that reflective practice traverses from doing reflection to being reflective. Reflective practice demands the ability to analyze situations and make judgments specific to the effectiveness of situational interventions and the quality of outcomes. Johns (2017) offers a typology of reflective practices that can be quite helpful in appreciating the transition of moving from reflecting as an activity to reflection as a state of being. In other words, the practitioner moves from the act of doing reflection to the state of being reflective. When doing reflection, the practitioner contemplates on a selected situation post-event to learn and grow so that future practice is better informed. Reflective practices are considered within a typology that includes: reflection-on-experience; reflection-in action; the internal supervisor that involves self-dialogue simultaneous with conversing with another as a sense-making and response process; and, a reflective practice type of being mindful. The reflective practices transition moves from a technical/rational mode to one of professional artistry (Johns, 2017, p. 7).

Johns's work on reflective practice challenges nurses to think differently about experiences that may typically be viewed as routine and yet, upon thoughtful reflection, are likely to be revealed as incredibly powerful. One particularly interesting quote that offers interesting fodder for reflection is shared by Johns (2013, pp. 4–5):

> There are no easy answers to the life problems that face patients and nurses who strive to care. When we think we know the solutions to complex situations, we endeavor to apply such knowledge, yet when we seek to impose control of events through applying such knowledge, we somehow miss the point. Practice is a mystery, drama unfolding. We may have had similar experiences but not this one. We draw parallels but it is not the same.

Typically, nurses are inclined to keep care practices the same, as there is comfort in routine. Long-established rituals provide security. Reflection encourages nurses to reveal and consider behaviors, feelings, and ideas that would not ordinarily be examined. For this reason, reflection facilitates professional development. It is also a time-consuming activity that cannot be forced.

Driscoll and Teh (2001) note that the benefits of reflective practice include helping practitioners make sense of challenging and complicated practice, reminding practitioners that there is no end to learning, enhancing traditional forms of knowledge required for nursing practice, and supporting nurses by offering formal opportunities to converse with peers about practice. There are also downsides to reflective practice:

Finding the time, being less satisfied with the status quo, being labeled as a trouble-maker, and having more questions than answers are a few of the challenges associated with the deliberate examination of practice (Driscoll & Teh, 2001).

Advanced nurses may want to consider the various reflective practice models and look for opportunities to connect with a view that is particularly appealing or, conversely, a model that challenges an individually held worldview. In general, the models encourage nurses to consider a situation in clinical practice. This situation may be positive or negative but should be important in some sense. After describing the event in writing, practitioners are encouraged to dissect the experience. Practitioners reflect on the emotions, thoughts, and beliefs underlying the experience. They consider the motivation underlying their action choices and think about the consequences of their behaviors. The reflective practitioner is urged to consider alternatives and to challenge assumptions. The final step in the process typically relates to identifying the learning that has occurred and applying this new knowledge in future situations.

Reflective activity is viewed as an opportunity to deliberately think about practice events; evaluate choices, reactions, and behaviors; consider alternatives; develop plans for improvement or identify learning needs; and follow this action plan in new or similar situations. Johns (2004) warned that stage models of reflection may support the belief that reflection occurs in a sequential fashion moving from step to step. He cautioned that although this approach may be helpful for practitioners new to reflection, in general, reflective practice does not follow a rote stage model. However, rather than offering critique of alternative models of reflective practice, Johns (2013) suggests that nurses should reflect on the models and develop insights into what might work best in practice.

Reflective practice is described as holistic practice because it is focused on understanding the significance and meaning of the whole experience (Johns, 2004). Johns recognized layers of reflection that progress from a reflection on experience to mindful practice, which are in juxtaposition with moving from "doing reflection" to "reflection as a way of being" (p. 2):

> *Reflection is defined as being mindful of self, either within or after experience, as if [there is] a window through which the practitioner can view and focus self within the context of a particular experience, in order to confront, understand and move toward resolving contradiction between one's vision and actual practice. (Johns, 2004, p. 3)*

Reflective practice may provide a means for connecting the art and science of nursing within a caring context. Reflective practice is an active process and supports the development of practical wisdom (Johns, 2004).

▶ Mindfulness as a Strategy to Promote Well-Being

Mindfulness is a type of meditative practice that may be viewed as a technique, strategy, intervention, or a way of life depending upon cultural influences and philosophical beliefs (Myers, 2017). Acute awareness of the present can help nurses experience relaxation, tranquility, and self-attentiveness. Myers (2017) asserts that cultivating mindfulness in deliberate fashion can promote self-care and assist nurses in promoting well-being, particularly given the stressful practice environments in which nurses provide care. Advanced nurses have challenging roles with stressors that are multifactorial and contribute to burnout and chronic stress responses. Developing mindfulness as a component of reflective practice takes time and a commitment to regular and frequent practice. There are many free resources that offer opportunities for nurses in advanced roles to support and encourage subordinates, colleagues, patients, and families to also learn to take advantage of the benefits afforded by mindfulness meditation (**TABLE 1-2**). Wise advanced nurses need to keep in mind Myers's (2017) admonition that if leaders expect their employees to care for patients in environments that are safe, supportive, respectful, and transparent, they "must care for their employees by supporting mindfulness practices that promote well-being, joy, and meaning in the workplace" (p. 265). Of course, advanced nurses who accept this challenge will need to be knowledgeable about reflective practice and mindfulness so that they can model these desired behaviors and practices for staff.

TABLE 1-2 Opportunities for Nurturing Mindfulness

Type of Resource	Web Address/Contact Information	Descriptions/Notes
Professional Associations/Organizations		
American Mindfulness Research Association	https://goamra.org/	Scientific database of references available for download. Links to mindfulness centers and programs.
Mindfulness Association	http://www.mindfulnessassociation.org/Home.aspx	Offers courses and resources with an emphasis on long-term, systematic training.
Center for Mindfulness in Medicine, Health Care, and Society	https://umassmed.edu/cfm/training/	The Oasis Institute is housed in the center and provides professional education and training. The center's website provides a rich repository of evidence-based recommendations, class options (online and onsite), and video resources as well as other learning supports and opportunities.

Type of Resource	Web Address/Contact Information	Descriptions/Notes
Mindfulness Everyday	http://www.mindfulnesseveryday.org/	Charitable organization that provides programs on mindfulness and mindfulness-based stress reduction for people of all ages.
Mindful	https://www.mindful.org/free-mindfulness-apps-worthy-of-your-attention/	A mission-driven nonprofit that publishes a bimonthly magazine, *Mindful,* and offers workshops, conferences, and networking opportunities to support mindfulness.
Applications for Electronic Devices (refer to Web address or app stores for details)		
Insight Timer (Newman, 2017)	https://insighttimer.com/	
Aura (Newman, 2017)	https://www.aurahealth.io/	
Omvana (Newman, 2017)	http://www.omvana.com/	
Stop, Breathe, and Think (Newman, 2017)	https://www.stopbreathethink.com/	
Calm (Newman, 2017)	https://www.calm.com/	
The Mindfulness App (Abate, 2017)	App store	
Headspace (Abate, 2017)	App store	
MINDBODY (Abate, 2017)	App store	
Buddhify (Abate, 2017)	App store	
Insight Timer (Abate, 2017)	App store	
Smiling Mind (Abate, 2017)	App store	
Meditation Timer Pro (Abate, 2017)	App store	

Nurses should consider that the tension between vision and current reality creates learning opportunities (Johns, 2004). This tension may be uncomfortable, but it offers the opportunity to face and solve the problems creating the anxiety state. Johns (2004) suggests that reflection is a learning process that may develop tacit knowledge. One vehicle for reflection is journaling, whereas others include poetry writing, sharing stories, and creating a portfolio.

▶ Professional Portfolios: Opportunities to Gather Personal and Professional Insights

The act of creating a professional portfolio provides an opportunity to reflect on experiences and establish insights that may inform future decisions specific to practice, education, and professional activities. Portfolio creation compels advanced nurses, as well as other nurses, to carefully consider a variety of potential items for inclusion and, in doing so, to contemplate the relative worth of each activity and the contribution of the parts related to the "whole" of the individual's practice. Advanced nurses also should evaluate the various portfolio components and identify strengths, challenges, and gaps in knowledge, expertise, or experience. The professional portfolio provides a context to examine subsets of practice with a focus on self-improvement and self-development. Just as with reflective practice, portfolio development requires self-awareness.

The professional portfolio has become an increasingly popular modality for reflecting on professional development, self-evaluation, creativity, and critical thinking. Portfolios are also useful to track expertise acquisition and to demonstrate competency. McColgan (2008) conducted a literature review to explore current thinking on portfolio building and registered nurses. The literature review revealed four themes: (1) portfolio use as an assessment method for validating competence; (2) portfolio use as a work-based reflective evaluation tool; (3) the relationship between portfolio building and lifelong learning; and (4) portfolio building as a strategy to motivate and develop nurses.

McColgan (2008) noted that while there is much theoretical discussion concerning the benefits and influences of the portfolio as a vehicle for promoting professional development, there is a lack of empirical evidence supporting these claims. The reflective activities associated with portfolio development intuitively seem connected to self-discovery, self-evaluation, and professional and personal growth; however, evidence-based practice does not prioritize intuition as an effective way of knowing (Duffy, 2007).

Differentiating Portfolios and Profiles

It is important to understand the basic premise of a professional portfolio and to appreciate the differences between a portfolio and a profile. The terms *portfolio* and *profile* are often used interchangeably but they are not the same product. A professional portfolio provides a record of professional development. It is a collection of evidence of products and processes documenting professional development and learning experiences (McMullan et al., 2003). A profile is derived from the personal portfolio and the materials selected for inclusion should vary according to the audience and the purpose. For example, a Nurse Practitioner applying for advanced practice role recertification might select a portable document format (pdf) of a published research study, continuing education certificates, and a transcript of a recent pharmacology course from the portfolio to include in a profile that is being submitted with a recertification application.

Portfolios in some form are often encouraged or required in undergraduate or graduate education programs (Alexander, Craft, Baldwin, Beers, & McDaniel, 2002; Joyce, 2005). They also offer opportunities for APRNs seeking credentialing when certification examinations in unique clinical specialty areas are unavailable. Some agencies use professional portfolios as tools that document the professional development necessary for advanced practice and, in some cases, validate excellent performance (Chamblee, Dale, Drews, & Hardin, 2015).

The UK requires a professional portfolio to demonstrate continued competency and current professional knowledge. Continued professional development (CPD) is required and is included in the portfolio (Bowers & Jinks, 2004). The portfolio is registered with the UK Central Council and addresses the need for some type of assurance that professional development has continued after basic training is complete. Professional nurses practicing in Ontario must also meet standards of mandatory portfolio management as part of its quality assurance program (College of Nurses of Ontario, 2008). The National Council of State Boards of Nursing (NCSBN) considered a proposal for nurses to initiate and maintain a professional profile referred to as the Continued Competency Accountability Profile (CCAP) (Meister, Heath, Andrews, & Tingen, 2002).

At this point in time, the CCAP is on hold, but NCSBN continues to work on developing methods for ensuring nurse competency to protect the public. One analysis paper published by NCSBN (2005) explored continued competence in nursing and the important issues and challenges associated with regulating competence and assuring the public that competence is, in fact, present. NCSBN identified the barriers to establishing a national system for competence regulation and described the various state-level efforts to address competence.

This background information is important for a few reasons. Competency is a hot issue that is likely to increase in its intensity as a focal point of professional practice regulation. Unsafe nursing practice poses public risk and, as a result, assurance of professional competence is a perpetual concern that requires consideration and regulation supported by states' consensus.

Variability across states regarding licensure and practice regulations is concerning and confusing to the public. Some states do not require continuing education, and some have varying title protections with differing licensure requirements and educational mandates. The Pew Health Professions Commission (1998) and Institute of Medicine (2011) raised similar concerns related to the state of self-regulation and the need to protect the public.

NCSBN defines competence as "the application of knowledge and the interpersonal, decision-making, and psychomotor skills expected for the nurse's practice role, within the context of public health, welfare, and safety" (2005, p. 1). Advanced nurses must give serious thought to strategies for demonstrating competence, particularly given the breadth and depth of the scope of advanced practice and the varying competencies and standards applicable to each advanced nursing role, whether an APRN role or a role associated with advanced certifications that build on recognized standards of practice. Portfolios may facilitate this process by encouraging reflection, strategizing, and documentation.

Contextualizing the Professional Portfolio

Keep in mind that a portfolio provides a record of growth and change. Think of a portfolio as an evidentiary collection of products and processes (McMullan et al., 2003). A portfolio showcases accomplishments and serves to display the unique experiences of an individual nurse's professional efforts and expertise (Chamblee et al., 2015). The idea of a professional portfolio originated with professionals who were expected to display their work in a portfolio (e.g., artists, models, and architects). Portfolios offer advanced nurses a chance to reflect on achievements, develop goals, and forge new insights. In some cases, a portfolio may be required for professional advancement. A portfolio is also useful for developing clinical career pathways (Joyce, 2005) and is frequently encouraged within academic centers as a vehicle for self-assessment and professional development.

Portfolio contents vary, but most include a résumé or curriculum vitae (CV), selected examples of individual or group projects, letters of recommendation or commendation, awards, transcripts, continuing education certifications, community service activities, publications, and presentation abstracts or handouts. Typical portfolio components may also include evidence that support an individual's experience with the appraisal of colleagues including mentoring, educating, and precepting. Evidence-based practice activities are also often included (Chamblee et al., 2015). In general, a professional portfolio is an excellent way to organize personal best work products for private perusal, while also serving as a vehicle for showcasing work efforts to future employers or to peer review panels. Portfolios can assist in self-evaluation or reflective practice strategies, and they provide a physical structure for organizing materials that support the premise of competency.

Organizing the Portfolio

The physical nature of the portfolio may exist as an electronic folder, expandable file folder, a three-ring binder, or any form that is portable, professional, and visually appealing. An electronic portfolio is likely the best choice given that it can be easily printed into hard copies. It is also readily backed up, secure, and conveniently shared with others via email, share services, or other modalities. Creating the portfolio in an electronic form suggests that the advanced nurse is comfortable with technology and has an appreciation for the benefits of keeping current with required skill sets.

Another less obvious benefit of an electronic versus hard copy portfolio is that credentialing applications are more efficiently submitted using copy and paste functions across electronic mediums. The American Nurses Credentialing Center (ANCC; http://www.nursecredentialing.org/) offers an individualized member's database that can be regularly updated and used to inform applications for certification examinations or certification renewals. This database serves as an electronic portfolio, including information about continuing education, academic credits, presentations, publications or research, preceptorship experiences, and professional service.

Advanced nurses should carefully consider the contents of the portfolio. If too much documentation is included without sufficient organization, it can become unwieldy and overwhelming, regardless of whether the portfolio structure is print or electronic. In general, view the portfolio as a valuable tool for formative assessment rather than summative assessment. Formative assessment is used to monitor professional progress and guide development, whereas summative assessment is used to measure proficiency or appraise performance. Portfolio perusal provides evidence of professional growth over time rather than providing a summary of advanced nurses' expertise or talents.

The Printed Portfolio

Jasper (1995) suggested that the portfolio resembles a scrapbook and noted that Benner's (1984) model of skill acquisition is compatible with the portfolio strategy. Meister et al. (2002) recommended that portfolios include a table of contents, provide section dividers, and use high-quality paper. Bright white paper greater than 90 brilliance with weight greater than 20 pounds will provide a professional look and feel to a hard copy portfolio. Even if the portfolio is housed in electronic form, keep the recommendations for hard copy portfolios in mind when printing select content areas. The intended audience is an important consideration. Do not assume that sophisticated technologies are always best. There are times when the intended audience may not have easy access to cloud storage, software platforms, or speedy Internet. In these events, a high-technology portfolio may elicit frustration from the intended viewer and an attractive, readily available hard copy portfolio may be the best option.

Binders are available for purchase in a wide range of sizes from 1/2 inch to 6 inches. In general, purchasing a heavy-duty binder is well worth the money. The rings of economy style binders tend to slip open or have gaps when closed, leading to portfolio disarray. Professional portfolios should be contained in a single binder. If there is a lot of documentation, purchase the heavy-duty, 6-inch binders. Anticipate paying $30 to $40 for this binder style.

When creating the portfolio in paper form, avoid handwritten work. Tables of contents and dividers can be easily created with a word processor. Professional work requires a standard font style. The sixth edition of the *Publication Manual of the American Psychological Association* (2009) offers suggestions for professional writing and identifies Times New Roman or Courier, 10- or 12-point font, as appropriate styles. Use black ink and avoid "word art," dramatic shading, or friendly borders. Although such artistry may be appealing in a creative arts project, they are inappropriate for professional work.

Plastic page covers or sheet protectors provide convenient, attractive protection for the portfolio contents. Several styles of sheet protectors are available. A heavyweight, diamond clarity type of protector will allow clear visualization of the covered documents without lifting print. Purchase the acid-free variety for archival quality. Remember that the portfolio is meant to provide formative evaluation data and will be useful for decades.

The Electronic Portfolio

Electronic portfolios have many advantages over traditional hard copy portfolios. They are easily revised, stored, shared, and protected. Selected documents and activities can be quickly shared and spell check, grammar check, and formatting tools are readily available and handy. As electronic devices become more accessible and technology skills become more requisite, electronic portfolios become more attractive.

The convenience and relatively inexpensive costs associated with compact discs (CDs), digital video discs (DVDs), and flash drives should encourage advanced nurses to consider developing an electronic portfolio rather than a paper copy. Electronically produced portfolios validate nurses' technology skills and suggest that the advanced nurse is technologically savvy. Certainly such an impression is important given the high-tech nature of many health care settings. Do consider that many notebooks, tablets, and other electronic devices are no longer built with CD or DVD drives. Although how an advanced nurse decides to store electronic data for easy access is a personal choice, it may be best to consider a cloud service or large file transfer system as an option for delivering portfolios to intended recipients. Doing so will avoid possibly vexing access issues.

Flash drives, also known as thumb drives or USB drives, are easily attached to key rings, attaché cases, or handbags and are conveniently shared. A thumb drive may hold up to 1 terabyte of data and is the size of a stick of chewing gum. Keep in mind that the greater the memory capacity, the more expensive the flash drive. A 1-terabyte drive may cost approximately $50. Lower capacity drives may be purchased at a more reasonable cost; however, it is important to select a flash drive that has the capacity to store the entire portfolio. The portfolio may demand significant memory if it includes videos, hyperlinks, presentations, and other multimedia files. Many electronic devices have USB ports making the flash drive a convenient and likely practical choice for physically transporting the electronic portfolio.

Electronic portfolios allow video, audio, and interactive components to be included in the formative data set. The multimedia presentation maximizes individualism and gives the reviewer a real look at the interactive and presentation skills of the advanced nurse. For example, a hard copy presentation built in PowerPoint software offers less information than the actual slide show with embedded files and hyperlinks. It is also possible to include a video stream of an actual slide show presentation that includes the advanced nurse interacting with the audience. The possibilities are practically endless and it is this sort of creative effort that builds on reflection. Keep in mind that few people will want to view numerous full-length presentations or program events. Rather, it is best to also reflect on the sections of a presentation that provide the richest opportunity to best represent the total work product.

The Web-Based Portfolio

There are an increasing number of Web-based commercial options for maintaining a professional portfolio. In general, the consumer begins by establishing an account for a set fee. Once the account is created, the advanced nurse uploads pertinent documents and enters data into the portfolio system. Data may be retrieved in the form of comprehensive or mini-portfolios, depending upon the situation. Initial data entry may be time consuming; however, once the account is established, portfolio maintenance is simple and very convenient. Web-based portfolio systems are also available for entire departments and institutions. Such a system can be very useful for Magnet certification and recertification processes.

The American Heart Association, Sigma Theta Tau International, the Academy of Medical Surgical Nurses, and multiple health care systems and agencies use electronic portfolio services offered through HealthStream (2017). This is one example of a talent management system that combines credentialing, education, and other administrative features using a comprehensive Web-based system. These types of systems are increasingly popular to provide standardized and timely documentation of education and credentialing as well as to centralize data collection and analysis with attention to improving various outcomes. While this is one example of a fee-based product, the benefits of a systemwide electronic portfolio are somewhat similar to the benefits of establishing and maintaining an individual professional electronic portfolio.

Potential Risks of Portfolio Assessment

Portfolios require reflective practice, a process of self-scrutiny. Ideally, this scrutiny includes peer review. It is very likely that in the process of self-evaluation or peer review, errors or weakness in practice may be identified. When a portfolio is used as a public document to renew professional licensure or regulation, as in Canada or the United Kingdom, it is possible that if an area of practice has been identified as "weak" within a portfolio and a nurse makes a mistake in this particular area of practice, potential defense from lawsuits may be problematic. At this point in time the concern is unresolved but recognized.

▶ Publicizing Professional Experiences and Expertise: The Curriculum Vitae and Résumé

Advanced nurses must develop and maintain a written log that showcases their education, work history, contributions to the profession, awards and honors, and other key components that demonstrate a richly engaged professional life. This record may be in the form of a CV or résumé. Many advanced nurses have both types of records available for relatively quick review. They differ from each other but both require constant maintenance and each has a unique role to play as advanced nurses progress in their professional development.

Competing with a Curriculum Vitae

A curriculum vitae (CV) is a comprehensive list of professional accomplishments. The term is derived from the Latin *curriculum* ("course of action") and *vitae* ("life") (Weinstein, 2002). The advanced nurse should view the CV as the "door opener" to opportunity. It should accurately reflect the accomplishments and interests of the advanced nurse while providing the viewer with a solid sense of the nurse's professional identity. The CV is a marketing tool as well as a record. The acknowledged four Ps of marketing include *product, promotion, price,* and *position.* Weinstein (2002) suggests that the fifth P is *portfolio.* It may be that a sixth P is worth acknowledging and avoiding—specifically, *padding* of the vitae. Cleary, Walter, and Jackson (2013) describe padding as "misrepresenting one's achievements or contributions to a particular field, with the aim of inflating one's record or role(s) for the purpose of securing an unfair advantage over others in competitive endeavours [*sic*]" (p. 2363). CV padding is usually more subtle than overt record falsification but is still a dishonest approach to self-representation (**BOX 1-1**). Advanced nurses should make certain that they regularly update their CVs and also carefully scrutinize the document to ensure veracity.

BOX 1-1 Padding the Curriculum Vitae

- Overstating work responsibilities, including supervisory and budgetary accountabilities
- Suggesting a greater contribution to a project, manuscript, research protocol than is accurate
- Listing published abstracts from podium presentations or poster presentations as though they are published manuscripts
- Claiming credit for student work products without fully acknowledging the actual percentage of contributed effort
- Listing committee memberships without having participated or engaged in the committee's work efforts
- Documenting works "in progress" or "under review" when the work has stalled or has been reviewed on several occasions without likely publication
- Failing to specify when professional activities have been invited or subjected to blind review
- Avoiding to note when positions are rotating appointments (e.g., taking turns) versus competitively elected roles
- Citing awards and recognitions without describing the selection process as noncompetitive, juried, peer reviewed, or student/staff initiated
- Documenting fellowships without sharing significant details, including competitive versus noncompetitive admission processes
- Taking credit for work setting projects that were group endeavors and overstating outcome improvements

TABLE 1-3 Résumé and Curriculum Vitae in Contrast

Résumé	Curriculum Vitae
Overview	Extensive description
One page in length—never more than two pages	Several pages in length. May be dozens of pages, depending on career length and productivity
Job application	Multiple uses including professional office, job application, awards, grants, presentations
Employment origins	Academic origins

The CV differs from a résumé (**TABLE 1-3**). There are general, customary guidelines for CV structure. Use a standard font and consistent font size. Although bold may be used, avoid designer fonts, colors, and elaborate spacing. Customary font styles include Times New Roman, Arial, and Courier in a 12-point size. Do not use a font size less than 10. Using spell check is critical.

CVs should be printed as one-sided documents usually on quality paper. In general, the advanced nurse will not err by selecting bright white paper of 92 or greater brilliance in 24-pound weight. Other paper forms are acceptable, including 100% cotton fiber; however, it is best to avoid pastel or tinted paper unless the color is off-white.

Create a header and include the last name with page number. Although it is acceptable to staple the pages together, there is still a possibility that pages will detach. A header or footer will make it easier to identify missing pages. Also, the advanced nurse may find it necessary to electronically send the CV, and a paginated header or footer will assist the recipient in keeping the document organized.

Structuring the Curriculum Vitae

Format the pages with the CV's headings flush with the left margins. Consider 1-inch margins or less. In general, begin with name, home address, and home telephone number and/or mobile phone number. Include the preferred email contact information. Make certain that each provided phone number is connected to a voice message that is professional and is readily identifiable as the message center for the applicant. Consider that the provided email address should be designed with return address information, including any quotations or expressions that have been added to the address that is appropriate and helpful.

Although some older publications recommend including a social security number (Hinck, 1997), given the possible distribution of the CV and the threat of identity theft, this is not a wise decision. Professional license numbers and certification credentialing should be included.

In writing, do not use pronouns. Use an active voice with appropriate tense and phrases rather than full sentences. For example, avoid, "I developed a research-based protocol for bladder ultrasound in lieu of bladder catheterization with annual savings of $165,000." Instead use, "Designed and implemented bladder ultrasound program with $165,000 annualized savings."

CV formatting varies and is primarily based on personal preference as well as the underlying purpose of the CV. For example, if the advanced nurse is submitting a CV to self-nominate for a key leadership position of a professional organization, the applicant may want to consider reformatting the CV to highlight the skills and experiences that are requisite for this type of opportunity. It is easy to revise and update word-processed CVs, but make certain to save revised files by the revision date for easy access.

There are many ways to structure a CV. Most list recent experiences first and move in a reverse chronological order. For example, in the education section, the highest degree earned is identified followed by the next highest degree. Do not include postsecondary school education prior to college. Include nondegree course work under continuing education or as a separate category.

Professional certifications should be noted on the CV. Certification as an APRN or as an advanced nurse with specialty expertise is increasingly important for practice, albeit inconsistently regulated at state levels or unevenly required across health care systems. The advanced nurse should note all types of certifications, including advanced cardiac life support (ACLS), cardiopulmonary resuscitation (CPR), chemotherapy, neonatal advanced life support (NALS), and any other relevant type of certified expertise. It may be useful to include the date of the most recent child abuse clearance and a criminal background check and offer to make these reports available on request.

These clearances save time and are increasingly expected, particularly when nurses are working with vulnerable patients or client populations.

All types of publications should be listed. Consider separating publication types: research versus nonresearch, and refereed, nonrefereed, invited, and newsletter contributions. List newsletter publications by professional organization, public organization, institution, department, or unit-based categories. Make certain to include published abstracts, but clearly identify the name of the conference proceedings and whether the abstract was accepted following peer review, blinded or nonblinded. Be clear about whether published abstracts pertain to competitively selected podium presentations at local, regional, state, national, or international venues versus poster presentations or group symposiums.

For the advanced nurse who has not yet published or has done so but scantily, consider this area as a possible area for development. There are beginning opportunities to publish, including book reviews, newsletters, and letters to editors. These first steps demonstrate an interest in writing and set the CV apart from those without publications in any form. In the meantime, if there is no publication credit, simply leave this topic off the CV. Do not include the heading and note "not applicable" or "none."

Grant applications, successful or unfunded but competitively scored, are important indicators of professional efforts. The type of grant should be noted—for example, federal, state, or local agency; competitive nature of the grant; funding request/award; contribution to the grant application endeavor if multiple people worked on the submission; and any other details that assist the reader in appreciating the significance of the grant. If there are multiple unfunded and poorly scored grant applications, it may be best to not include them on the CV. While they do demonstrate effort, there is a possibility that they also represent a lack of organization, writing ability, or appreciation for the priorities of the funding agency. Of course, the grants environment is very competitive and this context requires some consideration as well. Again, reflection is needed to make good decisions about what to include or exclude from the CV.

Professional organizations should be included on the CV. Note any leadership positions within an organization. The advanced nurse should critique the depth and breadth of the active membership organizations and contemplate joining a collection of organizations that represent a national nursing interest, clinical area of practice, local or regional organization, scholarly activity or research focus, as well as an organization that reflects a commitment to relationships, such as an alumni organization. Dues can become burdensome, so it is wise to select carefully. On the other hand, advanced nursing practice demands professionalism. It is difficult to demonstrate professional commitment without any type of nursing organization membership, particularly if there is a nursing organization that is solely designed to address the needs of nurses within the organization's specialty or to respond to policy or politics as the representative voice of nursing.

Honor society memberships should be included on the CV. Sigma Theta Tau, International is the worldwide honor society for nursing, and admission is competitive. Other honor societies should also be listed, including those that are outside nursing (e.g., Phi Beta Kappa or Phi Kappa Phi). Honor society memberships outside nursing are not uncommon, given the increasing numbers of nurses who enter the profession as second-degree students. Social sororities or fraternities may also be included if the nurse is actively involved.

Community activities, including leadership roles, should be documented on the CV. This area of the CV demonstrates citizenship and can be important in a competitive job search. Do not include trivial activities that contribute very little to the overall picture. For example, routinely donating money to a particular charity or tithing to the church are inappropriate to include on a CV. Serving on the church board of directors or volunteering with the Girl Scouts of America is important to include because each requires individual sacrifice and benefits a larger societal good in an organized fashion with recognized duties.

Do not include salary information or salary expectations on the CV. If the CV is in response to a potential job opportunity and salary information is requested or required by the employer, this information should be addressed in the cover letter.

If the advanced nurse has taught in a formal academic setting or participated in precepting or formal mentorships during clinical practical experiences, include a brief description of course responsibilities. For the experienced advanced nurse who has been involved in health care education, offer specific, factual information about program development and outcomes. If the nurse is a novice in the advanced field or new to the advanced role, consider including select educational activities that were part of the graduate educational program. Remember that appropriate CV style is terse rather than detailed and narrative so keep descriptions of graduate activities to a tightly woven minimum.

Designing the Résumé

The advanced nurse should keep in mind that résumés are quite different than CVs. A résumé is usually recommended as no more than two pages in length, although some suggest that the résumé can be too constrained when subjected to the two-page rule and should, instead, be crafted within whatever page length is needed to provide the required information. Advanced nurses should give the length serious consideration and if they make the decision to go with a resume that is longer than the generally accepted two-page limit, it is imperative that the résumé be succinct, actively voiced, tightly organized, and free of embellishments and unnecessary description. The résumé is meant to provide the necessary information without unduly burdening the reader by excessive length. Generally, the résumé represents a tightly constructed outline of educational background and work experiences with some sharing of professional activities. If more detailed information is needed, a CV may be helpful. Most academic positions require a CV, whereas business settings request résumés.

The employer-focused résumé differs from the traditionally formatted résumé in that it focuses on what the employer needs and wants from the potential hire. Résumés that are crafted with employers' needs in mind are designed to speak to the skills and competencies that are required of the successful applicant (Welton, 2013). Résumés can be devised in three formats, including chronological (organized by time in a sequential pattern of most recent to later events), functional, or a combination of the two (Welton, 2013). The chronologically organized résumé is the most common style and is likely the format that is less risky to submit given its familiarity to employers.

The résumé should begin with a header that identifies the name of the candidate, credentials, and preferred contact information. This section of the résumé is the only content that may be slightly larger in font size and in bold text. Otherwise, the résumé should be consistently formatted with a font size of 10 or 12. The credentials are important. They should be correctly listed; in other words, the credentials should reflect the actual license or earned certification. For example, if an advanced nurse is certified as an Adult Health Clinical Nurse Specialist through the ANCC examination, the correct credential is ACNS-BC to represent the appropriate board certification. The credential should not be shorted or revised to CNS. This requirement holds true for all types of advanced nurses, including those in APRN roles or those with advanced certifications (e.g., Nurse Executive Advanced-Board Certified [NEA-BC]).

The customary order of credentials is as follows: highest academic degree earned; highest academic degree earned in nursing; professional licensure; certifications; honorary awards and fellowships. The distinction between highest academic degree earned and highest academic degree earned *in nursing* is often a moot point as many nurses in advanced roles have earned master's degrees or doctoral degrees in nursing. However, there are many nurses who do earn their highest degrees in disciplines other than nursing. In this case, if the license or certification that the nurse carries requires a particular degree, it may be reasonable to avoid including the highest nursing degree in the credentials list, particularly if the list becomes cumbersome (**TABLE 1-4**).

TABLE 1-4 Examples of Résumé Credentials

Incorrect Credentials	Corrected Credentials	Explanation
Micah Ivers, M.S.N, B.S.N, NP, CCRN	Micah Ivers, MSN, RN, CRNP, ANP-BC, CCRN	Avoid periods. Use commas between credentials. Use the correct acronym of the earned certification credential. If CRNP is the license issued by the state and held by the candidate, it should be included.
Maria Rodriguez, DNP, MHA, BSN, RN, CRNA, FAAN	Maria Rodriguez, DNP, MHA, RN, CRNA, FAAN	The DNP degree requires the MSN or BSN so there is no need to include the BSN. The MHA (Master's Health Administration) is a nonnursing degree and may be included.
Frank Bruce, PhD, MSN, FNP-BC, CRNP	Frank Bruce, PhD, RN, CRNP, FNP-BC	Since an MSN is required for the FNP-BC certification, even if the PhD degree is in a nonnursing area (e.g., organizational behavior), it is common practice to avoid listing the MSN degree so as to avoid an overwhelming list of letters. If the state provides a required nurse practitioner credential designated as "Certified Registered Nurse Practitioner," the license should be included.

Welton (2013) suggests that it is best to avoid including doctoral degree candidacy status in the credential list. Although it is tempting for those who have nearly completed their doctorate to include PhD-C, PhD-Candidate, or DNP-Candidate, it is a highly controversial and, frankly, can trigger a negative reaction from employers, particularly those in academic positions. Candidacy status is only traditionally used by those in research degree programs who have successfully passed candidacy examinations and have transitioned into the dissertation phase. A second important point is that many people do not complete doctoral degrees, even those who have mastered the competency examinations. As a result, the candidacy credential is often viewed as a premature acknowledgment of degree completion and use of an implied degree that has not yet been earned.

It has been long-standing tradition to follow the résumé header with a statement describing the applicant's desired objective. These statements tend to lack impact because they address what the applicant hopes to obtain from the potential employer rather than responding to the needs of the person reviewing the résumé. The employer-focused résumé should offer a statement that describes the expertise and talents that the applicant has to offer to the employer, informed by the needs of the advertised position. Welton (2013) suggests that another opening approach is to provide a bulleted list or summary statement that describes the qualifications of the applicant based on the employment advertisement. This strategy potentially requires a résumé update with each submission but it may provide the sort of personalized, targeted approach that speaks to the employer who is looking for a specific skill set.

The education section typically follows the introductory information. Do not include high school data, including extracurricular activities. Do include all coursework, nursing and nonnursing, whether from a vocational/technical program, 2-year degree experience, and/or college education; include both undergraduate and graduate studies. In-progress educational endeavors should be included as well with an expected date of completion. Do not include anticipated degree programs if the plan of study has not yet been started. Welton (2013) recommends including the cumulative grade point average (GPA) if it is 3.0 or higher; however, keep in mind that most graduate programs require a maintained GPA of 3.0 or higher so a GPA that hovers close to 3.0 is actually not particularly impressive; rather, it is at or near the lowest required average. Generally, it may be wise to only include GPAs if they are exceptional overall. Otherwise, degree completion or continued enrollment in a program already support that the applicant has earned a satisfactory GPA.

For those advanced nurses who are new to their roles and have little work experience in their area of academic specialization, it is appropriate to include graduate student clinical/practice experiences, including graded projects and internship details. Once employment is found, the résumé is best served by deleting the graduate student experiences and focusing on employment projects and work experiences. Make certain to select important and quantifiable outcomes for each project that is listed on the résumé. Outcomes may be fiscal, quality based, productivity focused, or may relate to any number of focused areas of interest. Be specific but also remember to avoid padding the CV. Take ownership where appropriate and share credit as it should be shared.

Publications, presentations, research projects, and evidence-based practice endeavors should be included on the résumé. Depending on the richness of these experiences, it may be necessary to organize them using standard taxonomy. For example, research projects may be funded or nonfunded, and interdisciplinary or unit/department based. Publications are often organized by invited versus blind, peer-reviewed statuses. Alternatively, if there are very few publications, it is reasonable to organize by chronological date and provide information that describes the individual percentage of effort, type of published media, and selection process.

Once the résumé is constructed, including pagination, make certain to solicit critique from colleagues and, if available, from those with relevant expertise. Editing suggestions should be actively solicited from those with experience. It is useful to add the last name to a footer with the page number so that if the résumé pages and cover letter become separated, the potential employer can correctly reconnect the pages and in the correct order.

Disseminating the CV or Résumé

Make certain to craft cover letters that accompany each distributed résumé. If responding to a job solicitation via traditional mail, the cover letter is included with the résumé. Keep the letter brief and in pristine form. Typographical errors or grammar mistakes offer a quick excuse for application removal from the candidate pile; so, careful proofing is essential. Make certain that the cover letter speaks to the job requirements described in the advertisement.

The CV is often submitted in response to a query for background information or as an initial step in a job search, particularly in academic environments. The CV is sent electronically or in hard copy form, depending on the instructions of the request. In both instances, a cover letter is necessary. The cover letter to an electronically attached CV may be submitted as an email message.

If the CV is mailed in paper copy, the cover letter should be consistent with the CV in style and form. The paper or electronic cover letter should include an acknowledgment of why the CV has been forwarded. If there is specific information related to a job opening position number, name of an award, or request, this should be included in the letter. The cover letter should be brief but cordial. Acknowledge the availability of references on request and thank the reviewer for interest in the CV. The nurse should offer to be available for questions or if additional information is required.

One difference between an electronic cover letter and a paper copy cover letter is the addressee. Emails require an address, but this address is often unrecognizable as an individual's name. Given the succinct, abbreviated nature of email, a salutation of some form may not even be necessary, thereby releasing the advanced nurse from finding out the formal name and title of the intended recipient. If a salutation is preferred, a simple "Dear Employment Specialist" or "Dear Recruiter" may be appropriate.

Paper cover letters require a recipient name and address. The nurse needs to make certain that the addressee's name is spelled correctly and that the job title and credentials are also correct. If there is uncertainty as to any of this information, effort should be made to contact the organization and verify the addressee's information. If contact information is not available and a position title rather than an individual name is provided, the advanced nurse should begin the letter with an appropriate salutation. For example, if a CV is required by an organization for award consideration, the applicant may wish to begin the cover letter with "Dear Awards Committee Representative."

If the cover letter and CV or résumé are sent electronically and it is important to ensure that they have been received, use the email system *message options* functions (or use the Help function to search for "read receipt") to request a delivery receipt and a read receipt. The delivery receipt will acknowledge that the electronic message was received by the Internet Protocol address. The read receipt will ask the recipient to acknowledge that the CV was received. These options allow the sender to verify that the materials were received in a timely fashion.

If a CV or résumé is being mailed, particularly if they are related to an important professional opportunity, consider using certified mail. When certified mail is used, mail travels as first class, and delivery is confirmed. Certified mail is a smart choice for the advanced nurse who may need to substantiate that the CV was mailed and received. These confirmation and verification suggestions are applicable to any situation in which the nurse is committed to replying to a request for written materials or submitting completed work.

If the advanced nurse is looking for a position and is considering using a Web-based job search engine, keep in mind that electronic résumés will be found only via keywords that have been selected by a potential employer. Some applicant tracking systems search approximately the first 80 words of a document, so be certain to include critical phrases and terms early in the résumé. Avoid graphics, shading, italics, and underlining in electronic résumés; however, this suggestion is reasonable for résumés of any type.

Many resources are available for creating résumés. Advanced nurses interested in constructing a résumé should cautiously use these resources and request guidance from experts. Although many are Web-based and user-friendly resources, they can be difficult to revise and reformat. Software templates may also be difficult to reformat. Keep résumés and CVs clean and avoid creative fonts, colors, and styles, including bullet types. Developing the document without using a template may lead to a document that has greater utility and more efficient revising options. Some advanced nurses may choose to disseminate their open access publications by posting their CVs on the Web and using hyperlinks to connect to their work products (Kousha & Thelwall, 2014).

Providing References: Points to Consider

The advanced nurse should give careful thought to references. In general, employers are interested in hearing from individuals who can substantiate the character and abilities of the applicant. Most institutions have a standardized reference form, although reference letters may be acceptable. It is increasingly common for employing agencies to have policies in place about whether supervisors are permitted to provide references for current or previous employees and, if so, permissible information parameters. Some workplaces will not permit references while others may require that human resource department personnel generate any and all references. These rules are designed to protect the referring agency from liability but they can create challenges for the applicant and for the potential future employer.

Nurses who are new to their advanced roles may be uncertain as to whom to ask for a reference. Select an individual who can offer evaluative insight and who has a clear idea of the skill set required of the advanced role position in question. At times, graduate students will request references from professors who worked with the student during beginning graduate courses and who have little to share regarding advanced practice skills or professional attributes. This individual may not be the best referring choice and this poor choice may provide a reference letter that does not speak to the relevant talents of the applicant.

Instead, the advanced nurse applicant should consider requesting references from a previous preceptor, a faculty member with responsibility for evaluating end-of-program work, a recent employer, or a professional organization leader. It is useful to request reference letters before they are needed and include them in the professional portfolio. If references are gathered before the job search process, ask referring individuals if an employer, committee person, or admissions professional has permission to contact them at a later date for validation of the reference. Having written reference letters at the start of a process can save valuable time.

One helpful strategy that the applicant may wish to consider is to offer to the potential referring professional a copy of the résumé to assist with developing reference letter content. Another useful option is for the applicant to craft a one-page categorized bulleted list of key activities and accomplishments that are relevant to the position of interest so that the referring professional can handily view dates, activities, and brief descriptions to more readily craft a meaningful reference. Make certain to offer this supplemental tool and provide it only if the person agrees that it would be helpful. Providing a résumé is always acceptable and it may be provided with the reference letter template or form, if one is provided. If not, the résumé can be shared at the time of the request for the reference.

Contributing to the Meaningful Work of Professional Associations

There are so many professional organizations that it would be nearly impossible for an advanced nurse in any role or specialty to identify an area of clinical or leadership interest that is not represented by an organization. Generally, a Web-based search will identify appropriate professional nursing organizations. It is also useful to visit the ANA's website (www.nursingworld.org) or other large nursing organization's site and look for organizational links. The links will connect directly to other established, reputable organizations.

Part of the challenge of declining memberships may be that with the proliferation of organizations, nurses feel confusion and pressure specific to selecting the few organizations that are most compatible with their interests and priorities. Another reason for avoiding membership may be that family responsibilities compete for the scarce resources of a nurse's time and money. Given the busy nature of nursing work and the often simultaneous demands of family and other personal commitments, advanced nurses need to carefully craft a personalized strategy for involvement in professional organizations (**BOX 1-2**). In other words, it may be wise to carefully consider personally important aspects of professional association membership and, having prioritized these concerns, identify the most logical organizations for membership.

Professional associations offer members opportunities to develop new skills, network, and participate in relevant continuing education programs (Escoffery, Kenzig, & Hyden, 2015). Organizations can be a terrific vehicle for recruiting new employees or finding a new professional position. Opportunities to develop relationships with people who otherwise would have been inaccessible or unknown are also highly valued aspects of association membership. Fully engaging in a professional organization is a win-win situation for both the member and the organization. The member contributes to the life of the association and assists in supporting its goals while the organization uses its clout and resources to advocate for its members (Escoffery et al.,

BOX 1-2 Audit to Assist in Selecting a *Best-Fit* Professional Association Membership

The advanced nurse should consider each of these criteria:

1. Mission statement
2. Goals and objectives
3. Web-based resources
4. Membership fees
5. Ease of dues payment:
   a. Direct withdrawal from bank account (monthly/annually)
   b. Direct debit from credit card (monthly/annually)
   c. Annual dues by check
6. Continuing education opportunities
7. Journal resources: electronic versus hard copy?
8. Database access, including evidence-based practice resources
9. Professional activities, including conferences and workshops:
   a. Regional/local activities
   b. National activities
   c. International activities
   d. Relationships to other professional organizations
10. Volunteering options and ease of getting involved
11. Mentoring prospects
12. Leadership and networking possibilities
13. LISTSERV opportunities

2015). Membership and leadership in associations demonstrate the advanced nurse's commitment to the profession and illustrate the nurse's understanding of collective power and responsibility.

Stepping Up and Stepping In: Getting Organizationally Involved

Advanced nurses may be interested in becoming involved within an organization but may be a bit hesitant. This uncertainty is normal and understandable, but it is important to not allow reticence to impede participation. Organizations are eager to have interested, committed, and enthusiastic new members.

Professional organizations face many challenges. Many nursing organizations are experiencing stagnant or declining membership (White & Olson, 2004). Nursing societies are struggling with declining memberships, an aging nursing workforce, increasing expenses, and competition among professional organizations for both members and leaders. This trend is concerning for a number of reasons. Professional organizations provide opportunities for enhancing clinical expertise; keeping apprised of regional, national, and international issues; and developing professional networks. Most groups offer continuing education programs. Some are very involved in political action and have done good work in advancing nursing and societal health care agenda items.

When an advanced nurse joins a new nursing organization, the nurse should anticipate that active involvement can be easiest to initiate at the local level, if not geographically then organizationally. Local or regional groups are good places to volunteer as a committee member or to begin participation by attending meetings, offering time to assist at registration tables, or contributing on an as-needed basis. For those who cannot commit to a contribution of time and presence, encouraging others to join or donating monies has a positive impact on the association's fiscal health and energy.

Many national organizations have committees that are filled by appointments rather than elections. It is not uncommon for organizations to publish requests for participation. Members may be asked to submit a CV and a brief letter indicating interest in the committee work. As an example, the website for the Oncology Nursing Society (ONS, 2016) devotes a section of the member center page to opportunities for involvement in project teams, advisory panels, mentoring programs, or recruitment events. There are also opportunities noted in local chapters or special interest groups. ONS offers application forms (downloadable pdfs) on the website, which is very user friendly. The American Association of Critical Care Nurses also offers lots of information on its website, including a *Volunteer Opportunities* page that describes current needs and provides profile forms for application (American Association of Critical-Care Nurses, n.d.). These opportunities are wonderful networking vehicles for advanced nurses with an interest in acute and critical care. Other associations also solicit volunteers for any number of activities, but some are not as overt in their search. One such example is the American Nursing Informatics Association (https://www.ania.org/). A *volunteer* tab or section is not available on its website; however, a search using key word *volunteer* reveals opportunities for involvement. In addition to using the search tools available on organizations' websites, consider contacting the local chapter or national office and ask for information about calls for volunteers.

Connecting Professionally in an Electronic World

Listserv Opportunities

There is an increasing number of email lists, discussion boards, open forums, and chat opportunities for advanced nurses. One particularly useful tool for connecting with health professionals that share a common professional interest or practice area is the listserv. It is interesting to note that LISTSERV is a trademark for a product distributed by L-Soft International. For this reason, LISTSERV is capitalized. The term *listserv* is used in a variety of forms, but those groups using the LISTSERV product refer to it in the aforementioned style. Upon joining any type of email list, it is a good idea to print instructions for future reference or save a screen shot for convenient access to the participation "rules" of the list, including temporarily halting emails, disconnecting from the list, or rejoining. Instructions for joining always include the instructions for withdrawing from the list.

Generally, there is a moderator or owner of the list. Usually there is a contact person associated with the list to whom questions and concerns may be addressed. LISTSERVs specific to organizations do not typically require membership but do require an email address. Many lists are interprofessional and offer opportunities for engaging with a broad network of professionals. Lists vary in their audience of interest. Some lists address the needs of a particular group of nurses or health care professionals. For example, the CNS Listserv is designed to encourage connections and support shared expertise between CNSs. There are opportunities for nurse practitioners, specifically, to join a listserv and there are options for the broader group of APRNs to contribute to lists that address a broader range of subjects that relate to advanced practice. Other groups address particular subject areas; for example, the AHRQ recently initiated a TeamSTEPPS LISTSERV for professionals interested in exchanging ideas and needs specific to this particular program (Washington Patient Safety Coalition, 2016).

Some groups use the LISTSERV product (e.g., AHRQ). Others refer to their groups as a "listserv" and use a provider such as Yahoo to organize the group. Regardless of the provider or product, joining a list is easy. The LISTSERV product offers options for organizing and delivering the electronic mail. This feature can be useful when trying to minimize the number of daily emails or when working with vacation or part-time schedules. Many LISTSERVs offer the option of a daily summary rather than receiving individual emails. This is an important feature when receiving email via portable electronic devices such as cell phones or personal data assistants as the frequent email responses can be quite burdensome.

There are often guidelines for contributing to list discussions (**BOX 1-3**). Advanced nurses must be diligent about remembering the purpose of the list. In other words, each contributed message should relate to the overarching subject of the list. The connection may be weak but must be readily apparent. The advanced nurse must remember that the list is absolutely *not* for marketing or profiteering use of any sort.

List participants should carefully evaluate the content and wording of postings before clicking the *send* button. Many lists have significant numbers of members. Once the message has been sent, it cannot be retrieved. If each member follows the rules, the communications and connections can be useful and the networking opportunities cannot be beat. Advanced nurses often share policies, procedures, instruments, tools, product evaluations, experiences, and sage advice via the listserv.

Discussion Boards and Forums

Electronic discussion boards and forums are handy and informative. They offer access to a variety of colleagues, sometimes around the world, and can provide important

---

BOX 1-3   Listserv Rules of Engagement

Generic rules for polite listserv participation:

1. Use no commercial advertisements of any sort.
2. Remember that listserv participation is open to the world. There will be communication challenges related to diversity and language/communication differences. Try to be open minded. Avoid taking immediate offense, and give the benefit of doubt.
3. Avoid sending messages to the entire subscriber group that are relevant to only a select one or two. Send "thank yous" and other pleasantries to the relevant person only.
4. Do not post materials that are under copyright protection.
5. Do not attach files or hyperlinks to listserv comments.
6. Avoid use of inappropriate or generally offensive language or slang.
7. Do not post personal information to a listserv. Private contact should be handled through email.

networking when looking for ideas, data, expertise, speakers, and other contacts. Many professional organizations have discussion boards available for members. Registration is free with membership, and participants usually have a self-configured password provided after the registration process is complete.

Numerous electronic forums are also available for nurses that require registration without fees. One forum, www.allnurses.com, is reportedly the largest peer-to-peer nursing site across the globe with over 1 million members and over 1,700 posts each day from nurses around the world (Allnurses, n.d.). Discussion topics vary and are organized by subject. A variety of advertisements are posted on the website offering products, including education and employment opportunities, targeted to nurses. As mentioned, courtesy is required, and discussion board rules are clearly posted for review.

Essential Electronic Expertise

Technology skills are essential for employment in an advanced role. There is simply no way to effectively practice in today's health care environment without a basic understanding of commonly used software products. Technological competence in electronic mail, Excel, PowerPoint, Word, and Internet search strategies is particularly important. Database software familiarity may also be useful (e.g., Microsoft Access).

Technological competence is increasingly viewed as a routine expectation of advanced nurses. Abstracts for professional organization conferences as either poster or paper presentations increasingly mandate electronic submissions. Many organizations require the use of PowerPoint™ software as the presentation format and expect that presentations will be electronically forwarded to the conference committee to load the presentation for the conference and to develop conference CDs or for online viewing, synchronous or asynchronous. It is increasingly rare for organizations to use hard copy forms, and the ease of PowerPoint software makes other presentation media comparatively cumbersome and prohibitively expensive. As an example, 35-mm slides and overhead transparencies are not acceptable presentation formats at most national nursing conferences.

There are a variety of ways to develop software expertise. In-house educational programs are ideal. These programs are free to employees and are geared to the software and hardware used within the place of employment. The challenge lies in arranging the necessary time to attend. Community colleges and university settings offer credit and noncredit courses as do postsecondary technology schools. Online tutorials are available, and there are vendors that sell videotapes designed as user-friendly tools for learners who learn best through visual processes. Microsoft (www.microsoft.com) offers information related to tutorials and software program classes. YouTube (https://www.youtube.com/) is an excellent resource for instruction on technology. A simple search using "How do I use EXCEL?" retrieved over 5 million results.

Hardware familiarity is also valuable. Mobile tools like phones and tablets use android or iOS (i Operating System or Internet Operating System). Android is an open source software that permits users to download the base software at no charge and build on it. As a result, there are many different types of android devices and accessories. In comparison, iOS is an operating system for mobile devices that was created by Apple, Incorporated and is used in Apple products including iPhones and iPads. Products that use either Android or iOS operating systems are popular and incredibly powerful. Advanced nurses must work to develop expertise with mobile devices. Drug databases, clinical references, personal scheduling, wireless access, email options, and electronic medical record systems are increasingly designed for mobile devices. Most systems, whether android or iOS, are easy to use and intuitive. Many of the mobile programs and devices are accessible to desktops as well as the handheld devices making it easy to have uninterrupted data access.

▶ Certification: A Value-Added Enhancement

Nurses may notice that the terms *advanced practice nurse* (APN) and *advanced practice registered nurse* (APRN) are used interchangeably. APRN is the designated term used by the APRN Consensus Work Group and the NCSBN APRN Advisory Committee, otherwise referred to as the APRN Joint Dialogue Group (APRN JDG) report (2008). This group was charged with developing a regulatory model for APRN practice to ensure patient safety and to allow for patient access to APRN services. The model has significant implications for advanced practice. The model has been endorsed by many professional organizations and by NCSBN. State boards of nursing have not yet adopted this model into nurse practice acts; however, this model includes elements pertaining to licensure, accreditation, certification, and education (LACE) (APRN JDG, 2008). Advanced nurses of all types should carefully review the JDG report and consider how they need to position themselves specific to professional development, education, and certification within the context of their anticipated career trajectory. Conversely, advanced nurses with responsibility for personnel management and program planning or program operationalization need to understand the APRN Consensus Model so as to make decisions that are consistent with policy recommendations.

The JDG report defines an APRN as a nurse who has met educational criteria for one of the four APRN roles within at least one of the six population foci. Specialization provides depth, but the model specifies that the APRN cannot be licensed solely within a specialty area. For CNSs in particular, this proposal is quite a change and requires careful deliberation as they plan for their professional futures or nurse executives craft strategic workforce plans. For example, CNSs may identify themselves as specialized in "critical care" or "oncology" without regard for population. The APRN Consensus Model requires CNSs to be educated in at least one of the six population foci: family/individual across the life span, adult-gerontology, pediatrics, neonatal, women's health/gender-related, or psych/mental health (APRN JDG, 2008). The selected population of study would become the licensed population based on certification. Specialization would not be a component of licensure.

APRN Certification Opportunities

ANCC (2017) is a subsidiary of the ANA and is responsible for promoting worldwide excellence in nursing and health care through credentialing programs. It offers advanced role and APRN certification examinations. ANCC also provides individual portfolio creation and maintenance to facilitate future certification renewals. Certification examinations are not inexpensive but keep in mind that certification examination development is expensive. Examinations are not constructed for practice areas that are unpopular or underutilized because examination integrity necessitates a high number of users to support test bank development and test validity.

References

Abate, C. (2017). The best meditation apps of 2017. Healthline. Retrieved July 27, 2017, from http://www.healthline.com/health/mental-health/top-meditation-iphone-android-apps#1.

Agency for Healthcare Research and Quality. (n.d.). ePSS. Electronic preventive services selector. Retrieved July 28, 2017, from https://epss.ahrq.gov/PDA/index.jsp.

Alexander, J. G., Craft, S. W., Baldwin, M. S., Beers, G. W., & McDaniel, G. S. (2002). The nursing portfolio: A reflection of a professional. *Journal of Continuing Education in Nursing, 33*(2), 55–59.

Allnurses.com. (n.d.). About allnurses. Retrieved August 3, 2017, from http://allnurses.com/aboutus-info.html.

American Association of Critical-Care Nurses. (n.d.). Volunteer opportunities Retrieved August 3, 2017, https://www.aacn.org/nursing-excellence/volunteers.

American Nurses Association. (2014). Fast facts. The nursing workforce: Growth, salaries, education, demographics & trends. Retrieved July 27, 2017, from http://nursingworld.org/MainMenuCategories/ThePracticeofProfessionalNursing/workfor ce/Fast-Facts-2014-Nursing-Workforce.pdf.

American Nurses Association. (2018). Healthy nurse, healthy nation. Retrieved January 14, 2018, from http://www.nursingworld.org/HealthyNurse-HealthyNation.

American Nurses Credentialing Center. (2017). About ANCC. Retrieved August 3, 2017, from http://www.nursecredentialing.org/About-ANCC.

American Psychological Association. (2009). *Publication manual of the American Psychological Association* (6th ed.). Washington, DC: Author.

APRN Consensus Work Group and the National Council of State Boards of Nursing APRN Advisory Committee (APRN Joint Dialogue Group). (2008). Consensus model for APRN regulation: Licensure, accreditation, certification & education. Retrieved December 3, 2008, from https://www.ncsbn.org/FINAL_Consensus_Report_070708_w._Ends_013009.pdf.

Benner, P. (1984). *From novice to expert: Excellence and power in clinical nursing practice.* Menlo Park, CA: Addison-Wesley.

Bialous, S. A., Sarna, L., Wewers, M. E., Froelicher, E. S., & Danao, L. (2004). Nurses' perspectives of smoking initiation, addiction, and cessation. *Nursing Research, 53*(6), 387–395.

Bowers, S. J., & Jinks, A. M. (2004). Issues surrounding professional portfolio development for nurses. *British Journal of Nursing, 13*(3), 155–159.

Carper, B. (1978). Fundamental patterns of knowing in nursing. *Advances in Nursing Science, 1*(1), 13–323.

Casement, P. (1985). *Learning from the patient.* London; Routledge.

Centers for Disease Control and Prevention. (2014). Health care personnel and flu vaccination, internet panel survey, United States, November 2014. Retrieved July 28, 2017, from https://www.cdc.gov/flu/fluvaxview/hcp-ips-nov2014.htm.

Chamblee, T., Dale, J., Drews, J., & Hardin, T. (2015). Implementation of a professional portfolio: A tool to demonstrate professional development for advanced practice. *Journal of Pediatric Health Care, 29,* 113–117.

Cleary, M., Walter, G., & Jackson, D. (2013). Editorial: 'Is that for real?': Curriculum vitae padding. *Journal of Clinical Nursing, 22,* 2363–2365. doi:10.1111/jocn.12161

College of Nurses of Ontario. (2008). *Fact sheet. Quality assurance. Reflective practice.* Retrieved December 1, 2008, from http://www.cno.org/docs/qa/44008_fsRefprac.pdf.

Dearden, J. S., & Sheahan, S. L. (2002). Clinical practice: Counseling middle-aged women about physical activity using the stages of change. *Journal of the American Academy of Nurse Practitioners, 14*(11), CINAHL Database of Nursing and Allied Health Literature, 492–497.

Driscoll, J., & Teh, B. (2001). The potential of reflective practice to develop individual orthopaedic nurse practitioners and their practice. *Journal of Orthopaedic Nursing, 5,* 95–103.

Driscoll, J. (2007). *Practising Clinical Supervision: A Reflective Approach for Healthcare Professionals* (2nd ed.). London: Elsevier Limited.

Duffy, A. (2007). A concept analysis of reflective practice: Determining its value to nurses. *British Journal of Nursing, 16*(22), 1400–1407.

Escoffery, C., Kenzig, M., & Hyden, C. (2015). Getting the most out of professional associations. *Health Promotion Practice, 16,* 309–312. doi:10.1177/1524839914566654

HealthStream. (2017). Homepage. Retrieved August 1, 2017, from http://www.healthstream.com/.

Hinck, S. (1997). A curriculum vitae that gives you a competitive edge. *Clinical Nurse Specialist, 11*(4), 174–177.

Institute of Medicine. (2011). *The future of nursing: Leading change, advancing health.* Washington, DC: The National Academies Press. doi:10.17226/12956

Jackson, B. S., Smith, S. P., Adams, R., Frank, B., & Mateo, M. A. (1999). Health life styles are a challenge for nurses. *Image—the Journal of Nursing Scholarship, 31*(2), 196. Retrieved July 23, 2006, from OVID http://dbproxy.lasalle.edu:2249/gw2/ovidweb.cgi.

Jasper, M. A. (1995). The potential of the professional portfolio for nursing. *Journal of Clinical Nursing, 4*(4), 249–255.

Johns, C. (2004). *Becoming a reflective practitioner* (2nd ed.). Malden, MA: Blackwell.

Johns, C. (2013). *Becoming a reflective practitioner* (4th ed.). Hoboken, NJ: Wiley-Blackwell.

Johns, C. (2017). *Becoming a reflective practitioner* (5th ed.). Hoboken, NJ: Wiley-Blackwell.

Joyce, P. (2005). A framework for portfolio development in postgraduate nursing practice. *Journal of Clinical Nursing, 14,* 456–463.

Kousha, K., & Thelwall, M. (2014). Disseminating research with web CV hyperlinks. *Journal of the Association for Information Science and Technology, 65,* 1615–1626. doi:10.1002/asi.23070

Kreider, T. (June 30, 2012). The 'Busy' Trap. *The New York Times.* Retrieved February 18, 2018, from https://opinionator.blogs.nytimes.com/2012/06/30/the-busy-trap/.

McColgan, K. (2008). The value of portfolio building and the registered nurse: A review of the literature. *Journal of Perioperative Practice, 18*(2), 64–69.

McMullan, M., Endacott, R., Gray, M. A., Jasper, M., Miller, C. M., Scholes, J., & Webb, C. (2003). Portfolios and assessment of competence. A review of the literature. *Journal of Advanced Nursing, 41*(3), 283–294.

Meister, L., Heath, J., Andrews, J., & Tingen, M. S. (2002). Professional nursing portfolios: A global perspective. *MEDSURG Nursing, 11*(4), 177–182.

Miller, S. K., Alpert, P. T., & Cross, C. L. (2008). Overweight and obesity in nurses, advanced practice nurses, and nurse educators. *Journal of the American Academy of Nurse Practitioners, 20,* 259–265.

Myers, R. E. (2017). Cultivating mindfulness to promote self-care and well-being in perioperative nurses. *AORN Journal, 105,* 259–266.

Nahm, E. S., Warren, J., Zhu, S., An, M., & Brown, J. (2012). Nurses' self-care behaviors related to weight and stress. *Nursing Outlook, 60,* e23–e31. doi:10.1016/j.outlook.2012.04.005

National CNS Competency Task Force. (2010). *Clinical nurse specialist core competencies.* Executive summary 2006-2008. Retrieved May 22, 2018, from http://www.nacns.org/wp-content/uploads/2017/01/CNSCoreCompetenciesBroch.pdf.

National Council of State Boards of Nursing. (2005). *Meeting the ongoing challenge of continued competence.* Retrieved July 31, 2017, from https://www.ncsbn.org/Continued_Comp_Paper_TestingServices.pdf.

Newman, K. (2017). Free mindfulness apps worthy of your attention. *Mindful.* Retrieved July 27, 2017, from https://www.mindful.org/free-mindfulness-apps-worthy-of-your-attention/.

Oncology Nursing Society. (2016). Member center. Volunteer. Retrieved August 2, 2017, from https://www.ons.org/member-center/volunteer.

Pew Health Professions Commission. (1998). *Strengthening consumer protection: Priorities for health care workforce regulation.* San Francisco, CA: University of California, San Francisco Center for the Health Professions.

Royal College of Nursing. (2018). Revalidation requirements: Reflection and reflective discussion. Retrieved January 14, 2018, from https://www.rcn.org.uk/professional- development/revalidation/reflection-and-reflective-discussion.

Sarna, L., Bialous, S., Nandy, K., Antonio, A., & Yang, Q. (2014). Changes in smoking prevalences among health care professionals from 2003 to 2010-2011. *JAMA, 311*(2), 197–199. doi:10.1001/jama.2013.28487

Tobacco Free Nurses. (2017). Tobacco free nurses. Retrieved July 28, 2017, from http://www
.tobaccofreenurses.org

Washington Patient Safety Coalition. (2016). AHRQ launches TeamSTEPPS LISTSERV. Retrieved
January 14, 2018, from http://www.wapatientsafety.org/ahrq-launches- teamstepps-listserv.

Weinstein, S. M. (2002). A nursing portfolio: Documenting your professional journey. *Journal of
Infusion Nursing, 25*(6), 357–364.

Welton, R. (2013). Writing an employer-focused resume for advanced practice nurses. *AACN Advanced
Critical Care, 24*, 203–217.

White, M. J., & Olson, R. S. (2004). Factors affecting membership in specialty nursing organizations.
Rehabilitation Nursing, 29(4), 131–137.

Zuzelo, P. (2017). Smokers' guilt and shame. Reactions to smoking and to providers' cessation efforts.
Holistic Nursing Practice, 31, 353–355.

Zuzelo, P., & Seminara, P. (2006). Influence of registered nurses' attitudes toward bariatric patients on
educational programming effectiveness. *Journal of Continuing Education in Nursing, 37*(2), 65–73.

Zuzelo, P., Gettis, C., Hansell, M., & Thomas, L. (2008). Describing the influence of technologies on
registered nurses' work. *Clinical Nurse Specialist, 22*, 132–140.

CHAPTER 2

Communication Strategies and Tips to Achieve Desired Results

Patti Rager Zuzelo, EdD, RN, ACNS-BC, ANP-BC, CRNP, FAAN

Nurses practicing in advanced roles must be effective communicators. Many advanced nurses have people in subordinate roles reporting to them. Others may be in administrative positions with or without direct reports. All lead by example and through influence. Nurses in advanced roles need an effective, powerful, and positive repertoire of communication strategies. No matter the specific type of advanced role, skillful communication is the hallmark of the consummate nursing professional who is able to lead or contribute to interprofessional teamwork efforts, guide subordinates, accomplish department and systemwide charges, and ensure excellent rapport with patients and families, even those that may be particularly challenging! This chapter provides an overview of the more frequently used methods and modes of communication in health care settings. These communication vehicles include electronic mail (email), meetings, presentations, and print.

Nurses interact with a variety of people thereby requiring an appreciation for communicating with diverse personality types. Communication may take place on an individual basis during coaching, consulting, supervising, or interviewing. It may also occur in group venues during meetings and presentations. Advanced nurses should critique their communication style, develop their arsenal of communication techniques, and continuously improve their communication skills.

▶ Netiquette

Netiquette is a term used to refer to communicating via the internet (*net*) using good manners or rules of etiquette (*quette*). These recommendations apply to a variety of forms including email, discussion boards, Usenet, and listservs. Netiquette resources abound on the Web, and a simple search using the popular search engine *Google* retrieves over 48 million results. Advanced nurses interested in netiquette learning resources should consider beginning with a Web-based search and exploring recent materials that peak interest and offer relevant advice.

▶ Email

Email is an essential communication vehicle in work settings and for good reasons. It is much more efficient than voicemail and provides an electronic record of interactions. Email is more environmentally friendly than hard print memos and allows for a rapid exchange of information between individuals or within large groups. Many corporate systems provide smartphones and other handheld devices to employees, often depending on organizational rank, and these devices inevitably include email functions. Other agencies require that employees bring their own devices and while this sort of policy does come with corporate risks, it reduces startup costs for organizations and keeps employees readily connected via email.

Maximizing Email's Impact and Avoiding Its Pitfalls

The advantages of email contribute to its disadvantages. Email is easy and speedy. As a result, people tend to respond to emails in a reflexive fashion, hitting the "send" button before taking the time to thoughtfully consider their response. A habit of delaying immediate replies to awkward or challenging inbox messages avoids aggravation. Nonverbal and auditory signals are lost with email. The communication process is instant and potentially fraught with the danger of misunderstanding. The problems associated with the rapidity of email are worsened by the enormous volume of messages and the lack of human interaction during message exchange.

The lack of personal interaction encourages impulsivity and discourages social inhibitions. Firing off a caustic email message or replying to a message using sarcasm and unkind comments may be likened to road rage. The sense of isolation and anonymity in a vehicle encourages people to believe that they have been victimized and provides individuals who have poor impulse control an opportunity to retaliate in ways they might not use during face-to-face encounters.

Advanced nurses should think about the perils and advantages of email and establish personal guidelines for its use (**BOX 2-1**). Remember that workplace email is owned and controlled by the employer. As a result, employers have a vested interest in making certain that employees are using email appropriately and within the confines of the law.

Copyright, defamation, discrimination, and harassment regulations that apply to written communication also apply to email. A majority of employers monitor their employees, owing to concerns over potential lawsuits. A 2007 survey by the American Management Association (AMA) found that 66% of employers monitor employees' website visits, 65% block undesirable sites, and 43% review and retain email messages (AMA, 2018). Employers noted concerns about potential lawsuits and the role electronic evidence plays in determining litigious outcomes (AMA, 2008).

There is an innate tension between an employer's right to protect the agency's computer-mediated workplace communication (CMWC) and the employee's right

BOX 2-1 Smart Guidelines for Email Use

1. Verify your email settings. Make certain that settings promote efficiency while protecting email retrieval and verification.
2. Establish electronic file folders. Click and drag important messages into appropriate folders.
3. Develop a habit of reading messages and immediately deleting, electronically filing, printing, or forwarding them.
4. Use subject lines.
5. Forward and reply to messages selectively. Follow a need-to-know process to avoid cluttering colleagues' mailboxes.
6. Delete chain mail. Do not forward.
7. Generate a paper copy of important, irreplaceable messages that are sent or received. Alternatively, generate an electronic snip/screen shot/electronic image; save; backup file.
8. Do not leave email accounts open and accessible when the computer is unattended.
9. Read, review, and reread messages for tone and clarity.
10. Never send an angry email.
11. Avoid disrespectful comments; profanities; messages that promote gender/racial/sexual/prejudicial stereotyping.
12. Use delivery receipts and read receipts selectively.
13. Select high-priority designation infrequently.
14. Clear inbox of attached files, including pictures, video, and presentations, as soon as possible.
15. Make certain that attached files are not too large for the corporate system to handle before sending them (avoid system crashes).
16. Separate paragraphs with double spaces and keep text succinct.
17. Avoid bullying.
18. Avoid *reply all* unless there is a very good reason for responding to more than the sender.
19. Keep in mind that *bcc* refers to blind carbon copy. If an email is sent to you as a bcc, avoid responding or the others on the message will now know that you were blind carbon copied. Revealing your inclusion on the message could be problematic.

to privacy (Chory, Vela, & Aftgis, 2016). The most ubiquitous communication tool is email, although instant messaging, a text-based tool, is also popular and has significant utility plus associated risk (Chory et al., 2016). There are times when employers terminate employees for misusing email; in rank order, most firings occurred for the following causes: violation of company policy, unfitting or offensive language, excessive non-work-related use, and privacy breaches (AMA, 2008).

In general, the best way to approach email is to never send anything that is not appropriate for general viewing by the larger workforce group. There are no guarantees that email messages will not be forwarded. It is also wise to remember to log off email accounts when leaving computer terminals to avoid situations in which other people send out messages under the logged-in account name. Keep in mind that deleted messages may be retained on the workplace server. Recall that of the

43% of companies monitoring email, approximately three-quarters use automated technologies; and 40% assign this work to an employee (AMA, 2008). It is good practice to consider emails via work systems or managed in the work environment as public rather than private correspondence. The same caution holds true to text messaging and other social media communiques, including Twitter, LinkedIn, Facebook, or other platforms.

One final point regarding email and the right to privacy: When an employee accesses email at work using workplace computer monitors or work-owned equipment, even if it is a personal account (e.g., Gmail, Yahoo!), the employer should be considered to have the right to surveil these messages (Privacy Rights Clearinghouse [PRC], 2017a). There is case law to support employers' rights to access employees' email when open or used during work hours or on employer-owned computer terminals or equipment (PRC, 2017a).

Composing Email Messages

Many people use software to filter spam—unsolicited junk mail—from their inboxes. At times, spam filters block legitimate email messages. Blocking is more likely when the subject-line entry is not meaningful or is left blank. The sheer volume of email also encourages the use of spam filters as a way to reduce unimportant inbox messages. Advanced nurses should craft subject-line entries to accurately reflect the nature of the email message. Subject lines should be short and succinct.

Avoid forwarding chain letters through email. Keep in mind that many corporations and agencies have policies against chain letter distributions. It is also helpful to send messages only to people who really need to be in the communication loop. Sending replies to *all recipients* when it is not necessary for the entire group to read the response is impolite. It wastes server space and increases the volume of unnecessary inbox messages. Frankly, using the "reply all" feature triggers frustration and perturbed feelings from colleagues if the message does not have relevance to the group at large.

It is a good rule of thumb to keep email messages as brief and tightly written as possible. If there is a lot of information to convey, it may be best to craft a brief email message and attach a document that can be saved or printed. Make certain to ask permission before sending large electronic attachments or alert the recipient to the size of the attachment within the body of the email. Attachments allow mail recipients to quickly get through the message and return to the information-dense memo at a later time. There are options for sharing large files if the usual server does not permit sufficient space for transferring large amounts of data. These options include Google Drive (https://www.google.com/drive/), Dropbox (https://www.dropbox .com/), and other free sites that allow for large file transfers. Many Web-based sites (Dubey, 2017; Kaufman, 2013; Lowensohn, 2010) provide critique and details specific to free large file sharing tools and applications available to securely send and save files electronically (**TABLE 2-1**).

Advanced nurses should avoid electronically sending any sort of sarcastic or threatening messages. While this admonition may seem unnecessary, keep in mind that the challenge lies in accurately determining whether the recipient will *interpret* the message as threatening or demeaning. Without the opportunities of visual and auditory cues, misinterpretation is likely and such a reaction should be considered.

TABLE 2-1 Select Options for Sharing Large Files Online

Name	Web Address	Comments
Dropbox	https://www.dropbox .com	Free account signup provides 2 GB of free drive space. Upgrades are available.
DropSend	http://www.dropsend .com/	Files up to 8 GB may be sent for free.
File Dropper	http://www.filedropper .com/	Permits file sharing of up to 5 GB for free. As with other plans, fee-based plans are available for larger file transfers.
FilestoFriends	https://www.files tofriends.com/	Permitted to transfer large files of up to 1 GB for no fee.
JumboMail	https://www.jumbo mail.me/	Fastest growing cloud-based transfer service. Has an online media gallery to allow for viewing shared files on the download page before the files are downloaded.
Send This File	https://www .sendthisfile.com /solutions/overview.jsp	Has a free plan option as well as three levels of paid options—each with security features to keep large files secure.
TitanFile	https://www.titanfile .com/	Drag and drop features with secure sharing. Basic plan (free) permits uploading files up to 100 MB.
TransferBigFiles	https://www .transferbigfiles.com/	Free account signup for sending and receiving files up to 20 GB.
WeTransfer	https://wetransfer.com/	Free package provides easy access to transferring a maximum of 2 GB via email.

Emoticons, Emojis, and Acronyms

Emoticons, a typographical representation of a facial expression used in text-only media (Hern, 2015), may be used to convey the feeling associated with a message (**TABLE 2-2**). Emojis are actual pictures, often triggered by text symbols in a particular pattern or selected from a menu, that were designed to extend Unicode, the character set used by most current operating systems (Hern, 2015). There are also stickers that

TABLE 2-2 Emoticon and Select Emoji Examples

Emoticon	Meaning	Emoji
:-) or :)	Smile	😊
;-) or ;)	Wink	😉
:-O or :o	Astonished	😲
:-(or :(	Sad/Crying	😢
:-| or :|	Disappointed	😕

may be used in some social media applications, but sticker sets are unique to the particular platform. Some email services, for example, Microsoft Office 365 Outlook, provide emoji options for email use. Alternatively, as the sender crafts a message, if an emoticon is crafted, the system will provide emoji options in lieu of the text-based emoticon. When trying to find an emoji within certain software products, knowing the correct word to search on the menu is important. For example, a search on Microsoft's Office 365 Outlook will retrieve an *astonished* emoji option for insertion into email but using *surprised* in the menu bar will not yield an emoji. A quick Web-based search will provide the best keyword when searching for a specific emoji.

It may be appropriate to occasionally use emoticons to reinforce the intended emotion of an email; however, they should be used judiciously in the work environment. Similar to when a smiley or heart is placed above the letter "i" in a person's name, emoticon usage can convey playful or childlike behavior that may convey less sophistication and professionalism than the employment role or message requires. Some emoticons are sophisticated and not all are easily understood. Generally, do not use emoticons or an emoji in any sort of formal email. Reserve emoticon use for casual correspondence or to strike a particular tone; typically, only use them with a peer or with a subordinate if the message is positive ;-).

In general, it is best to keep email messages and replies brief. Some common acronyms are used in personal, and occasionally professional, emails that may be incorporated into workplace correspondence (**TABLE 2-3**). As with emoticons, it is important to make certain that selected acronyms are easily recognizable. A simple Web-based search using any common search engine provides many examples of frequently used abbreviations. Exclamation points may be useful to demonstrate emphasis or enthusiasm but make certain to use only one, as multiple exclamation points are unnecessary and may be perceived as irritating.

Be Electronically Judicious

A few final email caveats deserve emphasis. It is tempting to fire off a response to an incendiary email to immediately set straight the email recipient. As difficult as

TABLE 2-3 Select Electronic Acronyms	
Acronym	**Meaning**
BFN	Bye for now
IMO	In my opinion
BTW	By the way
LOL	Laughing out loud
HTH	Hope this helps
NRN	No reply necessary
TIA	Thanks in advance
AKA	Also known as
ASAP	As soon as possible

it may be, the advanced nurse *must* practice restraint. It is very important to take a time-out before responding.

Writing an immediate response may serve as a catharsis for the initial emotional response; however, once written, some knee-jerk messages should not be sent, particularly when written in anger. Most email software gives the user the opportunity to save replies as drafts. Take advantage of the option and save the response. Come back to the original message at a later time, read it again in a calm state, and try to determine whether the initial reaction was appropriate. Then, after reflection, review the drafted response.

Make certain that the written reply is a reasonable, rational, and fair retort. Remember that the response may be circulated to a broader audience or may precipitate an escalated *flame* response. Consider obtaining a second opinion on the initial interpretation or response. Alternatively, ask the sender a few clarifying questions.

Quote the original message and backtrack as appropriate. Backtracking involves the use of the karat right sign (>) in front of the words someone else wrote to symbolize quotations (Brinkman & Kirschner, 2012). Keep in mind that it takes less time to clarify an issue than it does to undo the damage associated with an inappropriate, rude, or angry electronic retort (see **EXEMPLAR 2-1**).

Select the Best Mode for Email Delivery

There are times when advanced nurses need to send a relatively important email that is deserving of immediate review. Similar to making a decision as to whether to send paper mail via first-class or priority mail, nurses need to think about whether an

EXEMPLAR 2-1 Taking the Electronic High Road

Richard is a nurse practitioner in cardiovascular (CV) care. He has been charged with responsibility for establishing clinical guidelines for managing patients with congestive heart failure (CHF). His multidisciplinary group—comprised of a cardiac fellow, medical resident, registered nurse, CV clinical nurse specialist, cardiologist, pharmacist, and other nonclinical professionals—has developed evidence-based guidelines that they believe are well suited to the patient population served by this particular acute care setting. The committee has worked for several months and has periodically communicated with various clinicians to solicit input. In preparation for rolling out the guidelines, Richard sends a brief, explanatory email with an attached guideline draft to the medical staff.

Within an hour, Richard receives an email response from a well-established cardiologist who has been practicing at the hospital for over 30 years. The physician, Dr. Smith, is livid with Richard and the committee and is incensed over the proposed guidelines. Dr. Smith's email response comments, "The practice of medicine cannot be reduced to a set of guidelines. I refuse to be dictated to by a nurse—go to school, become a doctor, and then try to tell me what to do. My patients trust me and I provide high-quality, individualized care. This guideline is yet another attempt to save money at the expense of our patients! I've made an appointment to speak with the Chair of Medicine and the Chief Nurse Executive (CNE) and will be offering your guideline as yet another example of how patient care is compromised at Get Well Hospital by supposed experts."

Richard's initial response is outrage. He quickly writes a scathing response pointing out the many opportunities for feedback during the guideline development process. Richard notes the importance of evidence-based guidelines and suggests that Dr. Smith would be aware of the importance if he was current in his practice. The email concludes with a hastily constructed, "Go ahead and talk with the Chair and the Chief Nurse. I was assigned this committee job and if my work is not up to par, someone else can do it!"

At this point, it may be wise to consider two possible conclusions.

The First Vignette

Richard hits the "send" button. For a few minutes, Richard feels satisfied in setting straight Dr. Smith. After calming down, Richard becomes increasingly anxious. Dr. Smith is an older physician with long-standing relationships and influence. Dr. Smith is usually rational, and although he can be cantankerous over patient care issues, he is genuinely concerned about his patients. Dr. Smith is considered a nursing champion and is recognized as such by most advanced practice nurses. In fact, Richard usually has an amicable, rather benign relationship with this physician. Richard pulls up his sent response and rereads it. He reads it several times and realizes that although the initial email from Dr. Smith was inappropriate and hostile, Richard has increased the stakes and likely worsened hostilities by replying in kind. He begins to think about the ramifications of this email. He considers the potential impact on his professional reputation as well as the adverse effect that his potential response could have on the evidence-based practice recommendations—work in which he and his colleagues are committed and fully engaged. Richard begins to plan a backout strategy for undoing the predicament in which he now finds himself.

The Second Vignette

Richard rereads his message slowly and looks at his computer screen. Written on a Post-It note is a simple reminder: "Vent it but don't send it" (Brinkman & Kirschner, 2012).

EXEMPLAR 2-1 Taking the Electronic High Road *(continued)*

Richard saves his response as a draft and leaves his office to get a cup of coffee. He tries to step back from the tone of Dr. Smith's email and consider the variables that may have led to such initial hostility. Richard decides to speak with a cardiologist colleague and get a second opinion.

A few hours later, Richard speaks with his colleague about the guidelines draft and the email response from Dr. Smith. Richard discovers that Dr. Smith is struggling to get insurance company approval for a medical therapy labeled as "experimental" for a middle-aged patient with end-stage CHF. The patient is doing poorly, and the pressure on Dr. Smith is great. One challenge confronting Dr. Smith is the inaccessibility of an insurance company physician to whom he could speak with about his concerns. Rather, the insurance company has connected him to a non-physician representative. The colleague recommends that Richard wait a few days and then approach Dr. Smith personally regarding the proposed guidelines and the angry email response.

Richard returns to his computer, reads his unsent reply, and hits "delete." He has vented his frustration using the computer as a sounding board and now feels calmer. Richard realizes that there was value in writing the response but that sending it would intensify a bad situation and create more work stress for him. Richard's decision does not mean that Dr. Smith is unaccountable for his response. Rather, Richard recognizes that perpetuating electronic hostility is a nonproductive use of his energies and may be counterproductive to the larger goal, approval of the CHF guidelines. Richard contacts the cardiology receptionist and schedules a meeting with Dr. Smith.

email should be sent with a priority notation. Avoid overusing this function. There are times when individuals use priority designations so frequently that the red font and exclamation mark associated with priority status lose their impact.

Other convenient functions associated with sent messages are the delivery receipt and read receipt options. A delivery receipt informs the sender that the electronic message has been received by the designated email address. The read receipt notifies the sender that the message has been read by the recipient.

A word of caution is needed, as some read receipt functions inform the recipient that a read receipt has been requested and ask for permission to notify the sender that the message has been read. If the recipient declines the notification opportunity, the sender will not know that the message has been read. This is why it may be a good idea to consistently send a delivery receipt notification request with a read receipt.

These options are available through most email software, although the function button locations vary. Use the help function feature if unable to locate the mail priority, delivery receipt, or read receipt functions. Some email systems, including a personal Gmail account, not connected to work or school do not have delivery or read receipt options unless upgrades are available.

Keep Email Organized

It is surprising how many advanced nurses do not use the helpful organizing functions available in most popular email software. The underutilization of filing options and the overuse of server memory can pose significant problems. Nurses should become familiar with the many varied options of the workplace email system to maximize efficiency.

Most email software allows users to select inbox and sent message functions. For example, some systems have an established default that saves copies of all sent messages. The sender is able to modify this default to individually select sent messages requiring a saved copy. This function reduces the number of individually saved messages. By reducing the number of saved message copies, the advanced nurse will also reduce server memory use.

Server memory is an important consideration for the entire email community of the organization. Attachments containing pictures, documents, and PowerPoint presentations can be very large files. It is important to review inboxes and check the size of each message file. Make certain to clear particularly large files as soon as possible using the *Save As* function and migrating the files to more appropriate locations. Then delete the email with the attachment.

Inbox messages can usually be read without deciding whether to delete or save the message. It may be tempting to quickly read messages without deleting or filing. This email practice can lead to cluttered inboxes making it difficult to retrieve important messages when needed at a later date.

Consider developing a pattern of inbox message scrutiny that relies on immediate decisions regarding deleting or filing. Email software provides options for creating a file directory. Advanced nurses can create files with short clear names that allow inbox mail to be categorized in a meaningful way.

Similar to the filing system popular in Microsoft Windows Explorer, most email platforms allow users to create a file folder, point and click on an email message, and drag the message to an appropriate folder. The individual message or folder can be reviewed and saved or deleted at a later date. Some email messages do not warrant filing and should be immediately deleted after review. Keep in mind that even when an email message is deleted, it likely remains on an employer system for an indefinite period of time. The message may appear to be eliminated, but it is likely backed up from within the system (PRC, 2017a).

There are times when servers crash, files become corrupted, and systems fail. With these scenarios in mind, advanced nurses should selectively print hard copies of vital email correspondence. Hard copies should be scarce or the nurse runs the risk of duplicating digital records without good reason. However, there are certainly isolated emails that should be saved and protected beyond ordinary digital filing. Advanced nurses may find that saving a particular email message in pdf or using a snip tool or screen shot tool to take a picture of the message provides a useful format for transferring important email into a relevant folder. For example, if an administrator sends a particularly positive email message to the advanced nurse, saving a copy of this positive feedback in a folder used to inform an annual self-evaluation is a good way to efficiently keep track. Likewise, a particularly egregious email message from a subordinate who is angry about a schedule concern might be an important document to save for latter review with the employee. Another reasonable rule of thumb is to view email as similar to hard copy files and, as with paper, discard email that is trivial or insignificant. Of course, shred sensitive hard copies of email when discarding them.

Email has certainly changed communication practices in all venues—including work and home. The advantages of rapid and convenient communication outweigh the disadvantages. The skillful advanced nurse will recognize the benefits of email and take full advantage of digital communication while remaining wary of its potential for misuse. Given that email is ubiquitous with access points across handheld and desktop devices, developing a reasonably sophisticated skill set, including coherent and consistent usage patterns, is an imperative component of efficient practice.

▶ Voicemail and Computer Usage Tips

Nurses in advanced roles of all types need to remember that telephone records, voicemail messaging systems, and computer terminal activities are employer owned and therefore not private. Employers have the right to access telephone usage records and may monitor calls, although some states do require employers to notify employees if calls will be recorded or monitored (PRC, 2017a). Voicemail messages may be backed up on magnetic tape in the event that call retrieval is necessary, making it difficult for an employee to know with certainty that calls have been deleted.

In general, employees should assume that workplace communications are not private. There are times when personal calls are necessarily placed during work time; however, advanced nurses may want to consider using a personal cell phone for these types of calls. Another important consideration to keep in mind is that inappropriate communication is neither acceptable nor wise, particularly during work hours. Voicemail messages may be forwarded, calls may be tracked, and computer usage may be monitored for both time on computer systems and specifics related to website activities. Monitoring telephone usage is legal, including tracking phone numbers that have been dialed.

▶ Personal Device Policies in the Workplace

Many workplaces have *bring your own device* (BYOD) policies and procedures. As mentioned, these programs have associated organizational benefits and risks. PRC (2017b) cautions that employees need to carefully review BYOD policies and procedures and ask questions before agreeing to participate. Mobile phones and other portable hardware, including tablets, are personal devices that are frequently used for work purposes.

There are many good reasons for BYOD opportunities. Employees often have a preferred technology; for example, they may work more efficiently using their iPhone rather than using a corporate-provided android phone. Preference and efficiency based on familiarity may also drive BYOD decisions around tablets or laptops. Many employees are interested in working remotely; and permitting the work-based use of personal devices supports offsite work. Employers appreciate BYOD policies because employees are likely more satisfied, employees are more readily accessible, and it is less expensive to permit BYOD practices than it is to purchase and maintain a portable technology inventory (PRC, 2017b).

Employers, including advanced nurses with supervisory responsibilities, do incur risks with BYOD programs. Once employees are permitted to transmit company data on personal devices or use work-issued devices for both corporate and personal use, the employer loses control of but not necessarily responsibility for data transmission and security (PRC, 2017b). Advanced nurses need to consider that BYOD agreements may include employer access to the employee's global positioning satellite (GPS) information; social media and passwords; phone call history; text, chat, and messaging history; video and photo files; and other access and communication histories. Using a device that is personally provided and owned does not guarantee a right to privacy (PRC, 2017b).

Nurses in advanced roles need to consider how to approach the use of personal technologies at work or employer-provided technologies at home. Carrying multiple devices can be inconvenient and physically cumbersome. On the other hand, there is significant responsibility associated with either approach to communication. Make certain that subordinates are fully informed as to the responsibilities of electronic devices. Keep in mind that the best approach is twofold: Use approved devices (BYOD or work issued) with no expectation of privacy; and consistently approach communication with professionalism and even-handedness. Advanced nurses need to carefully and deliberately consider the risks and benefits of both approaches to communication products and, if there is an option for work-issued devices, select the option that makes the most sense for their particular communication circumstances.

▶ Organizing Successful Meetings

Advanced nurses are often involved in committees as members or chairpersons. Successful meetings are chaired by effective people who purposively prepare to achieve deliberately selected goals (**BOX 2-2**). Disorganized, poorly planned meetings with no clear goals reflect poorly on the chair and discourage committee members from active engagement in group processes. Agendas drive meetings and agenda preparation is important.

Arranging the Meeting

Arranging a meeting time that works for multiple committee members can be a daunting task. If the advanced nurse has an administrative assistant available to handle meeting arrangements, it is certainly easier to coordinate a convenient date and

---

BOX 2-2 Meeting Preparation Checklist

Activity

1. Solicit agenda items from committee members.
2. Create an agenda with clear designations of work and responsibilities in preparation for the meeting.
3. Assign a recording secretary for the meeting and place assignation on the agenda.
4. Arrange for a meeting room and refreshments, if appropriate.
5. Distribute the agenda with a copy of the previous minutes. Note the room and time. Request répondez s'il vous plaît (RSVP), please respond, from committee members.
6. Provide a template for the minutes.
7. Make certain invited guests or committee members have necessary equipment ordered prior to the meeting (e.g., overhead projector equipment).
8. Prepare materials for duplicating. If electronic materials are used, send as email attachments with the agenda and old minutes. Make certain that committee members have at least 1 week to review materials, although 2 weeks is preferable.

time, but scheduling a meeting is still an arduous task. Many committee chairs find themselves relying on multiple emails, personal conversations, or telephone messages in an effort to winnow tentative dates and times for meetings.

There are Web-based scheduling systems that are convenient and free, providing that only basic services are required. DuPont (2014) suggests that several features should be considered when selecting a meeting scheduler application. Desirable features include synchronization capability with a variety of calendar applications. Another convenient feature is a polling option that provides committee members with the ability to select days/times that best work for them from a variety of options provided by the person scheduling the meeting. Some free schedulers provide an option for scheduling recurring meetings—for instance, if the advanced nurse is pulling together a committee that will meet on the first Monday of every other month.

One popular Web-based scheduler is Doodle (http://www.doodle.ch/main.html), which is useful for scheduling events or polling email recipients. Free accounts are available, and registration is optional. Premium accounts, available for a fee, offer advertisement-free services, contact information features, and customized branding. Another recommended application (DuPont, 2014) is World Clock Meeting Planner. This tool enables the advanced nurse to pick a time of day that works across national and international time zones (Thorsen, 2017). It does not schedule meetings, but it does provide an easy-to-use tool for making decisions about reasonable start times for all committee members across multiple time zones.

Agency and institutional email systems may also have embedded appointment schedulers that can be easy to use. However, these systems typically do not provide a polling feature that allows for the selection of a variety of convenient dates and times. This polling can make the difference between a well-attended and poorly attended meeting. Some schedulers will use a tool, perhaps Doodle, to find the best-fit date and time and will then send out the appointment using an in-house appointment scheduler system. No matter how the meeting date and time is determined, keep in mind that this first step is worth the effort. A well-attended meeting is more likely to yield the desired end product.

Agendas and Goal Setting

Agenda preparation provides an excellent opportunity for meeting planning. The chair should reflect on the main objective of the meeting, whether this is an agenda for a standing committee that meets on a regularly scheduled basis or a more impromptu ad hoc meeting. The agenda should be electronically distributed prior to the meeting. Avoid sending materials to committee members without providing sufficient time for members to review previous minutes or to accomplish pre-meeting activities. Generally, 1 week should be sufficient, particularly if goals and assigned tasks were reviewed at the conclusion of the previous meeting.

Include the date, start time, end time, and meeting location on the agenda. If there is an option to attend the meeting via a Web-based system, make certain to provide the electronic link and any login information. Use the subject line to identify the email as pertaining to the committee agenda and the date. This strategy assists members when they need to retrieve the agenda from their email. It is also helpful to send this information via an electronic calendar invitation that includes the Web-based link to the meeting and, if available, the attached agenda plus links to any other documents that may be needed for the meeting.

If recording responsibilities are shared by committee members, it is helpful to identify the meeting's assigned recording secretary on the agenda. This notification alerts the recorder of the need for a laptop, audiotape recorder, and timely arrival. Alternatively, if assigned recorders cannot attend occasional meetings, the onus for finding a replacement is on them. Make certain that the group is clear on these responsibilities. Assigning responsibility for minute taking without notice or cajoling members into taking minutes at the start of a meeting conveys a disorganized tone that may influence the dynamic of the committee group process, particularly in more formal meetings. The meeting chair should *not* be responsible for minute taking; rather, the chair should manage the meeting, facilitate discussion, solicit input, and pay attention. If the chair fills in as recorder because of a lack of volunteers, it is likely that dual responsibilities for chairing and recording will be to the detriment of performing either role successfully.

Consider the desired outcomes of the committee meeting and the preparation that is required of each committee member to accomplish the objectives. As noted, distribute materials as far in advance of the meeting as possible. Remember, members cannot get their work finished if they receive materials at short notice. Many chairs attach old minutes to the new agenda to draw the committee's attention back to previously discussed items that continue to require resolution or ongoing work. It can be useful to build an electronic repository for past minutes and agendas as well as for relevant documents that is accessible to committee members.

There are a variety of applications that facilitate electronic collaboration and enable sharing across devices within an identified membership group. SharePoint (https://products.office.com/en-us/sharepoint/sharepoint-server) is a popular Microsoft product that is designed to facilitate document sharing. Approximately 200,000 organizations and 190 million customers use this particular product (Microsoft Corporation, 2017). There are alternatives to SharePoint; and a quick Web-based search using any common search engine quickly reveals lists of options with evaluations and summaries of strengths and gaps. Most of these sites are laced with advertisements while others are supported by vendors of alternative products; however, they are a good place to begin if looking for a free or easily accessible sharing product.

Agenda building may be formal or informal. In general, customary activities lead to a finalized agenda. First, members should be asked to forward items to the chair for the agenda. Timing is important, so make certain to give the members enough time to think about important items but not so much time that the participant places the need for agenda items at the bottom of a to-do list and forgets to submit.

Second, provide committee members with a deadline for agenda items to avoid last-minute changes. The chair needs to decide whether it is acceptable to include late agenda items. Make certain to carefully discuss agenda items with the person submitting them to avoid any confusion. It is often helpful to denote who is responsible for a particular agenda item, if there is a point person, so that individuals are reminded of their specific responsibilities to the group prior to the meeting.

Conducting the Meeting

Most agendas follow a standard format (**BOX 2-3**). The meeting begins with a call to order. A specified person checks attendance and, depending on the type of committee, establishes that quorum is satisfied. A quorum is the minimum number of committee members required to conduct the business of the group. Usually a quorum is defined

BOX 2-3 The Agenda

Organization Name

Committee Name

Date of Meeting

  I.   Call to Order
 II.   Old Business
      A.   Reading of the previous minutes, revisions if needed, approval vote
      B.   Items are drawn from previous meeting's minutes
III.   New Business
IV.   Announcements
 V.   Adjournment

as a majority; however, this standard varies by committee. In committees with formal structures and processes, the quorum is usually established in the organizational bylaws. Without a quorum, the status quo cannot be changed. If there is not a quorum, any decisions requiring votes, including motions, need to wait until a quorum is available.

The chair may follow the call to order with a brief review of the measurable objectives set for the particular meeting. This strategy focuses the group on the tasks at hand and facilitates a shared consensus about the intent of the meeting. The call to order and brief introduction is usually followed by old business. The usual first item of old business is the review of the past minutes, revisions if required, and a vote for approval.

New business items are discussed next, followed by announcements. The meeting concludes with instructions regarding the scheduling of the next committee meeting, if an additional meeting is necessary. The meeting concludes with a formal adjournment by the chairperson. A final point is that the agreed-upon agenda is not immutable. If there is a need to adjust the agenda at some point during the committee meeting, it is customary to allow a revision, providing that a majority consent to the revision. Advanced nurses employed by agencies or assigned to committees that strictly follow parliamentarian rule should review Robert's Rules Newly Revised (RRNR) (Robert, Honemann, Balch, Seabold, & Gerber, 2011) specific to actions necessary for agenda revision; RRNR does permit modification if rules are followed.

Documenting the Work of the Committee

Committee minutes are critically important. Similar to the popular premise underlying nursing charting, if it is not documented, it was not done—minutes document the work and accomplishments of the committee. They provide a context for evaluating the efforts of the committee. Minutes keep people current with the committee's work by allowing new members, supervisors, and members who miss an occasional meeting to be apprised of the committee's work. Minutes also demonstrate the work of the committee to ensure that accreditation requirements are being addressed and met. Accurate and sufficiently detailed minutes also support handoffs from one chairperson to the next. There are times when minutes are needed to provide evidence that rules and procedures have been followed. In short, think of minutes as a data source that provides historical data, details current plans, and tracks progress toward goals, objectives, and committee mandates.

The recording secretary, or in lieu of an established secretary, the chairperson is responsible for tracking minutes. Minutes should be documented using a word processor during or immediately following the meeting. An electronic record and paper copy should be saved. Losing minutes can be a significant problem, particularly when accreditors want to determine that organizational requirements have been met. Make certain that minutes are departmentally or centrally housed rather than leaving responsibility for minutes with a particular person. There are many times when recording secretaries leave agencies and committee records are lost or inaccessible.

At the conclusion of the committee year—usually the fiscal, calendar, or academic year—minutes may be saved to a labeled compact disc–read only memory (CD-ROM) for easy retrieval and/or to the cloud or organizational hard/home (h) drive. CDs are convenient during accreditation visits, as missing minutes can be easily replaced and surveyors can quickly scan minutes, providing that a CD-ROM drive is available. Cloud or h-drive storage is the most efficient option but there are times when cloud access is not that convenient, particularly for non-employees such as external reviewers or auditors. Eliminating paper copies of minutes beyond 1 year can substantially reduce hanging file clutter, and CD copies protect and backup server memory capacities. Another suggestion is to maintain for 1 year hard copies of minutes and supporting materials in a 5-inch binder that may be easily transported to meetings and accessed quickly if a computer network is unavailable.

It may be helpful for committee chairs to develop a standard format for the minutes. Providing a written or electronic template (**BOX 2-4**) can ensure that minutes are recorded consistently between meetings. If recording responsibilities are shared and rotated among committee members, having a template can be a real time saver and is often appreciated by the recorder. If the meeting's recorder prefers taking handwritten minutes, a template can make it easier for the administrative assistant to follow when word processing.

BOX 2-4 Template for Minutes

Name of Organization
Name of Committee
Date of Meeting

Present:
Excused Absences:

Agenda Item	Discussion	Outcome/Responsible person/ Due date

   I.   Call to Order
  II.   Old Business
      a.   Agenda item
 III. New Business
      a.   Agenda item
 IV.   Announcements
  V.   Next Meeting Date/
      Time/Location

Respectfully submitted
Recorder signature
Recorder name

Isolating a column specific to outcomes related to each item of business facilitates follow-through and assists in keeping agendas lean. Once an item is concluded with a final outcome, it is not necessary to carry the item onto the next agenda. Making clear who is responsible for any carried item of business helps to establish accountability among committee members. Both the recorder and the chairperson should ensure that each agenda item has an agreed-on outcome or action plan. It is vital that the chairperson lead the group and determine end points and responsibilities for the work of a committee. Too often committee discussions are abstract or broad without resolution or measurable outcomes. Compelling an outcome or action plan for each agenda item ensures that members leave the meeting with a clear sense of their assignments.

Minutes are used to construct the next meeting's agenda. Old business items for the agenda are retrieved from the previous sets of minutes. New business items should be new to the work of the committee. Minutes provide the necessary data for subsequent agendas. The cycle perpetuates itself, so organizing minutes is well worth the time and effort.

Maintaining Order

Asserting control is crucial to ensuring the best use of people's time and achieving the meeting's aims. Establishing an agenda is one control mechanism. Asking open questions to stimulate discussion, closed questions to narrow discussion, and directed questions to encourage participation are communication strategies that enhance control and assist in getting work finished (Banks, 2002).

Applying RRNR (Robert et al., 2011) is another control strategy that brings order from potentially chaotic meeting situations. Many advanced nurses have participated in meetings that strictly or loosely follow *Robert's Rules*. As an aside, the rules were originally developed by Henry Martyn Robert in 1876 (Robert's Rules Association [RRA], 2011) after presiding over a church meeting and realizing that he did not know how to effectively use parliamentary law.

Robert was an engineering officer in the regular Army and lived in a variety of places in the United States. He found that different parts of the country had different interpretations of parliamentary procedure, and so he wrote *Robert's Rules of Order*. These rules are now in their 11th edition and are used by many organizations and governments in its current form, RRNR, as parliamentary authority (RRA, 2011).

There are many RRNR tools that can be useful to new and established chairpersons. User-friendly resources include laminated charts, dummy versions that present the rules using simple explanations, quick-start guides, and others. Following an established set of rules avoids many within-committee disagreements and establishes a useful air of professionalism that allows for debate and dialogue while ensuring that all members have a voice.

Advanced nurses working within committee structures or leading committee efforts are well advised to have a basic working knowledge of RRNR and to consistently follow select procedural rules to avoid potential chaos (**BOX 2-5**). The rules are very formal and inalienable and so are probably less appropriate for casual meetings or small groups. One specific example might be to allow committee members to speak only after recognition from the chair. This rule prevents members from interrupting others or boisterously dominating a meeting. It also facilitates difficult conversations by directing members to the chair rather than to a member when disagreements

---

BOX 2-5 Basic Strategies for Maintaining Order

1. Establish a deadline for submitting items to the chair for agenda consideration.
2. Develop a thoughtful agenda appropriate to the length of available meeting time.
3. Distribute the agenda 5 to 10 business days prior to the meeting, depending on the frequency of meetings.
4. Attach the previous meeting minutes to the new agenda.
5. Create a minutes template for the recorder. Include an action/outcomes column with identification of the responsible committee member.
6. Follow select parliamentary rules of order in consistent fashion during every meeting and with each committee member, regardless of role or perceived status.
7. Be transparent about the use of parliamentary procedure and review these rules with committee members so that each member is familiar with expectations (consider developing a handout for new members to acquaint them with the "rules of the game").
8. Summarize the action plan and members' responsibilities at the meeting's conclusion.
9. Follow up the meeting with electronic reminders of agreed-on action items and the upcoming meeting date.

---

arise. Disallowing interruptions can make a positive difference when some members are virtually attending and trying to distinguish between speakers or when meeting activities are being recorded.

In conclusion, advanced nurses are involved in many sorts of committees, either as members or as officers. Chairing a committee is rewarding work that has the potential to become frustrating if requisite skills are undeveloped. Keeping the group focused, maintaining reasonable control, and ensuring documentation of the committee's work are a few functions of committee chairs. Preparation is key and can make the difference between a productive committee and an inefficient committee. In general, advanced nurses of all types are well suited to committee work given their expertise in nursing process and communication.

▶ Communicating Professionalism

The term *professional presentation* usually conjures a vision of a nurse expert standing in front of a filled room presenting a topic of interest. Sharing work and promoting scholarly practice are certainly integral to professionalism. It is important for advanced nurses to recognize that each day and in every work or practice encounter they present themselves to individuals and groups in both informal and formal settings. Communicating professionalism is a critical component of an individual's advanced role practice.

Whether presenting to a group or presenting oneself to others as a professional, understanding the nature of professional behavior is imperative. The word *professional* is used in all types of venues, just as *unprofessional* is used to connote some type of behavior or characteristic that is less than that desired of a true professional. The underlying assumption is that the professional ideal is a shared concept. In fact, advanced nurses probably have divergent views on professionalism. Nurses know what professionalism is when they see it but may have a difficult time agreeing on its attributes.

Grove and Hallowell (2002) offered an interesting perspective on professional behavior based on their research. They explored what it means to behave as a professional in the United States and uncovered that behaving professionally is a balancing act between contrasting cultural values.

In addition to the seven balancing acts (**FIGURE 2-1**), professional behavior includes presentable appearance, reliability, conscientiousness, and a nonjudgmental disposition (Grove & Hallowell, 2002). This model provides an interesting perspective and helps make sense of the tensions advanced nurses experience as they try to juggle between the contrasting cultural values. It also helps nurses better appreciate the challenges experienced by foreign nurses, medical residents, and other health care professionals as they attempt to navigate the health care system.

For example, most nurses realize that health care professionals are conscious of hierarchy while they also recognize that American society is based on egalitarian premises. This idea may explain why advanced nurses and staff may engage in friendly banter with attending physicians and may interact as colleagues when discussing patient care, yet may refer to attending physicians using the title "Doctor," whereas attending physicians refer to most nurses on a first-name basis without a formal prefix (e.g., "Mrs." or "Mr."). Even nurses with completed terminal doctoral practice degrees in nursing are often referred to on a first-name basis by staff, contrary to the

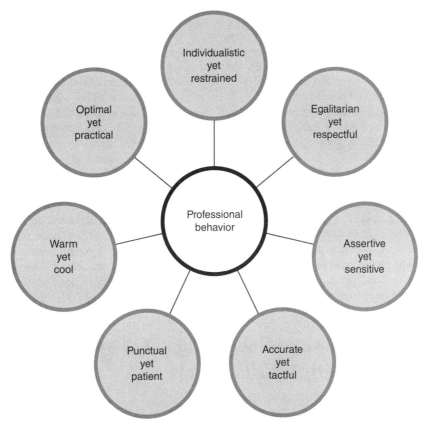

FIGURE 2-1 Seven Balancing Acts of Professional Behavior in the United States.

Data from © Grove, C., & Hallowell, W. (2002). Published by GROVEWELL LLC. Available at: www.grovewell.com/pub-usa-professional.html

titles of physician-colleagues. The difference in communication style is anecdotally attributed to social status and traditional female versus male roles; however, the Grove and Hallowell (2002) model suggests that people in the United States are generally conscious of hierarchy, and friendly equality should not be confused with social prestige awarded to and expected by people based on income, education, and history.

Advanced nurses are expected to be warm and friendly while being careful to not become so chummy with staff or other health care professionals that they lose the ability to wield influence or supervise practice in efforts to accomplish goals. The difficult aspect of Grove and Hallowell's (2002) contrasting values is that there are no absolutes. Attempting to describe to the new manager or to the graduate student enrolled in an advanced role or advanced practice nursing program that being punctual is good and holding staff accountable for punctuality is appropriate but that this timing expectation needs to be tempered with patience begs the questions, "How much patience?" and "When is late too late?" An awareness of Grove and Hallowell's (2002) seven balancing acts can attune nurses to the necessity of gauging the reactions of colleagues specific to these behaviors and learning the expectations of the organizational culture in which the advanced nurse is employed or practices.

A final thought about professionalism relates to professional titling. Many advanced nurses have completed doctoral studies and it is anticipated that the number of doctoral-prepared nurses will increase. As greater numbers complete doctorates, questions increase in frequency related to whether non-physician providers may or should use the title "doctor" in clinical practice settings.

In part, these discussions are in response to concerns about patients and others incorrectly attributing the title of doctor as signifying a physician. Likely these discussions have also been fueled by uncertainties about potential shifts in power, influence, and income opportunities. It may also be that the health care system is in a state of flux that is straining the cultural value of *egalitarian yet respectful* (Grove & Hallowell, 2002). The American Association of Colleges of Nursing (AACN) asserts that the title of doctor is not the domain of any single profession and those with an earned Doctor of Nursing Practice (DNP) degree are justly entitled to use the title "Doctor" (AACN, 2014).

Perhaps historical hierarchies are in the midst of gradual evolution. Professional persistence and consistent messaging about earned academic titles and their appropriate use in practice settings, including the necessary partnering of clearly stated license types, should be employed by the consummately professional advanced nurse. This individual works to display assertive yet sensitive, accurate yet tactful communication styles and behaviors to assure interprofessional colleagues that "a candle loses nothing by lighting another candle" (Brainy Quote, 2018). Talking points developed by AACN (2006) may have utility for the advanced nurse looking for counsel on this topic.

▶ Surviving and Flourishing in a Work World Filled with Difficult People

Advanced nurses are usually effective communicators. They work well with others and have a clear grasp of the basic principles of communication and group processes. Nurse in advanced roles are often asked to intervene in situations that involve difficult patients, staff, or health care colleagues based on their communication prowess. Nonetheless, most advanced nurses would concur that there are many times in real-world practice when working nicely with others requires the patience of a saint!

The Nurse Lament: Why Cannot Everyone Get along?

It is a simple truth that no one gets along with everyone. Advanced nurses may find themselves assigned to committees, working groups, and task forces with colleagues whom they do not prefer. Brinkman and Kirschner (2012) described 13 different types of difficult behaviors people can exhibit when under stress that can vary depending on context and relationship. They offer the "Lens of Understanding" (2012) (**FIGURE 2-2**) for viewing interpersonal dynamics and understanding the focuses and needs of these differing types during normal periods and during times of increased demands. The copyright figure is available for download from R & R Productions, Incorporated following email registration at http://www.dealingwithpeople.com /dealingwithpeople.shtml.

The Lens of Understanding is constructed with a cooperation zone and four primary foci of intents: "get the task done; get the task right; get along with people; and get appreciation from people" (Brinkman & Kirschner, 2012, p. 18). As stress is

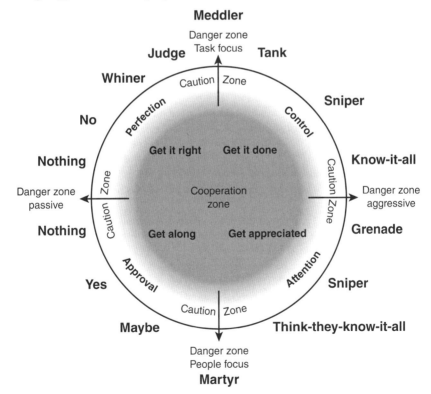

FIGURE 2-2 The Lens of Understanding

applied to the system, the four basic types of behavior begin to further differentiate into their more extreme condition. For example, the individual who at a particular time is motivated to be appreciated by colleagues at work may exhibit attention-seeking behaviors during stressful working group activities. With continued stress, this person snipes at the chairperson or becomes explosive and grenade-like. Brinkman and Kirschner (2012) make the point that behaviors change with intent. An advanced nurse concerned with getting along with her team at one particular point in a project may shift focus to getting a project done right or, perhaps at another juncture, prioritize getting the project done or begin to require feeling some appreciation from team members. The intention shifts result in behavior changes. Recognizing where the leader's or team members' behaviors are positioned within the lens can assist in responding in the best ways possible to colleagues' actions.

The Lens of Understanding is an excellent resource. Nurses in graduate courses have been encouraged to read Brinkman and Kirschner's (2012) book, and they rave about its helpfulness. Nurses have shared that they developed a better appreciation for the motivations underlying the behaviors of difficult people. Many times, they have also discovered that *they* are the difficult ones at work. Some have used the recommendations to better connect with family members as well, thereby reducing their personal stressors in ways that may have a positive effect on overall well-being, resulting in more effective work behaviors.

The four basic intents underlying the difficult behavior categories are general but useful. The advanced nurse may be able to identify colleagues who are primarily focused on getting assigned tasks completed. They want to know what is required and accomplish it as efficiently as possible. These sorts of colleagues can be quite useful on committees, as they tend to take responsibility for completing work and help to keep the group moving. However, once the stakes become greater, these get-it-done colleagues can become aggressive and act as know-it-alls (Brinkman & Kirschner, 2012).

Using the Lens of Understanding, the advanced nurse may be able to better understand why, when this task-focused person is placed under stress with deadlines or seemingly insurmountable workload, the person may become pushy and aggressive (Brinkman & Kirschner, 2012). Their comments relate to the task at hand. They are not interested in chitchat. Rather, they want the job finished. Whether it is finished to the desired quality standard of the get-it-right colleague is not as much a priority as completing the work.

This typology is an interesting tool for group exercises and self-reflection. It is interesting to apply the Lens of Understanding to work groups and to family. If, for example, the advanced nurse has a get-it-right focus and seeks perfection when developing a clinical algorithm in partnership with other professional colleagues, there may be interpersonal challenges if this nurse is obligated to work with a get-it-done colleague who wants to finish the algorithm without waiting for additional references or reviewing more data. Brinkman and Kirschner (2012) offer many suggestions for facilitating group processes and promoting healthy interpersonal dynamics based on this typology.

High-Stakes Conversations

Nurses practicing in advanced roles regularly engage in high-stakes conversations with a variety of health care personnel and stakeholders. These exchanges are described as "crucial conversations" (Patterson, Grenny, McMillan, & Switzler, 2012, p. 1) because they are high-stakes discussions involving two or more persons with varied opinions and strong emotions (Patterson et al., 2012). Advanced nurses may find it difficult to effectively handle these dialogues, preferring to avoid them or experiencing anxiety because they recognize that they do not have the necessary skill set to achieve a successful outcome.

There are resources available to assist with developing and enhancing the communication tools necessary for important conversations (Patterson et al., 2012) and the conversation techniques that facilitate jointly understood commitments to accountability (Patterson, Grenny, McMillan, & Switzler, 2013). Mastering the ability to transcend habitual, ineffective responses to high-stress conversations is imperative, particularly when working with teams composed of various types of professionals and practitioners. High-performing advanced nurses must know how to confront administrators, physicians, and high-powered colleagues without committing professional suicide (**EXEMPLAR 2-2**).

 EXEMPLAR 2-2 Ensuring Accuracy with Tact

Bernie Ward, MSN, RN, CDE, is a Nurse Educator in the staff development department of a community hospital charged with establishing a community diabetes outreach program and assisting nursing staff in efforts to improve inpatient diabetes management. In particular, Bernie's job is to guide the nursing staff to a higher quality of diabetes nursing care. Bernie had 12 years of experience as a certified diabetes educator (CDE) at a local teaching hospital prior to accepting this job at Smithville Hospital. She has been at Smithville Hospital for 7 months. Bernie is smart, conscientious, and reliable. She has a good reputation in general but is warily regarded by the medical-surgical nursing staff, who see Bernie as a relative outsider who may report them if diabetes care is amiss.

During a meeting, Bernie is asked to comment on the progress made toward meeting the established inpatient goal of 100% compliance with nursing documentation specific to medical nutrition therapy and self-monitoring of blood glucose for patients admitted with diabetes mellitus as a primary or secondary diagnosis. Bernie shares the lack of progress on one particular nursing unit as compared to two others. She accurately notes that the nurses on the more successful units, 4 West and 6 South, are eager to learn and seem pleased with the opportunity to improve their teaching and documentation, whereas "the nurses on 2 North are pretty disagreeable. It's difficult to get anything done on that unit simply because the nurses are generally disinterested and annoyed by the suggestion that they need to do things differently. The nurses page me for all the patient teaching and seem to be really uncomfortable providing instruction that even beginning nursing students are able to handle."

Bernie believed her appraisal of the 2 North staff was accurate and fair. However, she was not tactful. The CNE was present at this multidisciplinary meeting and felt that her leadership was reflected poorly by Bernie's comments. This particular unit had experienced administrative turnover several times in the past 2 years and was now managed by an inexperienced nurse manager. The unit's census had been running high due to the closure of an adjoining unit, and staff was frustrated. These circumstances did not justify the lack of attention paid to meeting the standards for diabetes mellitus nursing care; however, the lack of progress shared by the educator was perceived as tactless due to the abruptness of the criticism and the lack of explanation related to the context of the perceived inadequacy of nursing care.

Following the meeting, the CNE met with Bernie privately to share her assessment of Bernie's unprofessional behavior. Bernie was dismayed as she believed her brief

(continues)

EXEMPLAR 2-2 Ensuring Accuracy with Tact *(continued)*

explanation was candid and balanced, although it may have been less tactful than necessary. The CNE reinforced with Bernie that as a result of her indiscreet comments, the new nurse manager and the staff of 2 North were going to feel further alienated from Bernie. The CNE reiterated her expectation that Bernie balance honesty with tact and appreciate the impact that accurate but tactless comments could have on the dynamic of the nursing group in which Bernie needed to effect change.

Advanced nurses often work in teams. Some teams work in a parallel fashion, drawing information from each other without developing a common understanding of the issues that could affect the group's work or the problem at hand. Other teams are interprofessional, using inclusive language to share information and collaboratively work toward a commonly understood end (Sheehan, Robertson, & Ormond, 2007). Learning to discover or invent a mutual purpose (Patterson et al., 2012) may contribute to effective teamwork, particularly for teams striving for a collaborative approach to problem solving.

To successfully build a repertoire of strategies designed to persuade others, avoid anger and hurt feelings, and establish a safe conversational context within which to discuss high-stakes concerns, advanced nurses must first understand their personal reactions to difficult encounters and learn to monitor their responses to stress (Patterson et al., 2012). Nurses should take stock of their strengths and challenges related to difficult conversations and crucial confrontations by soliciting feedback from valued peers and supervisors. Using self-help resources and attending continuing education programs may also be useful strategies. Patterson et al. (2012) point out that many people, including advanced nurses, see only two options when in the midst of a crucial conversation (or a crucial committee meeting with a high-stakes agenda item!). These two options—either speak up and create enemies or silently suffer and contribute to a bad decision with a potentially catastrophic outcome—are labeled the "fool's choice" (Patterson et al., 2012, p. 22) because there is a viable and important third option, effective dialogue. Advanced nurses need to reflect on their style under stress and consider personal reactions to difficult conversations. One option that may be a useful catapult into this contemplative self-evaluation is the "Your Style Under Stress Test" (Patterson et al., 2012). After completing the test, advanced nurses should consider how to incorporate this new self-knowledge into their crucial conversation skill set.

Another ubiquitous communication problem plaguing health care systems and contributing to advanced role stress relates to bad behavior, performance violations, and broken pacts. Patterson et al. (2013) refer to this problem as issues of crucial accountability. It can be challenging to respond to broken promises with a sense of curiosity rather than hostility. Trying to figure out why colleagues do what they do rather than do what they are "supposed to do" or "have promised to do" is a tall order, particularly given the stressful context within which advanced nurses tend to practice and lead.

Patterson et al. (2013) offer recommendations designed to establish a safe tone at the start of the accountability conversation. They emphasize the importance of mutual respect during this conversation as the players work to establish a mutual purpose. The wise advanced nurse will need to avoid harsh conclusions or behaviors that encourage the colleague to feel uneasy and unsafe. These communication skills take practice and, again, require self-reflection and personal critique. Advanced nurses should take advantage of opportunities to master these sorts of communication processes and look for in-house or external coaching resources that may be useful to improve communication skills.

Avoiding Naïveté When Navigating Dangerous Waters

Advanced nurses must be strategic in their interactions with other health professionals, including physicians. Working strategically requires excellent communication skills, a talent for handling difficult situations without an aggressive or withdrawn stress response, and a keen sense of organizational politics. It is not uncommon for advanced nurses to experience workplace challenges and, at times, failures because of an inadequate appreciation for strategic alliances.

"How to Swim with Sharks" (Cousteau, 1987) is a wonderful piece that offers opportunities for personal reflection as well as lively discussion (**EXEMPLAR 2-3**). Use this piece as a stimulus for frank group discussion and also to illustrate some of the characteristics inherent in a very political environment. It can be interesting and informative to consider the applicability of the various rules to life in the waters of health care.

 EXEMPLAR 2-3 Swimming with Sharks: A Reflection and Discussion Opportunity

How to Swim with Sharks: A Primer
Voltaire Cousteau

Foreword
Actually, nobody wants to swim with sharks. It is not an acknowledged sport and it is neither enjoyable nor exhilarating. These instructions are written primarily for the benefit of those, who, by virtue of their occupation, find they must swim and find that the water is infested with sharks.

It is of obvious importance to learn that the waters are shark infested before commencing to swim. It is safe to say that this initial determination has already been made. If the waters were infested, the naïve swimmer is by now probably beyond help; at the very least, he has doubtless lost any interest in learning how to swim with sharks.

Finally, swimming with sharks is like any other skill: It cannot be learned from books alone; the novice must practice in order to develop the skill. The following rules simply set forth the fundamental principles which, if followed will make it possible to survive while becoming expert through practice.

Rules
1. **Assume all unidentified fish are sharks.** Not all sharks look like sharks, and some fish that are not sharks sometimes act like sharks. Unless you have witnessed docile behavior in the presence of shed blood on more than one occasion, it is best to assume an unknown species is a shark. Inexperienced swimmers have been badly mangled by assuming that docile behavior in the absence of blood indicates that the fish is not a shark.
2. **Do not bleed.** It is a cardinal principle that if you are injured, either by accident or by intent, you must not bleed. Experience shows that bleeding prompts an

(continues)

EXEMPLAR 2-3 Swimming with Sharks: A Reflection and Discussion Opportunity *(continued)*

even more aggressive attack and will often provoke the participation of sharks that are uninvolved or, as noted, previously, are usually docile.

3. Admittedly, it is difficult not to bleed when injured. Indeed, at first this may seem impossible. Diligent practice, however, will permit the experienced swimmer to sustain a serious laceration without bleeding and without even exhibiting any loss of composure. This hemostatic reflex can, in part, be conditioned, but there may be constitutional aspects as well. Those who cannot learn to control their bleeding should not attempt to swim with sharks, for the peril is too great.

   The control of bleeding has a positive protective element for the swimmer. The shark will be confused as to whether or not his attack has injured you and confusion is to the swimmer's advantage. On the other hand, the shark may know he has injured you and be puzzled as to why you do not bleed or show distress. This also has a profound effect on sharks. They begin to question their own potency or, alternatively, believe the swimmer to have supernatural powers.

4. **Counter any aggression promptly.** Sharks rarely attack a swimmer without warning. Usually there is some tentative, exploratory aggressive action. It is important that the swimmer recognize that this behavior is a prelude to an attack and takes prompt and vigorous remedial action. The appropriate countermove is a sharp blow to the nose. Almost invariably this will prevent a full-scale attack, for it makes it clear that you understand the shark's intention and are prepared to use whatever force is necessary to repel aggressive actions.

5. Some swimmers mistakenly believe that an ingratiating attitude will dispel an attack under the circumstances. This is not correct; such a response provokes a shark attack. Those who hold this erroneous view can usually be identified by their missing limb.

6. **Get out of the water if someone is bleeding.** If a swimmer (or shark) has been injured and is bleeding, get out of the water promptly. The presence of blood and the thrashing of water will elicit aggressive behavior even in the most docile of sharks. This latter group, poorly skilled in attacking, often behaves irrationally and may attack uninvolved swimmers and sharks. Some are so inept that, in the confusion, they injure themselves.

7. No useful purpose is served in attempting to rescue the injured swimmer. He either will or will not survive the attack, and your intervention cannot protect him once blood has been shed. Those who survive such an attack rarely venture to swim with sharks again, an attitude which is readily understandable.

   The lack of effective countermeasures to a fully developed shark attack emphasizes the importance of the earlier rules.

8. **Use anticipatory retaliation.** A constant danger to the skilled swimmer is that the shark will forget that he is skilled and may attack in error. Some sharks have notoriously poor memories in this regard. This memory loss can be prevented by a program of anticipatory retaliation. The skilled swimmer should engage in these activities periodically and the periods should be less than the memory span of the shark. Thus, it is not possible to state fixed intervals. The procedure may need to be repeated frequently with forgetful sharks and need be done only once for sharks with total recall.

9. The procedure is essentially the same as described under rule 4: a sharp blow to the nose. Here, however, the blow is unexpected and serves to remind the shark that you are both alert and unafraid. Swimmers should take care not to injure

EXEMPLAR 2-3 Swimming with Sharks: A Reflection and Discussion Opportunity   *(continued)*

the shark and draw blood during this exercise for two reasons: First, sharks often bleed profusely, and this leads to the chaotic situation described under rule 6. Second, if swimmers act in this fashion, it may not be possible to distinguish swimmers from sharks. Indeed, renegade swimmers are far worse than sharks, for none of the rules or measures described here is effective in controlling their aggressing behavior.

10. **Disorganized and organized attack.** Usually sharks are sufficiently self-centered that they do not act in concert against a swimmer. This lack of organization greatly reduces the risk of swimming among sharks. However, upon occasion the sharks may launch a coordinated attack upon a swimmer or even upon one of their number. While the latter event is of no particular concern to a swimmer, it is essential that one know how to handle an organized shark attack directed against a swimmer.

   The proper strategy is diversion. Sharks can be diverted from their organized attack in one of two ways. First, sharks as a group, are prone to internal dissension. An experienced swimmer can divert an organized attack by introducing something, often minor or trivial, which sets the sharks to fighting among themselves. Usually by the time the internal conflict is settled the sharks cannot even recall what they were setting about to do, much less get organized to do it.

   A second mechanism of diversion is to introduce something that so enrages the members of the group that they begin to lash out in all directions, even attacking inanimate objects in their fury.

   What should be introduced? Unfortunately, different things prompt internal dissension of blind fury in different groups of sharks. Here one must be experienced in dealing with a given group of sharks, for what enrages one group will pass unnoted by another.

   It is scarcely necessary to state that it is unethical for a swimmer under attack by a group of sharks to counter the attack by diverting them to another swimmer. It is, however, common to see this done by novice swimmers and by sharks when under concerted attack.

Little is known about the author, who died in Paris in 1812. He may have been a descendant of Francois Voltaire and an ancestor of Jacques Cousteau. Apparently this essay was written for sponge divers. Because it may have broader implications, it was translated from the French by Richard J. Johns, an obscure French scholar and Massey Professor and director of the Department of Biomedical Engineering, The Johns Hopkins University and Hospital, 720 Rutland Avenue, Baltimore, Maryland 21203.

Cousteau, V. (1987). How to swim with sharks: A primer. *Perspectives in Biology and Medicine, 30*(4), 486–489. © The Johns Hopkins University Press. Reprinted with permission of The Johns Hopkins University Press.

Reproduced from Cousteau, V. How to swim with sharks: A primer. Thorac Surg Clin 21 (2011) 441-442. © 2011 Published by Elsevier Inc.

▶ Excellent Interviews: Knowing What to Ask and How to Ask It

Conducting an effective interview is a skill that can be developed with effort and practical information. It is not uncommon for advanced nurses to lead or participate in interviewing applicants for varied employment positions. As shared governance processes become more widespread, staff is increasingly involved in interviewing and may require the guidance of an advanced nurse. It is important to have a basic understanding of interview processes, including the permissibility of certain types of questions. Conducting a successful interview not only leads to the acquisition of useful, accurate information from applicants, it also facilitates relationship building and assists in avoiding litigious situations.

Selecting people for leadership positions based on a demonstrated solid clinical skill set is no longer sufficient to ensuring quality patient care outcomes. Nurses need to be able to work as team members. Communication skills are critical. Nurses must be technically proficient and able to acquire information using the World Wide Web, electronic databases, and other library or research tools using a variety of hardware including handheld devices, smartphones, and desktop computers. Generally, health care providers of all types need an understanding of evidence-based practice and quality improvement processes, and appreciation for the health care system's focus on the triple aim (i.e., improving the patient experience of care, improving populations' health, and reducing costs) (Institute for Healthcare Improvement, 2017). These areas of expertise may or may not be informed by past clinical experiences. The key point is that interviewing proficiencies are important because stakes are high.

Evaluating job candidates for these necessary skills sets is difficult under the best of circumstances but particularly so when interviews are unplanned or casually managed. It may be helpful for advanced nurses who are involved in pre-employment interviews to consider developing an interview query path before conducting the interview. Soliciting input from staff and colleagues for structured interview guidelines supports consistent interviewing processes within the department. An interview tool that encourages collection of objective data based on the stakeholders' priorities will ensure that priority data are collected while also allowing for objective comparisons between candidates (Pearce, 2007).

Even with a structured interview format that has been endorsed by the interview team, there will be differences in interviewers' judgments as to a candidate's desirability. Graves and Karren (1996) suggest four causes of idiosyncratic interview decisions (**BOX 2-6**). These idiosyncrasies may explain how several advanced nurses interviewing a candidate for an open advanced role position can have divergent views of the applicant's suitability for the job.

Possible explanations for differing conclusions may be that each interviewer has a personal preference for a personality or communication style. Some may be looking for a particular type of past experience, whereas another is more concerned about the type of institutions in which the applicant has previously worked. Sometimes interviewers' abilities to digest and synthesize information differ, and this difference influences interview decisions. Others are intent on detail and do a fine job of recalling detail as compared to others who struggle with remembering information.

There is evidence to suggest that physical attractiveness plays a role in hiring decisions and that particularly handsome men are more frequently offered subsequent interviewing opportunities than are plain-looking men (Ruffle & Shtudiner, 2015). However, attractive women are comparatively penalized for their good looks. The researchers suggest that additional investigation is necessary but offer that a mixed interview group of men and women may aid in evening out this bias. Another potential intervention to enhance objectivity is to have applicants submit de-gendered resumes or curricula vitae to avoid sex-based assumptions and critique in an effort to level the playing field prior to the interviewing experience (Ruffle & Shtudiner, 2015). Some of these issues may be resolved by proactive discussions preceding interviews on

BOX 2-6 Etiologies of Idiosyncratic Interview Outcomes

1. Divergent views among interviewers about the qualities of the model applicant.
    - The CNS believes that the ideal applicant will be energetic and enthusiastic with management experience. Specific degree attainment is not a priority concern.
    - The NP determines that the ideal candidate will have solid practice experience in gerontology with a completed Doctor of Nursing Practice degree.
2. Interviewers with differing recall and processing abilities.
    - The nurse manager struggles to recollect interview details specific to each candidate.
    - The informatics specialist recalls minutiae about each applicant and prefers to review this data with interviewing colleagues.
3. Preferences of interviewers for a candidate that shares the interviewer's attributes and characteristics.
    - The staff educator speaks quickly and has an outgoing personality. Candidates that demonstrate these characteristics are consistently rated more highly than those who are quiet and deliberate in their verbal communication.
    - The CNL is methodical and prefers to listen before offering comments. She does not prefer applicants who are boisterous and quick-responders.
4. Interviewers' affinity for a candidate that behaves in a similar fashion to the individual interviewer.
    - The nurse anesthetist enjoys interviewing applicants that are not "up tight" and that demonstrate relaxed, fairly casual behaviors during the session.
    - The nurse executive is reserved and his behaviors are formal and deliberate. He connects best with candidates that are similarly formal and reserved.

what skills, experiences, and attributes are most highly preferred. Employing crucial conversation skills during these discussions to assure open, honest dialogue offers the best possibility of fairness.

Graves and Karren (1996) note that idiosyncratic differences also relate to whether interviewers react intuitively versus analytically to interviewing decisions. They suggest that intuitive judgments may be less accurate and are probably more difficult to defend. Advanced nurses may want to collaborate with interview colleagues to develop checklists or data collection forms that would be helpful during the interviewing decision process. These forms would differ depending on the position.

Demographic similarities may also influence interview decisions (Graves & Karren, 1996). When applicants share traits and experiences with the interviewer, they have commonalities and connect on a variety of levels. This connecting experience is different when two people have very little in common.

The interviewer's interpersonal skills also affect interview decisions (Graves & Karren, 1996). Personable, engaging interviewers who know how to draw information from applicants elicit more detail from candidates than interviewers with fewer people skills. Inappropriate comments, joking, and personal observations may also influence the interview outcome; however, there is variability in what people label as inappropriate behaviors or comments. It is wise to avoid any sort of questionable communications during an interview.

Given the potential for variability in recommendations for hiring or promoting based on interviewers' characteristics and style rather than the qualifications of the candidate, it is important for the nurses involved in interviewing processes to develop some type of guidelines for group and individual interviews. After all, the organization is adversely affected when less noteworthy candidates are hired instead of qualified candidates with potential.

In addition, developing guidelines and developing query paths based on collective input encourages the professional development of all concerned. Frank discussions help clarify values and compel people to articulate what is important to them. Graves and Karren (1996) offered five action steps for improving interview decisions (**BOX 2-7**). Advanced nurses should consider the usefulness of these action steps for interviews of all types, including interviews for promotions and in-house transfers.

Once an interview structure has been determined and general guidelines have been established, teaching people how to effectively interview is very important. Make certain to begin the interview on time and ensure that the candidate is comfortable. If there are several interviewers, remember to introduce the applicant to each group member and explain the interview process (Pearce, 2007).

Developing questions before the interview helps to avoid inappropriate and potentially litigious situations. However, during the course of a structured interview, it is not uncommon for the interviewer to deviate from the query path and explore areas that have been raised by the candidate. Education programs should address the limits to questions and the rationales for the restrictions.

Falcone (2008) shared 96 effective interview questions that can be used during the pre-employment interview. These questions may be modified to meet the needs of the health care organization (**BOX 2-8**). Falcone (2008) recommended asking behavioral questions. These types of questions require quick thinking and self-analysis. Falcone

---

BOX 2-7 Action Steps for Improving Interview Decisions

Step 1—Develop selection criteria.
Determine the knowledge, skills, and abilities required to perform the job, as well as any characteristics needed to function in the broader organizational environment.
Determine which of these criteria are most important.
Step 2—Determine how criteria will be assessed.
Determine which of the criteria can be assessed in the interview and which should be measured using other techniques.
Step 3—Develop an interview guide.
Develop a semistructured interview guide to assess any criteria identified in Step 1 and determined to be suitable for assessment in the interview in Step 2.
Step 4—Train interviewers.
Train interviewers to use the interview guide and teach them how to have positive interactions with applicants.
Step 5—Monitor the effectiveness of interviews.
Collect data on the job performance, job satisfaction, and retention of new employees. Evaluate and reward managers based on their selection decisions.

BOX 2-8 Potential Interview Questions

1. Tell me about your greatest strengths and assets. What are the three most important attributes or skills that you would bring to this health care system if you were hired to this position?
2. Describe your most positive work experience. What supports were in place that aided you in having this experience?
3. What was your least favorite position? Describe the features that you found lacking.
4. What makes you stand out among your peers?
5. What has been your most creative work achievement?
6. How would your coworkers and colleagues at your current position describe your interactions with them? How would they describe your work performance? (Heathfield, 2018)
7. How would your current supervisor describe your work patterns and contributions to the unit/department? What would your current supervisors/ team members say makes you most valuable to them?
8. What aspects of your current position do you consider most crucial?
9. What will you do differently in your present position if you do not get this position?
10. What kind of mentoring and teaching style do you have? Do you naturally delegate responsibilities or do you expect staff to come to you for added responsibilities?
11. How would you describe the amount of structure, direction, and feedback that you need to excel? Describe your ideal work environment.
12. How do you approach your work from the standpoint of balancing your professional career with your personal life?
13. What other types of positions and health care organizations are you considering right now?
14. Give me an example of your ability to facilitate progressive change within your nursing unit or department.
15. Tell me about your last performance appraisal. In which area were you most disappointed?
16. Tell me about a time when you had to overcome a major obstacle to accomplish an important goal or obligation. How did you approach the situation?
17. Why are you leaving your current employer/position/unit?
18. How do you believe that your current skills will contribute to the accomplishment of our company's goals and mission as stated on our website or in company literature? (Heathfield, 2018)

Data from Paul Falcone, AMACOM. © 1997

(2008) recognized two categories of behavioral questions: self-appraisal and situational. An example of a situational question geared to nursing practice is, "Tell me about a time when you took action on a clinically significant problem without getting the nurse manager's or supervisor's prior approval." Falcone (2008) offered rationales for each of the suggested questions, red flags that warrant concern or follow-up, and response analyses.

Some questions cannot be asked during an interview (**BOX 2-9**). These restrictions are nonnegotiable. Inappropriate questions include asking about a candidate's age. Asking about college graduation is acceptable because it is not age related; however, queries about high school graduation are not permitted. Other inappropriate question topics include specifics about disabilities, previous arrests, bankruptcy, marriage, child-rearing plans, ethnicity, and religion. Military status is protected and cannot be used to make decisions about employment.

BOX 2-9 Interview Questions That Must Be Avoided

1. What is your maiden name so that I can check your references and nursing license history?
2. Would your religion prevent you from working weekends?
3. Are you married? Are you planning on having children in the near future?
4. How many days were you sick last year?
5. Have you ever been arrested?
6. Your name is interesting. What is your family heritage?
7. Do you smoke?
8. I see that you are in the Army Reserve. How often are you deployed for training?

There are ways to obtain the information that is needed for the job interview without violating privacy conditions. For example, the interviewer is permitted to ask whether a candidate will be able to meet the attendance requirements of the job (ED Management, 2008; Falcone, 2008). Remember that candidates tend to avoid self-blame when considering why a job was not offered. Gratuitous comments and inappropriate questions reinforce the possibility that discrimination contributed to the decision to not extend employment to the candidate (ED Management, 2008).

Keep in mind that while there are no federal laws protecting candidates based on gender identity or sexual orientation, there are some state and local laws that do afford these protections. At least 22 states bar discrimination based on sexual orientation. Most afford similar protections to transgender people (Eckholm, 2015). Many corporations and other organizations have policies in place that include sexual orientation protections. Most Fortune 500 companies have sexual orientation policies and a majority also include gender identity. More than half of the 100 largest American corporations expect their suppliers to follow LGBTQ-inclusive workplace policies (Human Rights Campaign [HRC], 2017). It is very important for advanced nurses to protect the rights of all candidates, particularly those who are likely marginalized in some way, during pre-employment processes. Developing interviewing skills that are evidence based and consistent with current laws is a necessary skill for all advanced nurses involved in hiring internal and external candidates as well as those who participate in promotion processes.

▶ Social Media Networking Opportunities: Exploring New Connections

The most popular social networking websites (SNW) include LinkedIn, Facebook, Snapchat, Instagram, YouTube, Reddit, Google Plus, Pinterest, Ask.fm, Flickr, Meetup, Myspace, and Tumblr (ebizMBA, 2017). LinkedIn and Facebook are widely used across the globe for connecting professionally and personally. Nikolaou (2014) used surveys to explore how SNWs are used in job searches and how recruiters use these tools to attract and recruit candidates. Although many people use SNWs for enjoyment, LinkedIn is particularly designed to provide access to networking opportunities. These networks can be useful when searching for a new employment possibility or looking for connections to advantageous professionals.

There are also opportunities to connect with potential employers or actively looking candidates via job boards (e.g., Monster, ZipRecruiter, CareerBuilder, and Indeed). Job search engines differ from job boards. These search engines provide listings from multiple sources, so there will be duplicates. Using both options is often wise when seeking good candidates or when searching for a new employment opportunity (Doyle, 2016).

▶ Conclusion

Most advanced nurses work in demanding practice settings filled with diverse personalities, multiple agendas, and limited resources. Wielding influence in this type of environment requires excellent communication skills, both verbal and nonverbal, that can be quickly and readily transferred from one type of situation to another. Advanced nurses interact with people possessing varying degrees of social prestige and privilege. They rapidly transition from colleague status to subordinate, supervisor, coach, mentor, leader, practitioner, and friend. Those who aspire to succeed in meaningful ways will continue to develop their communication skill sets.

Advanced nurses with and without formal rank often use influence to affect outcomes, enhance positive work environments, and promote quality care. Whether sending emails, chairing committees, interviewing applicants, facilitating group processes, or intervening in distressing or awkward group dynamics, the effective advanced nurse demonstrates finesse and aplomb through consistently professional communications. This chapter reviews communication basics with the goal of assisting the advanced nurse with the procedural, structural, and process information necessary to begin building a repertoire of effective communication strategies.

References

American Association of Colleges of Nursing. (2006). News from AACN: AACN talking points in response to the AMA's resolution 211. *Journal of Professional Nursing, 22*, 265. doi: 10.1016/j .profnurs.2006.08.001

American Association of Colleges of Nursing. (2014). DNP talking points. Retrieved January 15, 2018, from http://www.aacnnursing.org/DNP/About/Talking-Points.

American Management Association. (2008). 2007 electronic monitoring and surveillance survey. Retrieved August 9, 2017 from, http://www.amanet.org/training/articles/2007-electronic -monitoring-and-surveillance-survey-41.aspx.

American Management Association. (2018). The latest on workplace monitoring and surveillance. Retrieved January 15, 2018, from http://www.amanet.org/training/articles/the-latest-on-workplace -monitoring-and- surveillance.aspx.

Banks, C. (2002). Taking the hot seat. *Nursing Standard, 16*(47), 96. Retrieved February 5, 2006, CINAHL Database of Nursing and Allied Health Literature.

Brainy Quote. (2018). James Keller quotes. Retrieved January 15, 2018, from https://www.brainyquote .com/quotes/authors/j/james_keller.html.

Brinkman, R., & Kirschner, R. (2012). *Dealing with people you can't stand. How to bring out the best in people at their worst* (3rd ed.). New York, NY: McGraw-Hill.

Chory, R. M., Vela, L. E., & Avtgis, T. A. (2015). Organizational surveillance of computer- mediated workplace and communication: Employee privacy concerns and responses. *Employee Responsibilities and Rights Journal, 28*, 23–43. doi:10.1007/s10672-015- 9267-4

Cousteau, V. (1987). How to swim with sharks: A primer. *Perspectives in Biology and Medicine, 30*(4), 486–489.

Doyle, A. (2016). Difference between a job board and a job search engine. *The Balance.*
Retrieved August 18, 2017, from https://www.thebalance.com/difference-between-a-job -board-and-a-job-search-engine-2061865.

Dubey, R. (2017). 15+ excellent free large file sharing tools to securely send and share large files online. *TechReviewPro*. Retrieved August 10, 2017, from https://techreviewpro.com /free- large-file-sharing-tools-send-large-files-online-4575/.

DuPont, P. (2014). The 16 best meeting scheduler apps and tools. Retrieved August 11, 2017, from https://zapier.com/blog/best-meeting-scheduler-apps/

ebizMBA. (2017). Top 15 most popular social networking sites. Retrieved January 15, 2018, from http://www.ebizmba.com/articles/social-networking-websites.

Eckholm, E. (2015). Next fight for gay rights. Bias in jobs and housing. *The New York Times.* Retrieved August 18, 2017, from https://www.nytimes.com/2015/06/28/us/gay-rights-leaders -push-for-federal-civil-rights-protections.html.

ED Management. (2008). Interview questions are dangerous territory. *ED Management, 20*(2), 21–22.

Falcone, P. (2008). *96 great interview questions to ask before you hire* (2nd ed.). New York, NY: AMACOM.

Graves, L. M., & Karren, R. J. (1996). The employee selection interview: A fresh look at an old problem. *Human Resource Management, 35*(2), 163–180.

Grove, C., & Hallowell, W. (2002). The seven balancing acts of professional behavior in the United States. A cultural values perspective. Retrieved January 15, 2018, from http://www.grovewell .com/pub-usa-professional.html.

Heathfield, S. (2018). Best interview questions for employers to ask applicants. *The Balance.* Retrieved April 25, 2018, from https://www.thebalance.com/best-interview- questions-for-employers-to-ask -applicants-1918483.

Hern, A. (2015). Don't know the difference between emoji and emoticon? Let me explain. *The Guardian.* Retrieved August 10, 2017, from https://www.theguardian.com/technology/2015 /feb/06/difference-between-emoji-and- emoticons-explained.

Human Rights Campaign. (2017). An important step toward workplace equality. An executive order on federal contractors. Accessed August 18, 2017, from http://www.hrc.org/resources /an-important-step-toward-workplace-equality-an- executive-order-on-federal-c

Institute for Healthcare Improvement. (2017). Initiatives. The IHI triple aim. Retrieved August 18, 2017, from http://www.ihi.org/engage/initiatives/TripleAim/Pages/default.aspx.

Kaufman, L. (2013). The best free programs and online services for sending and sharing large files. *How-To Geek.* Retrieved August 8, 2017, from https://www.howtogeek.com/133761 /the-best-free-programs-and-online-services-for- sending-and-sharing-large-files/.

Lowensohn, J. (2010). How to save and share ridiculously large files. CNET. Retrieved August 10, 2017, from https://www.cnet.com/how-to/how-to-save-and-share-ridiculously-large- files/.

Microsoft Corporation. (2017). *SharePoint.* Retrieved August 14, 2017, from https://products.office .com/en-us/sharepoint/collaboration.

Nikolaou, I. (2014). Social networking web sites in job search and employee recruitment. *International Journal of Selection and Assessment, 22,* 179–189. doi: 10.1111/ijsa.12067

Patterson, K., Grenny, J., McMillan, R., & Switzler, C. (2013). *Crucial accountability. Tools for resolving violated expectations, broken commitments, and bad behavior* (2nd ed.). New York, NY: McGraw-Hill.

Patterson, K., Grenny, J., McMillan, R., & Switzler, C. (2012). *Crucial conversations. Tools for talking when stakes are high* (2nd ed.). New York, NY: McGraw-Hill.

Pearce, C. (2007). Ten steps to conducting a selection interview. *Nursing Management, 14*(5), 21.

Privacy Rights Clearinghouse. (2017a). Workplace privacy and employee monitoring. Retrieved January 15, 2018, from https://www.privacyrights.org/consumer-guides/workplace- privacy-and-employee -monitoring.

Privacy Rights Clearinghouse. (2017b). Bring your own device (BYOD) . . . at your own risk. Retrieved January 15, 2018, from https://www.privacyrights.org/consumer- guides/bring-your -own-device-byod-your-own-risk.

Robert, H. M., Honemann, D. H., Balch, T. J., Seabold, D. E., & Gerber, S. (2011). *Robert's rules of order newly revised* (11th ed.). Philadelphia, PA: DeCapo Press; Perseus Books Group.

Robert's Rules Association. (2011). Short history of Robert's rules. Retrieved August 1, 2017, from http://www.robertsrules.com/history.html.

Ruffle, B., & Shtudiner, Z. (2015). Are good-looking people more employable? *Management Science, 61.* 1760–1776. https://doi.org/10.1287/mnsc.2014.1927.

Sheehan, D., Robertson, L., & Ormond, T. (2007). Comparison of language used and patterns of communication in interprofessional and multidisciplinary teams. *Journal of Interprofessional Care, 21*(1), 17–30.

Thorsen, Steffen. (2017). Home. Retrieved August 11, 2017, from https://www.timeanddate.com/.

CHAPTER 3

Executing Effective Performance Appraisals: Energizing Employees and Improving Practice

Patti Rager Zuzelo, EdD, RN, ACNS-BC, ANP-BC, CRNP, FAAN

Nurses are frequently and regularly involved in performance evaluation processes, including self-appraisals, colleague assessments, postmortem team process reviews, and, at times, formal reviews of subordinates, supervisors, and new employees. While managers and administrators typically provide feedback that follows established reporting mechanisms based on a bureaucratic chain of command, many nurses in advanced roles participate in performance appraisals without having line authority; in other words, many do not have organizationally subordinate employees reporting directly to them. Advanced nurses practicing in various direct and indirect care roles are often asked to contribute to formal employee evaluations and may also be responsible for participating in action plans designed to improve individual employee job performance or to substantiate the need for employee dismissal or continued hire. These are important and potentially high-stakes activities for the organization and for the appraised employee.

Learning to execute effective performance appraisals is an important indirect care skill that influences direct care processes and outcomes. Effectively evaluating job execution relies on honest and authentic communication and a genuine interest in leading the collective team and its individual members to an improved level of performance. Effective appraisers want to see employees grow and succeed. Personal development is also important and advanced nurses need to practice self-reflection and self-critique so that they, too, can grow and improve in their contributions to care processes and outcomes.

Advanced nurses of all types participate in informally evaluating performance on a day-to-day basis. They provide feedback, recommend colleagues for additional responsibilities, address patient care problems related to nursing performance, and frequently give nurses a "thumbs up" or "thumbs down" related to the quality of their care practices. These informal performance appraisal encounters often contribute to formal performance reviews.

Many people are intimidated by evaluation processes and would prefer to avoid appraisal activities. Performance appraisal discomfort is a problematic concern in human resource management (Gbadamosi & Ross, 2012). Advanced nurses may feel uneasy with perceived conflict between their roles of coach/mentor and judge when appraising staff. Gbadamosi and Ross (2012) observe that performance appraisal discomfort effects may include more lenient appraisal ratings than warranted and less variability than is correct among subordinates' formal evaluations. Evaluators may give higher ratings in an effort to avoid difficult face-to-face conversations with employees whose performance warrants lower scores. Poorly performing employees do not always readily concur with critical feedback, and this situation may be very uncomfortable to the appraiser thereby contributing to evaluator avoidance tactics.

There are important dos and don'ts associated with formal evaluation processes. Advanced role nurses need to confront the challenges associated with performance appraisal and learn to view evaluation processes as opportunities to establish relationships, support motivated colleagues, or redirect disengaged or frustrated nurses. Skilled evaluators have the potential to significantly contribute to the employment environment and affect positive change at individual and team performance levels.

From a practical perspective, performance appraisals are here to stay, regardless of the organizational model within which advanced nurses practice, so it is important to learn how to make them work for the benefit of all concerned. This chapter addresses performance appraisals, including self-evaluation, employee evaluations whether satisfactory or unsatisfactory, and peer review. Succession planning is also discussed given its close relationship to evaluation and goal setting. Strategies, techniques, and human resource guidelines are offered; and exemplars provide coaching opportunities for self-instruction and group discussion.

▶ Employee Evaluation

There is little evidence to support the premise that performance appraisals actually improve performance (Zemke, 1991). Hewko and Cummings (2016) suggesting that when performance management and evaluation (PME) is examined through the lens of critical theory, findings reveal that health care system PME activities potentially encourage a compliant, dependent, and passively oriented workforce that focuses on technology. It may be that typical PME systems support a perpetually reinforced system of inequitable power structures. Usual PME activities include established definitions of performance expectations, measurements, and application partnered with feedback (Hewko & Cummings, 2016).

Of note is the question of whether nurses require their performance to *be* managed. There is little proof that this is a true proposition. It is also interesting to consider that management tends to incorporate two approaches, hard and soft (Hewko & Cummings, 2016). Hard tactics refer to those that direct, control, and rule; soft methods represent those that guide and lead. The hard versus soft approach varies depending on the context of the interaction and, perhaps, the goal of the discourse.

Hewko and Cummings (2016) suggest that encouraging a passive, compliant, and dependent workforce is counterintuitive given health care system challenges and the need for independent thinkers with initiative and autonomy. This critical analysis of performance appraisal is worthy of consideration. Advanced nurses should, perhaps, think about the attributes and behaviors that they are attempting to nurture and encourage via performance appraisals and keep their focus on encouraging nurse traits that support assertive, independent, and autonomous professionalism.

The Effectiveness of Performance Appraisal

Performance appraisal may be less effective than hoped because it focuses on a uniform set of behavioral expectations that fail to consider unique and desired individual strengths and characteristics (Van Woerkom & de Bruijn, 2016). There is concern that employee performance evaluation may focus on highly variable behavioral criterion and disregard areas in which the employee performs in excellent fashion. As a result, employees often devalue appraisals and feel frustrated with these annual processes.

Van Woerkom and de Bruijn (2016) assert that employees should be cheered to maximize their strengths and, in this way, perhaps achieve superb job performance. It may be that a strengths-based performance appraisal that focuses on strategies an employee might use to maximize contributions to health care system goals would be a more uplifting, empowering, and successful approach than traditional strategies to capitalize on valuable attributes and talents in the health care system workplace. Van Woerkom and de Brujin (2016) make the additional point that a workplace that encourages inclusivity and full participation is more likely supported by a strengths-based performance appraisal system than a linear, nonindividualized criterion-based system.

Recognizing the limitations of the traditional annual performance review, goal setting may be one of the most useful aspects of performance improvement processes providing that the conditions are right. Goal-setting theory (Locke & Latham, 2002) was formulated on the idea that conscious goals affect action. Front-line managers and nurses in advanced roles may not have access to the learning and development needed to become skilled goal-setting advisors to employees. The heavy workloads associated with advanced practice roles are also barriers to developing the managerial skill set needed for effective performance appraisal (Kellner, Townsend, Wilkinson, & Lawrence, 2016).

Many advanced nurses likely prefer their practice-focused work, and because this is the work that is usually rewarded and supported in care-centered settings, performance appraisal techniques and front-line managing skills are often deficiently addressed. Balanced and accurate evaluative input from advanced practice registered nurses (APRNs), educators, staff development specialists, managers, and clinical nurse leaders (CNLs) is critically important to the relevance and accuracy of staff evaluations, including associated goal setting; and this input may affect whether individual nurse performance flourishes.

What Do Performance Appraisals Actually Accomplish?

The performance appraisal process has multiple purposes, including rewarding and recognizing good employees, coaching nurses and ancillary staff who are having difficulties, staying in touch with staff, and avoiding legal trouble in the event of employee disciplinary actions, up to and including termination. Work performance appraisals have utility when making personnel decisions related to promotions or transfers (Chandra, 2006) and also to support succession planning, an activity that is often deficiently addressed in hospital settings (Kellner et al., 2016). Keep in mind that performance appraisals are formative, intended to support ongoing performance growth. Assessment is summative. This distinction is important. When nurses in advanced roles work with staff and colleagues to appraise performance, the goal is to encourage growth from the vantage point of the employment role and mutual perceptions and goals. The partnership is similar to that of a learner and a mentor. When advanced nurses participate in summative assessment, the goal is to judge. Oftentimes, nurses in advanced roles are more comfortable mentoring than judging but both activities are necessary and important.

Performance evaluations are useful when evaluating new hires for purposes of making judgments as to whether the employee meets required standards set for the end of the probationary period. This particular evaluation is critically important to the new hire and to the organization as it is best to make decisions about continued employment early in the employment relationship rather than after an employee has been officially endorsed as acceptably performing at end orientation. Advanced nurses of many types may have opportunities to participate in orientation activities and are wise to keep evaluative responsibilities in mind when interacting with the new employee during this probationary period. Educators, staff development specialists, and clinical nurse specialists (CNSs), in particular, often have good rapport and close working relationships with front-line staff, providing these advanced nurses with opportunities to contribute personalized and accurate assessment data to performance evaluations.

Performance Appraisal as a Factor in Performance Management

Performance appraisal may be viewed as one component of comprehensive performance management. Shaneberger (2008) suggests that performance management consists of eight elements:

1. An accurate, well-written job description
2. Initial competencies that describe the knowledge and skills required of the nurse
3. Appropriate orientation to the role and its expectations
4. Goal setting and performance planning
5. Annual competency assessment
6. Coaching, mentoring, and recognition
7. Performance evaluation conducted by the employee and by a peer
8. A performance enhancement plan

Managing performance as a strategy for elevating its quality is certainly a noteworthy goal. Siriwardena and Gillam (2014) assert that quality improvement science approaches may be applied to individual practice performance to improve it. They offer recommendations for incorporating quality improvement science techniques into the appraisal process based on Norfolk's RDM-p model, integrating relationships, diagnostics, management, and professionalism (RDM-p) (Siriwardena & Gillam, 2014).

Relationships are viewed as central to clinical work. Effective practice relies on skilled communication techniques and processes. Diagnostics refers to gathering, interpreting, and appropriately prioritizing information necessary for solid decision making. Management pertains to effectively monitoring the self in terms of performance and personal health. Professionalism is considered the glue of individual practice as it is evidence of a commitment to best practice (Siriwardena & Gillam, 2014). Showing respect, acting responsibly, and demonstrating ethical and moral behavior are cornerstones to performance excellence.

The performance management elements (Shaneberger, 2008) and the RDM-p model (Siriwardena & Gillam, 2014) offer guidance for managing, critiquing, and improving performance. Performance appraisal should ideally occur within the context of a management system that provides necessary structural, procedural, and functional elements while also nurturing, nudging, and sustaining individual performance improvements. Nurses in advanced roles need to partner with new and established colleagues to work toward continuous improvements in individual and team performances.

Preparing for the Appraisal

Advanced nurses need to think about staff performance appraisals before they happen. A proactive stance will provide the data necessary for a fair and well-informed evaluation. In some ways, employee performance appraisal is similar to the nursing process. Both processes involve assessment, diagnosis, goal setting and intervention planning, evaluation, and a feedback loop to continue surveillance and persist in adjusting or continuing planned interventions to achieve desired goals (**FIGURE 3-1**).

Collecting Data to Inform the Appraisal

Collecting appraisal data is critical to a fair evaluation. Employees have both strengths and weaknesses. Recognizing both types of performance goes a long way toward demonstrating to the employee and the collective employee group that the advanced nurse acted fairly and with professional intentions. In the rare event of employee-initiated grievances or lawsuits related to the outcomes of an evaluation, fairness, balance, and due process are essential. Of course, ensuring just and evenhanded critique is also the right thing to do. An employee evaluation is a test in the eyes of the law as it reflects a decision that affects an individual's status in the organization (Zemke, 1991). The organization must be able to confidently assert that this test was nondiscriminatory and unbiased.

Various strategies may be used for collecting and organizing evaluation data. Keep an electronic or hard copy log (DelPo, 2005) that details memorable incidents, patient care exemplars, projects, leadership activities, or other job-related occasions that showcase behaviors relating to performance. Consider constructing a spreadsheet

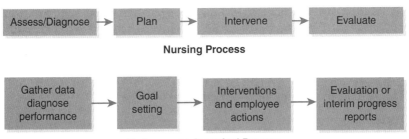

FIGURE 3-1 Similarities Between the Nursing Process and Performance Appraisal Processes.

that enables the user to quickly add and retrieve information. Make certain to ask staff to share information on an ongoing basis about their involvement in professional organizations, continuing education, and community-based activities. Take advantage of email and request that staff periodically share information and updates. Electronic communication is easily filed away in individual computer-based folders or printed in hard copy form for traditional files. Staff should be encouraged to take the initiative and proactively share appraisal data.

Electronic record keeping is often a popular mode of appraisal data collection; however, paper-based files do have advantages. Hanging files labeled with each employee's name are useful in preparation for the written evaluation. Take the time to file or scan letters from families, patients, colleagues, and administrators. Save flyers from in-service programs that the employee has presented or attended. Keep copies of documentation that demonstrate the employee's charting habits. Photocopies, scanned documents, snips, or computer printouts are easy to save but make certain to remove any patient identifiable data. Maintain retrieval data in case chart retrieval is necessary, again, attending to patient privacy.

Smartphones can be valuable tools for data collection. Audio recording and quick reminder notes to avoid forgetting critical incidents or particularly stellar occasions of work efforts are two examples of how smartphones demonstrate utility. Using the camera feature to record flyers or Health Insurance Portability and Accountability Act (HIPAA)–compliant documentation can save time and prevent missed documentation opportunities.

There are times when nurses practicing in advanced roles notice either an exceptional effort or a troubled behavior exhibited by colleagues or subordinate staff. At these times, it is important to give immediate evaluative feedback. Do not wait for the annual review period. If oral feedback is offered, make certain to document the conversation in writing and place it in the employee's file. Facts of events, positive or negative, are important to the written annual evaluation or to support possible disciplinary action at some future point (DelPo, 2005). Keep in mind that formal performance assessments should never come as a surprise to the employee. Rather, data informing the assessment should be familiar to the employee as should the associated critique.

Make certain to document anecdotal information as close to the event's occurrence as possible. Do not procrastinate on describing events. Certainly do not delay documentation and then attempt to pass off these notations as having been made at the time of the incidents. Not only is this a dishonest tactic, but it also jeopardizes the integrity of performance appraisal. Credibility and veracity are important, particularly if the end result of the appraisal is disputed by the employee.

Performance appraisals must be consistent with written job descriptions. Make certain to have copies of job descriptions and nursing department standards, guidelines, and protocols available for review, if needed, during the appraisal encounter. Reviewing materials together is a good opportunity for both staff and advanced nurses to become reacquainted with job expectations and professional development opportunities.

Documenting Appraisal Findings

Describing observed behaviors or expectations in written form can be challenging. Employees expect unique evaluations that are pertinent to their individual contributions or practice patterns. Comments should relate to observable, measurable activities and outcomes. Developing a repertoire of varied comments and observations using a variety of wording and phrases emphasizes the individuality of the written evaluation and promotes an understanding that appraisals have been uniquely tailored to each nursing employee (**TABLE 3-1**).

In other words, try to avoid a "cookie cutter" approach to written evaluations. Each written evaluation should be reasonably unique and personalized. It is deflating for an employee to share with a colleague a particularly positive comment or enthusiastic phrase of endorsement that was offered by the evaluator only to hear, "The same thing was on my evaluation!" Various published resources provide helpful suggestions and templates for documenting and describing behaviors. These resources may be helpful to nurses in advanced roles who are contributing to a performance appraisal.

Keep in mind that most employees, including nurses, perform in an *average* fashion. The notion of *average* has important implications for performance review. In general, average performance is an expected or typical level of job execution. Average or standard performance satisfies job expectations, meets practice standards, and is a reasonable and usual level of employee functioning. The expected level of performance should be detailed in the job descriptions of the employing institution.

TABLE 3-1 Examples of Individualized Evaluative Feedback

Positive Evaluative Comments	Evaluative Comments That Document Need for Improvement
■ Attends to important patient care details ■ Dresses and grooms neatly and consistently with dress code requirements ■ Effectively organizes staff assignments during periods of increased acuity ■ Offers assistance to colleagues on consistent and regular basis ■ Shows friendly demeanor that encourages collegiality ■ Contributes to positive group dynamics by demonstrating consistently professional communication style ■ Accommodates unit-based care needs by adjusting schedule whenever possible ■ Frequently shares evidence-based practice information with colleagues ■ Contributes to positive team-building efforts by remembering staff birthdays and celebrating important occasions	**NOTEWORTHY INCIDENTS:** ■ Required several reminders to remove acrylic nails and gel polish. ■ Called in sick the day before two major paid holidays. **NOTEWORTHY PATTERNS:** ■ Returns late from agreed-upon break times. ■ Displays inconsistent handwashing practices ■ Wears inappropriate footwear that is inconsistent with dress code requirements ■ Gossips during shift report about nursing and team colleagues ■ Uses profanity or vulgarity during interactions with team members and within hearing range of patients and families

Describing job performance as *ordinary* or *standard* or suggesting that an employee's quality of work is *consistent with the mean* is not often perceived as a particularly flattering description; however, it is likely the most accurate depiction for most staff members. Typical performance is more difficult to evaluate than atypical or extreme performance. As a result, evaluative ratings tend to be less accurate when they pertain to average work performance (Chandra, 2006).

In comparison, exceptional performance is an exception from the norm. Consider that if each employee performs at a level deemed as exceptional, this superior level of functioning then becomes the mean or average. Exceptional performance is atypical and unique. Behaviors evaluated as such may be positive or negative. Assisting nurses to identify areas in which they excel versus those that satisfy required standards is an important responsibility of advanced nurses. This sort of coaching contributes to staff developing realistic self-appraisals and contributing to productive evaluation encounters. Shepard (2005) noted, "There are superstars in the workforce, and there are derelicts. The vast majority of the workforce falls between these two extremes" (p. 4). This observation is true for the nursing workforce just as it is for the workforce at large.

Many health care systems tie financial remuneration and incentives to job performance. If the advanced nurse regards *every* employee as exceptional rather than most as average and some as underperforming, resource allocation can become unfair. Likewise, if nurses are evaluated poorly to ensure that available dollars are not exceeded due to rightfully high performance assessment scores, the performance appraisal system becomes falsified. In fact, associating financial incentives with performance evaluations is one area in which evaluators routinely cheat to make the system work to satisfy their own purposes (Zemke, 1991). These manipulations contribute to the skepticism that many employees have about performance appraisal systems. Of course, institutional manipulations also may occur when dollars are capped and nurses are scored to satisfy the capped limits rather than to reflect true performance ratings. Staff members often identify these maneuverings as dishonest and their perceptions can contribute to negative feelings about evaluation systems.

One interesting caveat is that performance evaluation determinations should take into account nurse disposition and structural and situational factors. Swift, Moore, Sharek, and Gino (2013) point out that it is common practice to attribute too much of an employee's success to ability and personal attributes and too little to structural and situational circumstances that placed the individual in the position to be successful. The concern with this inflated appraisal is that employees who benefit from practicing in favorable situations may be more likely to be highly appraised and rewarded, including promotion, than equally skilled but less advantaged peers. Advanced nurses need to consider the ease with which success was achieved (**TABLE 3-2**). One interesting strategy for dissecting attributes from context is to reflect on a modification of Lewin's attributional equality statement (Behavior equals a function of [Disposition and Situation] to Disposition equals [Behavior minus Situation]) (Swift et al., 2013).

Make certain that there is documentation readily available to support evaluative comments. When the advanced nurse is contributing to or taking the lead on constructing a negative performance appraisal that may lead to employee suspension or termination, the evaluator should seek the advice of institutional human resource personnel before the actual appraisal session to verify that necessary documentation is in order and to ensure that the written evaluation is consistent with personnel

TABLE 3-2 Discerning Between Ease of Circumstances Versus Influence of Talent

Situation	Facilitating queries: Ease of circumstance?	Facilitating queries: Influence of talent?
The nurse reports that there has been a decrease in medication administration errors of 75% since implementing walking rounds as a reporting strategy between shifts. The nurse designed and led the walking rounds initiative.	■ Is the reduced number of errors the result of under-reporting? ■ Is a reduction of 75% a positive finding or does this reduction reflect a concerning trend? ■ Were other units also implementing walking rounds and did this trend influence the receptivity of staff to the unit-based project? ■ Were other nurse colleagues involved in the walking rounds initiative? ■ How did staff enthusiasm and talents influence this outcome? Who was the *driver* of the practice change? ■ Was nursing administration actively supporting walking rounds as a required change in reporting practices?	■ Did the nurse directly affect unit staff resistance to this project? ■ Was there resistance or was the staff eager to participate in walking rounds? ■ Did the nurse positively engage colleagues and facilitate this change in practice? ■ How much of the walking rounds initiative was accomplished because of the talents and efforts of this nurse versus because the "time was ripe" on the unit?
A nurse practicing as a staff development specialist is responsible for new hire orientation. Three of five new nurses have resigned from the institution before successfully completing orientation activities.	■ What are the local hiring conditions? ■ How are new hires treated by those staff assigned to preceptorship roles? ■ Is there collaboration between staff development and unit-based management?	■ Have there been similar occasions of attrition during previous orientations under this particular specialist's leadership? ■ What other performance indicators are available for consideration specific to this specialist?

(continues)

TABLE 3-2 Discerning Between Ease of Circumstances Versus Influence of Talent *(continued)*

Situation	Facilitating queries: Ease of circumstance?	Facilitating queries: Influence of talent?
The specialist is applying for a promotion to a new role.	■ What are the institutional attrition trends for this same period of time? ■ To where did these new hires transfer/seek new employment? ■ Were the resigning nurses hired to their first choice of unit/department and was this a concern for these hires? ■ What was the performance level of these new nurses at the point of resignation? ■ Is exit interview data available for review?	■ Was the specialist aware of any concerns with this particular orientee group and, if so, how were these issues addressed prior to the resignation? ■ Was feedback from the staff partnered with the orientees and the specialist? ■ Has the specialist identified possible areas for future improvements and developed a possible action plan? ■ How has the specialist attributed responsibility for the attrition?

policies, procedures, and practices. Seeing preliminary guidance may prevent litigation or grievances. Even if such a response is not prevented, it is certainly best if the appraisal has been vetted by an objective human resource expert.

Ensure Consistency Between Job Descriptions and Performance Appraisals

Job descriptions and institutional goals and objectives should drive performance appraisals. Nurses' practice should be compared to these established standards and not necessarily to the level of peer group performance. There are times when advanced nurses need to consider the day-to-day execution of job responsibilities of nurses who are performing better than, consistent with, or below the norm of staff practicing on the particular work unit. If an average functioning nurse works within a group of high performers, the written appraisal should reflect this average, but satisfactory, level of activity. Of course, it is reasonable and desirable to encourage this nurse to capitalize on the availability of above-average and excellent colleagues so as to enhance professional development. If pay increases are influenced by documented appraisal outcomes, the financial rewards should be less for the average performing nurse than the monies awarded to the more productive peers.

Job Descriptions or Job Standards

Job descriptions typically have results standards and behavior standards. A results standard is a description of a result that is expected from any employee who holds a particular job (DelPo & Guerin, 2003). For example, an RN might be required to present two unit-based educational programs each year using a variety of presentation strategies and supported by a minimum of two evidence-based practice resources. Alternatively, the nurse is likely expected to maintain current cardiopulmonary resuscitation certification or other types of credentials.

A behavior standard is a description of how nurses should behave while getting work done. For example, the health care agency administration may have prioritized patient and family satisfaction. A behavior standard related to this focus might be that nurses will respond to all patient and family requests with courtesy and professionalism and in a timely manner. Job description standards, results, and behaviors should be periodically reviewed with staff, particularly if there are new initiatives and revisions. Job standards are the foundation of the performance appraisal, in partnership with job goals (DelPo & Guerin, 2003).

Types of Appraisal Forms and Processes

Performance appraisal systems vary by institution, and these systems may have idiosyncratic processes and functionalities. Most systems are paper based in some aspects but Web-based and software systems are available and increasingly common given potential cost savings and efficiencies. A quick Web-based search reveals hundreds of software appraisal systems promising increased productivity, reduced costs, simplified scoring, and enhanced tracking. These systems provide opportunities to mine performance appraisal data to inform robust human resource tracking enterprises. High frequency appraisal methods incorporate a variety of components and approaches, including self-evaluation, peer review, portfolio compilation, multisource feedback (including 360-degree feedback), and employer–employee encounters that may be paper based and institutionally home *grown*.

Administering the Effective Evaluation

Once the performance appraisal has been documented based on careful consideration of performance within the context of expectations, the evaluation needs to be shared with the employee or, in the event of peer review, the colleague.

Arranging the Evaluation Interview

Employees should receive advance notice of the evaluation time, date, and setting to allow ample time for planning and data gathering. Providing the opportunity for a period of self-reflection prior to the evaluative event is important and courteous. Conducting an appraisal session on the run is not conducive to product goal setting or relationship building. Employees need to feel valued, and good planning facilitates this sentiment. The meeting should be held in a private, comfortable setting without distractions.

Depending on their roles, advanced nurses may be directly involved in these sessions as either the sole evaluator or as a partner to the nurse manager or administrator.

Each party should be comfortably positioned; and if there are two evaluators, then efforts should be made to eliminate a possible impression of "two against one" during the appraisal gathering. It is usually more appropriate for the nurse with line authority to control the meeting with input offered by the other advanced role nurse when requested.

Delivering the Appraisal

The expression "Keep it real" refers to the importance of authentic and honest relationships and communications. Authentic relationships are built on candor and mutual respect. If the advanced nurse avoids sharing performance problems with a nurse or colleague, this individual will be unaware of what is needed to improve performance. Ignoring deficiencies or sharing the circumstances of problems with uninvolved colleagues without directly informing the person who is involved eliminates opportunities to share perceptions and work through incorrect assumptions or judgment errors. The fundamental rule of performance appraisals is that they must be honest, even if this honesty contributes to discomfort.

Avoid Biases

A biased performance appraisal refers to an inaccurate distortion of performance measurement (MSG Experts, 2017). Advanced nurses should be aware of these biases so as to safeguard against incorporating these inaccuracies into the appraisal process or individual performance evaluations. Primacy effect, halo effect, horn effect, excessive leniency or stiffness error, central tendency or middle-path error, personal biases, spillover effect, and recency effect collectively encompass the wide range of potential performance appraisal biases (**TABLE 3-3**). Some of these particular biases may be unfamiliar to advanced nurses, but lack of awareness does not protect the evaluated nurse from the adverse effects of appraisal misrepresentation or misjudgment.

Stick with the Facts, Not the Persona

Nursing is a people profession. Personality *does* count as it affects key relationships, including those with patients, families, coworkers, and administrators. There are many different communication styles and highly variable work patterns that contribute to high-quality outcomes. In other words, there is not one path to excellence. When the advanced role nurse is compelled to engage in work with people who have markedly different personalities and preferences, it may be necessary to reflect on whether the coworker's style is personally unappealing or if the team member's style is genuinely inappropriate or ineffective within the context of professionalism. If a performance problem is directly related to a nurse's conduct, focus on the behavior and offer specific details. As an example, consider, "You have offered negative comments during taped shift reports specific to patients' weight, alcohol addiction, or family circumstances on at least five occasions in the past 6 months. This behavior is unacceptable and must immediately stop." Focus on the behaviors and the results of these behaviors. There is nothing to be gained by negative comments about the nurse's personality or disposition; rather, focus on the behaviors that require correction or improvement.

TABLE 3-3 Performance Appraisal Biases and Exemplars

Type of Bias (MCG Experts, 2017)	Exemplar
Primacy effect: First impressions are excessively influential on subsequent performance appraisal decisions.	The clinical nurse leader (CNL) is interacting with a small group of senior nursing students. One student arrives late and appears disheveled and angry. He does not apologize for the disruption and interrupts the group to share complaints about the hospital parking situation. The CNL perceives that this student is rude and unprofessional. Three months later he is hired to the unit and the CNL is assigned responsibility for guiding his orientation experience. Although his preceptor reports that his performance is on par with that of the other newly hired graduate nurses and his communication skills are above average, the CNL documents his interpersonal skills and professional demeanor as requiring improvement. The CNL's initial encounter with this nurse continues to dominate her appraisal of his professionalism.
Halo effect: One particularly valued positive attribute triggers a high evaluation overall on performance parameters that are actually unrelated to the single positive quality.	A registered nurse is very attentive to the nurse practitioner (NP) during walking rounds. The nurse is enthusiastic and the NP enjoys the opportunity to interact with this inquisitive colleague. When asked to provide evaluative feedback about this particular nurse and her direct care skills, the NP appraises the nurse as "exceeds expectations" in all performance areas, even those that are unrelated to the NP's interactions during walking rounds.
Horn effect: A quality that is perceived as negative by the evaluator is used to inform the performance evaluation across a number of criteria, some unrelated to the particularly concerning attribute.	The nurse manager is asked to participate in the evaluation of an interprofessional colleague that the manager views as having a dismissive and abrasive communication style. The nurse manager subsequently appraises this colleague as below average or needing improvement in performance areas that include clinical decision making, organizational skills, and technical skills because the manager dislikes the colleague's communication style.

(continues)

TABLE 3-3 Performance Appraisal Biases and Exemplars

(continued)

Type of Bias (MCG Experts, 2017)	Exemplar
Central tendency: All nurses perform at average levels and individual differences are not considered.	The staff development specialist is charged with evaluating the performance of experienced nurses who have completed a critical care mentoring program. The specialist evaluates each of the nurses as "meeting requirements" and documents verbatim commentary on each of the appraisal forms.
Personal biases: Allowing partialities and prejudices to play a role in rating performance behaviors.	A nurse administrator is uncomfortable with people who are not heterosexual. Lesbian, gay, bisexual, transgender, queer, and intersex (LGBTQI) nurses typically receive harsh evaluative feedback as compared to that shared with heterosexual staff. This same scenario is applicable to biases related to race, faith, socioeconomic status and circumstances, and other demographic characteristics. Alternatively, biases may also advantage particular employees over others if the evaluator has strong preferences that subsequently have a positive influence on appraisal outcomes.
Spillover effect: Present performance is evaluated as consistent with past performance without consideration of actual behaviors.	A nurse informatics specialist is evaluating members of a technical work group that provides help desk assistance. One employee has been earning low evaluation scores from users as a result of documented occasions of delayed response time and antagonistic responses to requests for help. The specialist has worked with this employee for 8 years and provided excellent evaluations for the first 5 years. The specialist continues to highly appraise this employee because the work quality was good the first 5 years and there is no reason to assume that the work is not good now in spite of user feedback
Recency effect: The most recent behavior drives the appraisal and earlier performance is neglected or dismissed.	A clinical nurse specialist (CNS) is chairing an interprofessional work group that includes a physical therapist (PT) that has been a poor contributor to the group work effort for most of the year. During the final 2 months of the project, the PT develops an educational program for the work group that represented the group nicely to hospital administration. The CNS evaluated the PT's annual contribution to the group as exceeding expectations and all other behavioral criterion were assessed as above average despite the many issues related to nonparticipation throughout most of the appraisal period.

Positive behaviors should be considered when appraising performance. Aslan and Yildirim (2017) observe that employees who master difficult challenges and successfully manage demanding tasks are more valuable than those who are impatient or demonstrate behaviors that negatively affect the team. Positive attributes enhance institutional energy and increase its effectiveness. Aslan and Yildirim (2017) explored contextual performance and nurses' behaviors and feelings of job satisfaction on this particular performance domain. Behaviors that support a contextual performance are those that enable teams to effectively function. Those who proficiently perform within the context of the work environment are those who share information, help others, demonstrate organizational loyalty and commitment, volunteer, and support organizational priorities. These are important attributes and behaviors as they contribute to a positive and appealing work environment.

Aslan and Yildirim (2017) examined the relationship between contextual performances, personal characteristics, and job satisfaction of hospital nurses (N = 500). The sample was drawn from two hospitals in Turkey. Instruments, including a contextual performance scale developed by the researchers, demonstrated validity and reliability. Findings support that when nurses like their jobs, they tend to be more agreeable than those who are dissatisfied with their employment circumstances. The ways that nurses contribute to contextual performance are important and are worthy of discussion during performance evaluations. Although influenced by personality, contextual performance is also driven by job satisfaction. Nurse leaders may not be able to impact personality but certainly can exert influence on satisfaction.

Goal Setting

Job goals vary among employees. They are developed mutually by the employee and the appraiser and should be considered in relation to an employee's gifts, challenges, and aspirations. Aspirational goals contribute to meaningful performance evaluation.

Goals must be specific, realistic, challenging, and measurable. When people are asked to do the best job possible, they rarely do so. The request is too arbitrary and intangible and could be satisfied by a wide range of acceptable performance levels (Locke & Latham, 2002). Goals should not be ambiguous; rather, they must be specific and clearly understood. During any type of performance appraisal that involves goal setting, advanced nurses should focus on exactly what is required of the nurse. For example, "Start change of shift report at the correct time and finish it no later than the scheduled stop time" is much clearer than "Give a better shift report."

When goals are individually determined, nurses who believe that they are able to accomplish the agreed-upon tasks set higher goals than those with less confidence in the ability to successfully meet the goals (**BOX 3-1**). These same highly confident people are more committed to the agreed upon goals, use better strategies for reaching the goals, and are more receptive to critique along the way (Locke & Latham, 2002). So, include nurses in goal setting and create specific goals that are attainable with effort and persistence. Research findings suggest that the most important agents of high and low productivity include employees themselves, immediate supervisors, and the organization's resources. If performance appraisal is going to influence changes in practice patterns, it will do so via these agents. Nurses practicing in advanced roles without direct-line authority are important resources and certainly have the potential to contribute to employees' individual and collective goals.

BOX 3-1 Goal-Setting Tips

1. Include the employee in goal development. The nurse who participates in the goal-setting process will probably have more success in goal attainment.
2. Goals provide focus. Without established goals, nurses are distracted by less important activities.
3. Goals are energizing. High goals lead to greater effort.
4. Nurses need the tools, support, and strategic planning necessary for successful goal attainment.

Goals should include deadlines. If there is a date by which a behavior, project, or assignment must be completed, be explicit. Goals must be realistic. Impossible goals discourage employees. Goals should not be so easy that they require little effort, but established goals should take into account the limitations and realities of the practice environment (DelPo, 2005).

Once mutually agreeable goals have been established, make certain to ask the nurse what he or she needs to be successful. Perhaps the nurse will set a goal of "certification in specialty area within 9 months" or "participate as a preceptor to a new nurse" or "develop expertise in evidence-based practice (EBP) demonstrated by development of a unit-based interprofessional project." Each of these exemplars demonstrates a need for input from nurses with advanced expertise. There are many opportunities for advanced nurses to contribute to goal development and attainment, and these opportunities will be highly valued by those nurses in need of expert coaching and mentoring.

▶ Postperformance Appraisal Communication and Reflection

At the conclusion of each performance evaluation session, ask the appraised person to provide feedback about the quality of the experience, including the presession preparation and anticipated postsession guidance opportunities (**BOX 3-2**). Consider that there are frequently shared common appraisal mistakes posted on social media and easily retrieved that should be avoided at all costs (**BOX 3-3**). Acknowledge the effort that each nurse or team member has contributed to the organization. Ask for suggestions from subordinates and colleagues related to the supports that they need to successfully meet goals. Be clear to acknowledge personal responsibility in this process and encourage employees to provide updates on a regular basis, perhaps quarterly, as to how they are progressing toward the mutually agreed upon outcomes. Emphasize opportunities for guidance and partnership.

Avoiding a Successful Wrongful Discharge Suit

Wrongful discharge is a common basis for litigation. Although employers have the right to fire employees, it is illegal to fire when the job termination is based on discrimination of protected classes—specifically race, religion, sex, or age. In some localities and states, it may be illegal to terminate employment based on gender or sexual orientation.

BOX 3-2 Postperformance Appraisal Queries

1. Were you provided with sufficient guidance and support throughout this appraisal process?
2. Was there ample time for preparation?
3. Did you have the records that you needed for a sufficient self-evaluation process?
4. Was the appraisal session physically comfortable?
5. What, if any, feedback was surprising to you? Had you discussed the scenarios or behaviors previously with the manager or other evaluator?
6. What suggestions do you have regarding the appraisal process?
7. What are your expectations following the performance evaluation? How, specifically, might the evaluator and other advanced nurses and colleagues support you in goal attainment?
8. As a result of the appraisal experience, what recommendations do you have for annual record keeping, monitoring, and feedback?

BOX 3-3 Frequently Described in Social Media as Performance Review Errors

1. Brief and unplanned discussion that avoids specific details about previous performance and does not offer opportunities for meaningful goal setting.
2. Glowing annual reviews followed by unexpected layoff or termination with the suggestion that performance required some improvement.
3. Recency effect: A recent event dominates the appraisal review and the remainder of the performance year is ignored (Jackson, 2012).
4. No preparation on the part of the evaluator. Some cut and paste from one performance review year to another.
5. No scheduled appraisal because "my door is always open."
6. No recognition for a job well done.
7. No acknowledgement of the extra responsibilities and load that have been assumed due to vacancies and "right-sizing."
8. Fake evaluative feedback. Either being told that the performance has been "great" or "terrible" without truthfulness.
9. No periodic follow-up or loop closure. Goals should be periodically checked and progress or lack thereof should be analyzed.
10. Little to no attention paid to future plans, including career goals.

Paper trails and real-time documentation are absolutely essential to demonstrate that an employee has been afforded progressive discipline and fair consideration.

Documentation should accurately reflect the reality of the evaluation process. In other words, advanced nurses, including nurse managers and administrators, must be careful to offer evaluative input that is honest, reasonable, and free of bias. Make certain to avoid treating an appraisal session as a disciplinary session. Performance evaluations should be kept private and each person should be afforded the opportunity to appeal evaluative feedback and measurement. Since corrective action is presumably addressed immediately following the concerning behavior, there should be no surprises during a scheduled evaluation session. Nurses should know where they stand before they walk into the meeting room.

Seek Out Information and Develop Appraisal Expertise

Advanced nurses with an interest in improving their evaluation skills should seek direction and suggestions from the many printed resources on this subject. There are often education and training programs at work sites specific to performance evaluations. Nurse leaders, including those who mentor and support nurses across a variety of roles, should take advantage of these opportunities if they will be regularly contributing to formal appraisal processes.

▶ Appraising Deficient Performance with Success as the Goal

There are many types of employee problems, including low productivity, performance deficiencies including incompetence, insubordination, interpersonal problems that affect the work environment, excessive absenteeism, drugs and alcohol, theft and dishonesty, violence, disrespectfulness, and immorality. Many advanced nurses in practice, education, or administrative roles are directly involved in addressing staff productivity and performance issues. They may be peripherally involved in reporting other employee problems as either a direct observer or a confidant of staff. As a result, advanced nurses need to have an understanding of and appreciation for the complexities of assisting nurses who demonstrate performance proficiency deficits.

Evaluating the Unsatisfactory Performer

Advanced nurses are often involved with appraising the performance of a nurse or staff member who is practicing below expectations. CNSs, CNLs, managers, educators, staff development experts, and nurses engaged in mentoring and supervising are often viewed as coaches and clinical experts. As a result, they may need to work with struggling nurses to develop performance-based remediation plans. Struggling nurses may be established practitioners who have transferred to a different practice area requiring new skills, nurses demonstrating performance deficiencies caused by difficult life circumstances, or new nurses having difficulty meeting the challenges of orientation programs. The nurse who is new to the clinical setting or new to practice is significantly different than the nurse who has experience but begins to demonstrate low performance in key areas.

The Struggling New Employee

Before beginning the written performance appraisal, advanced nurse evaluators should begin by meeting with the employee and discussing the nurse's perspective, including concerns, worries, and suggestions. Do not assume that the nurse has *chosen* to perform poorly. Care must be taken to avoid arguing or eliciting defensive posturing. In general, although the evaluator and employee may have differing opinions on the quality of performance, examples of behaviors should be discussed in matter-of-fact language that includes the outcomes of these behaviors. Quotations, charting, medication administration records, and patient/family complaints and compliments should be reviewed.

This reflective process should include discussion specific to the orientation structures and processes (**FIGURE 3-2**). Many institutions arrange supervised experiences with a preceptor to guide new employees. These arrangements may be referred to as orientations or mentorships and may be arranged as unit-based, dedicated education unit, department, or academy-type activities. The basic structure and processes tend to be fairly similar across nursing care settings: (1) Develop a structured orientation

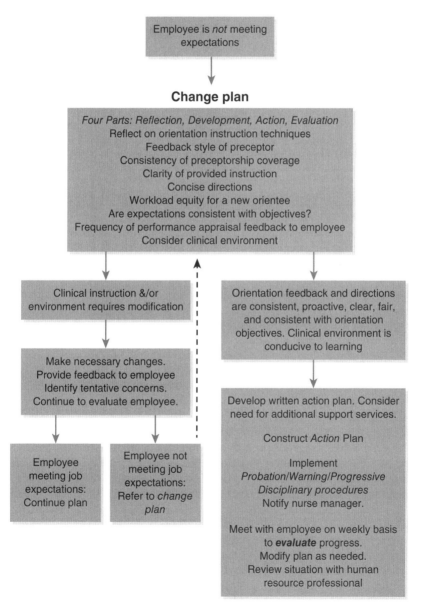

FIGURE 3-2 Struggling Employee Evaluation Algorithm.

program that includes behavioral objectives and opportunities to evaluate feedback; (2) assign one or more individuals to work with the new nurse; (3) gradually increase employee independence; and (4) evaluate at probationary period end and make a decision on whether to continue the employment.

In this type of arrangement, the preceptor wields significant influence on the quality of the orientation and the outcomes of the experience. It is important to consider the skill of the preceptor and the relationship between the new employee and the preceptor. In some cases, this relationship does not click, and, as a direct result, the new employee is unsuccessful.

Conflict may exist in nursing student–preceptor relationships (Mamchur & Myrick, 2003), and it makes sense that this same conflict may manifest itself in new employee–preceptor relationships. The advanced nurse must keep an open mind when considering this possibility and recognize that it is also possible that the preceptor is being wrongfully blamed for the lackluster performance of the new hire.

Workload equity may also be a concern. New hires should be able to anticipate a reasonable workload that provides for learning opportunities and guidance throughout the day. Perhaps a heavy workload, increased patient census, or high acuity has prevented the new employee from doing a good job. It is not uncommon for preceptors to juggle orientation responsibilities while also managing a full patient assignment. This divided attention may adversely affect the new employee's access to guidance through the system.

New employees deserve regular, objective feedback that is offered to them privately and that includes both positive and negative behavior exemplars. Preceptors should treat evaluative data as confidential, shared only on a need-to-know basis. If orientees are not receiving objective feedback, they have no legitimate opportunity to improve or succeed. If performance is discussed outside the preceptor–orientee relationship with employees who have no right or need to know, then the orientee is being sabotaged with legitimate grounds for formal complaint. The preceptorship relationship should be based on trust and good intentions to encourage the new employee to share questions and concerns. New hires cannot identify clinical skill deficiencies or learning needs if they do not feel safe.

The appraiser should also critique the clinical environment with the employee. Make certain that the new hire feels comfortable and supported. If not, specific areas must be identified and behaviors must be addressed. If there are challenges or intimidating exchanges with other professionals, including the medical staff, these issues must also be remedied.

Another possible explanation for poor performance may be substance abuse. Employees who abuse drugs and alcohol may demonstrate diminished job performance, reduced productivity, lateness, or absenteeism. If the new employee demonstrates these behaviors, make certain that they are accurately documented and inform the employee that these behaviors will be brought to the attention of the appropriate administrator. Established employees may have in-house support options for addictions that are unavailable to newly hired nurses during the probationary period. Exploring program options in this case should be the responsibility of the new employee in consultation with human resources.

If an advanced nurse notes slurred speech, alcohol on breath, changes in pupil size, or uncoordinated motor movements, document the findings and speak with the employee. The situation should be immediately addressed. Patient safety is the imperative obligation. There are times when behaviors are the result of prescribed medications. Notify the administrator and follow through with institutional policy. Remember to address the results or potential outcomes of alcohol and drug-related behaviors, particularly if these behaviors are occurring after work but are affecting the quality of the employee's work performance.

Responding to the Issues. After reflecting on the circumstances of the new employee's unsatisfactory performance and speaking with both the orientee and the preceptor, the advanced nurse must decide how to proceed. These assessments and discussions should be documented. Share the data and conclusions with the appropriate administrator.

If the problem lies with the work environment or the preceptorship arrangement, correct these problems and establish a date for performance reevaluation. A change in preceptor assignment or targeted education may move the orientee back on track. If these changes correct the performance deficiencies, the orientation plan should continue with the revisions in place.

On the other hand, perhaps careful scrutinizing of the preceptorship relationship, work environment, and workload reveal that the system does not sufficiently reveal the root of the problem. Rather, evaluation reveals that the performance deficiencies directly relate to the skill set, disposition, or motivation of the orientee. In this case, the advanced nurse needs to participate in developing a remediation plan to address these issues or needs to support both the employee and the manager during the termination process.

Developing the Action Plan. Evidence suggests that the most effective remedy for poor performance is to focus on the future rather than the past. Focusing on the past is unproductive because performance cannot be undone and because such a discussion is likely to encourage arguments due to differing perceptions of past events (Zemke, 1991). Once it is clearly established that the new employee is performing at an unsatisfactory level, it is common for the appraiser and, perhaps, an advanced nurse colleague to participate in developing an action plan.

The action plan's intent is to specify behaviors, target dates, and steps that the employee is required to fulfill to achieve required outcomes. The plan's focus is to provide opportunities for the employee to master requisite job expectations. The appraiser must remember that this is a private event for the new employee. A remediation plan must be handled sensitively and in such a way that the employee receives needed support and learning experience opportunities without bearing the brunt of the curiosity and gossip of coworkers and members of the health care team.

The employee should clearly understand that if established goals of the remediation plan are not met, the employee will be discharged. Remember to make certain to evaluate, remediate, and reevaluate within the time limits of the probationary period. If this is not enough time to give the employee a reasonable time for improvement, consider extending the probationary period in consultation with human resources.

After the Action Plan. Remediating the struggling employee can be a time-consuming activity. The advanced nurse will probably work with an administrator, perhaps a nurse manager, when completing the initial written appraisal. Once this evaluation has been shared with the employee and an action plan has been developed, the evaluator or other involved advanced nurse may be responsible for coordinating and monitoring the employee's progress. Good organizational skills and effective communication strategies are essential during this period.

The primary advanced nurse preceptor should schedule interim meetings, preferably with the nurse manager or evaluator in attendance. These interim meetings are intended to measure the progress the employee has made toward the action plan goals and to solicit input and feedback. Generally, probationary periods are short. Schedule interim evaluations frequently enough that the employee receives feedback and suggestions in a timely fashion relative to the amount of time remaining in the probation. Meetings may be scheduled weekly or biweekly, depending on employee shift patterns.

Interim appraisal sessions are also good opportunities to "check in" and really listen to this new employee. Keep in mind that this process is anxiety producing for any employee and particularly for a new employee. Be ready to give specific feedback and practical suggestions. Have genuine dialogue about the expectations. If they require plan revisions, do so within reason. Make certain that the employee has early notification of the scheduled interim review sessions. Encourage the nurse to prepare for the review and to consider suggestions for strategies, supports, and resources that might be helpful to the employee as he or she continues to develop skills.

Some institutions have formal mechanisms for documenting interim reviews, whereas others leave the format to the discretion of the evaluator. In general, it is wise to come to the interim review with written documentation. Share feedback from coworkers, patients, and families. If the employee has demonstrated improvement and goals appear attainable, make certain to share this positive feedback but do not offer guarantees of continued employment. Remember that the employee needs to demonstrate continual and consistent growth as measured against the agreed-upon goals.

If the employee continues to demonstrate an unsatisfactory level of performance, continue to provide objective examples of concerning behaviors and skill deficiencies. Offer assistance where appropriate while making certain that final responsibility for job performance lies with the employee. Remember that there are times when probationary periods should not be extended. There may be other viable alternatives for this struggling employee. As an example, perhaps the new employee is struggling in a high-acuity intensive care unit but may perform satisfactorily in an inpatient or outpatient area. This may be a reasonable suggestion if the employee's performance deficiencies relate to technical skills or an identified realization that the demands of the high-acuity practice area are inconsistent with the new employee's interests.

During the interim evaluation session, keep in mind that demeanor is important. It is not uncommon for the struggling employee to view these sessions as threatening. This is not an unreasonable perspective, given that continued employment requires a satisfactory level of performance. The advanced nurse is obliged to treat the employee with respect. Hostility or frustration is inappropriate, and expressions of such may escalate into personal attacks.

When meeting with the employee, keep the office or conference room door open but schedule the evaluative discussion in a reasonably private area. Ultimately, the decision to terminate a new employee is an administrative decision. Input from the advanced nurse or nurses who have closely engaged with the struggling employee is likely critical to the process and is usually an important consideration when making the determination of whether to continue the employment relationship (**EXEMPLAR 3-1**).

EXEMPLAR 3-1 The Partying Orientee

Josie is a newly hired RN on a medical-surgical nursing unit. The advanced nurse educator, in this case, an experienced RN with a graduate degree in nursing education, is responsible for developing an orientation program and tracking employees' progress through this program. The nurse educator arranges for a consistent preceptor to work with Josie. The preceptor is an experienced mentor. The preceptor informs the nurse educator that Josie frequently goes out following the 3–11 shift and claims to "party late." The preceptor is concerned that this lifestyle is destructive and that Josie appears fatigued and distracted during patient care experiences.

The nurse educator shares these same concerns but recognizes that Josie's lifestyle choice is outside the purview of the employee–employer relationship and to address this concern with Josie would be an intrusion into her personal life. However, the educator is concerned about patient safety and job performance and recognizes that these concerns are work related and necessary to raise with Josie if patient safety may be compromised. If Josie demonstrates a pattern of lateness, poor performance, clinical errors, or absenteeism, the educator and preceptor will note the specifics, document details, and share with the responsible administrator. Given Josie's self-reported alcohol intake and late nights, there may be an opportunity to discuss potentially needed employee assistance programs. Mutual goal setting may assist Josie with improving her performance, redirecting her focus, and, if needed, seeking professional supports or guidance.

The Struggling Established Employee

When a nurse has been practicing satisfactorily and then begins to demonstrate problems with productivity or practice quality, the advanced nurse is often the first person to whom staff turns for advice. This advanced nurse may be a CNS, CNL, NP, staff educator, nurse manager, charge nurse, or even a nurse faculty member or researcher. Losing a nurse is expensive in terms of both dollars and human cost, particularly a nurse who has previously practiced as an effective member of the health care team. The advanced nurse should consider a variety of possible explanations for the performance deficiencies, including possible changes in the nurse's personal life or work environment (**TABLE 3-4**). As mentioned, substance abuse is always a concern and should be considered and ruled in or out early in the process.

The best initial strategy is to collect preliminary information before approaching the nurse. There is a possibility that the advanced nurse has been misinformed about the employee's performance. Observe the nurse during clinical practice. Review charts and documentation and develop a clear sense of whether there is an actual performance issue.

After preliminary data review, approach the employee in a thoughtful and considerate fashion. If the appraiser has an established relationship with the employee, having a private discussion in a relaxed environment over lunch or coffee may be an effective approach to this difficult conversation. Remember that patient safety is paramount. If the employee is providing safe care but care that is less organized or productive than usual, the performance problem may be easier to address than if patient safety is at risk because potentially compromised safety requires swift response that errs on the side of eliminating avoidable risk.

TABLE 3-4 Possible Explanations for Compromised or Inadequate Performance

Work Challenges	Intrapersonal Problems	Relationship Difficulties
■ Discrimination or harassment ■ Overwhelming physical demands ■ Fast-paced workload demands ■ Changing technologies	■ Substance abuse ■ Changes in vision or hearing ■ Alterations in physical health or stamina ■ Mental health concerns ■ Worries ■ Crisis in faith ■ Economic stressors	■ Divorce ■ Death ■ Conflicts with family, friends, coworkers, supervisors ■ Fear of violence

Consider the institutional resources that may be available to the nurse. Many health care systems have employee counseling programs and employee assistance opportunities that can help staff with problem solving for a wide range of issues. Encourage the nurse to take advantage of available services. Consider including the nurse manager in a conversation to share possible changes in scheduling or shift rotations to accommodate the employee's issues. For example, there are times when nurses who are struggling with difficult family circumstances find that weekend 12-hour shifts or a permanent evening or night shift can help with financial worries or remedy a need for predictability. Again, keep only appropriate personnel informed and involved in the process as designated by policy.

▶ Self-Regulation and Peer Review

Peer evaluation or peer review is associated with activities that require self-regulation within the context of professional practice. Self-regulation strengthens the nursing profession's credibility in society and builds a sense of personal and professional responsibility (McAllister & Osborne, 1997) within the nursing rank and file. Scholarly journals use blind peer-review processes to review manuscripts submitted for publication consideration. Peer review is also used for grant reviews, tenure and promotion decisions, conference abstract submissions (Dougherty, 2006), accreditation processes, and to supplement performance evaluations. Peer-review processes are used to facilitate student learning (McAllister & Osborne, 1997). There is also opportunity to use a nursing peer-review committee structure and process to conduct root cause analyses in a nonpunitive manner (Spiva, Jarrell, & Baio, 2014).

Peer-review processes place practice evaluation squarely in the hands of the professional. Professionals should be evaluated by their peers, specifically colleagues with similar competence and possessing clear understanding of practice demands and standards. Briggs, Heath, and Kelley (2005) reported that certain states expect some form of peer review. Also, when peer-review processes are required for advanced practice nurses (APNs), some state boards of nursing stipulate that the review must be conducted by a similarly licensed APN practicing in the same clinical area. The peer-review process may also be statutorily required as part of fact-finding activities related to a nurse's conduct (Walters, 2000).

Peers should be evaluated against established, written standards (Briggs et al., 2005; McAllister & Osborne, 1997), regardless of the motivation for the peer review. Journals, foundations, organizations, accrediting agencies, universities, and employment settings have performance standards. Peer-review conflicts often relate to the interpretation and application of standards as well as conflicts that arise from contentious communications and perceived unfairness.

Connecting Evaluation Processes to Role-Specific Job Descriptions

It is challenging to participate in valid performance appraisal processes if there is an absent or tenuous relationship between the performance evaluation system and the job description. Many nurses in advanced roles experience role challenges as a result of amorphous scopes of practice within the institution and lack of clarity about role differentiation. CNSs and CNLs, as well as other sometimes more fluid advanced roles, may experience both role ambiguity and role confusion. There are often occasions when differences between CNS and CNL expertise, role responsibilities, and competencies are not clearly understood by nurse colleagues or administrative personnel. Staff development, staff educators, and quality improvement professionals may experience similar challenges. Job descriptions may be inappropriate and may loosely categorize CNSs, in particular, as APRNs, staff development or clinical educators, or administrators. CNLs may be confused with CNSs or mistakenly labeled as advanced practice nurses. Staff educators often have varied educational and experiential backgrounds that can contribute to job description challenges; some have graduate degrees in nursing while others lack nursing-specific advanced degrees. Such ambiguity presents challenges beyond the performance appraisal concern and may contribute to role strain and job dissatisfaction. The performance appraisal process should directly relate to the job description that is informed by the needs of the organization as influenced by the larger health care environment and as determined by state practice regulations.

Advanced nurses should scrutinize their job descriptions and ensure that the descriptions accurately describe the role and its responsibilities. If the job description requires modification or needs to be crafted from scratch, advanced nurses should use any and all available resources that specifically relate to their role and work to create a relevant description of employment requirements, job responsibilities, and outcomes (**BOX 3-4**).

Peer-Review Performance Evaluations

Peer-review processes are useful to include in the performance appraisal of all categories of nursing staff members. Data sources that inform these processes should be selected based on the role and responsibilities of the nurse. Traditional methods of performance evaluation can be problematic for nurses in advanced roles, particularly when supervisors/directors do not regularly observe advanced nurses' work. Staff nurses have these same concerns regarding the legitimacy of appraisals. Devising a peer-review system may help alleviate some of these issues, although the very nature

BOX 3-4 Suggested Strategies for Job Description Development

1. Request copies of relevant job descriptions from networking colleagues accessible through listservs or discussion boards. Many professional nursing organizations have associated listservs.
2. Connect with advanced nurses through relevant specialty organizations and request copies of job descriptions relevant to the practice area and type of work setting.
3. Explore the literature for materials that differentiate types of advanced practice roles and use this evidence to inform and support the proposed job description.
4. Include coworkers in the process. Consider that advanced nurse roles may have differing priorities and job expectations depending upon the department and specialty. Make certain to provide opportunities to validate and modify drafted job descriptions using the input of those nurses practicing in the roles, internal stakeholders, and, perhaps, outside experts.

of peer review can stimulate nurses' anxieties as they worry about confidentiality protections and the potential for disparaging comments.

Canadian nurses are required to participate in continuing competence programs (CCPs) to ensure that nurses are current and competent in professional practice (Mantesso, Petrucka, & Bassendowski, 2008). CCPs often integrate reflective practice as a vehicle for self-assessment (Association of Registered Nurses of Newfoundland and Labrador [ARNNL], 2015). One aspect of reflective practice is peer feedback.

Nurses are varyingly receptive to peer feedback depending upon locus of control, a personality variable (Mantesso et al., 2008). Giving and receiving peer feedback requires a conversation between colleagues that emphasizes dialogue and development. Advanced nurses should consider working with staff to develop peer feedback opportunities that may enhance nursing practice. Locus of control may be an important variable to consider when planning continuing development programs for staff with both internal and external control foci since nurses with external locus of control may be more anxious during feedback processes when compared with the more assertive and confident internally controlled nurse (Mantesso et al., 2008).

Establishing peer-review processes takes planning. Review tools need to reflect job expectations, values, and required competencies. When developing a peer-review process, advanced nurses should solicit stakeholder input, establish the criteria against which the nurse will be evaluated, and create the process for reviewer selection (Briggs et al., 2005). Staff should participate in selecting appraisal items and developing guidelines, including the number of peer appraisals per staff member, role of self-evaluation, reviewer selection criteria, and confidentiality protections (Mathews, 2000).

There are numerous ways to structure peer-review processes and format evaluation tools. Some review systems are fairly unstructured, whereas others use guiding questions or very specific review criteria (Briggs et al., 2005). Advanced nurses should examine a variety of structures and processes and choose a format that is best suited to nurses' needs within the particular organization. Briggs and colleagues (2005) cautioned that peer review differs from traditional, annual performance evaluations. Often, peer review supplements the standard review process.

Identifying colleagues to serve as reviewers is an important activity. There are pros and cons to physician inclusion. Certainly, if physicians or other interprofessional colleagues are included, they need to have an accurate understanding of different nursing roles and how these roles vary in responsibility and scope of practice. Reviewers need to be informed of the process and boundaries of the evaluation program and will require education and training.

When designing a peer-review process, advanced nurses need to have frank discussions about whether reviewers should be anonymous or known. Anonymity may facilitate honest and candid feedback. At times anonymity can also allow for aggressive, mean-spirited reviews. Briggs and colleagues (2005) commented that individuals often express the belief that they have the right to know who is reviewing their work. There are times when a reviewer or the reviewed nurse might want additional information or clarification; however, in an anonymous process, this option is not possible.

Peer review implemented as an open process with identified, known reviewers has different associated concerns. Reviewers may feel pressure to provide positive feedback. Some reviewers may worry about retribution when an honest review reveals performance deficiencies that are shared with the reviewed peer. These types of concerns should be openly discussed, guidelines should be established, and education should be provided.

Peer review is a legitimate source of data that facilitates self-development. Vuorinen, Tarkka, and Meretoja (2000) examined nurses' experiences with peer evaluation and its potential impact on professional development. RNs (N = 24) employed on an intensive care unit in Finland completed questionnaires with five open-ended questions pertaining to peer review. Content analysis revealed that peer review assisted nurses in better understanding their actions. Peer feedback offered the reviewed nurses alternative ways of looking at and conducting their work. The respondents evaluated peer evaluation as positive and collaborative.

While peer review certainly offers positive opportunities for personal and professional growth for individuals and for teams, it is not a risk-free endeavor. Siedlecki (2016) describes the ethics of peer review and identifies avoidable ethical pitfalls, including confidentiality violations, developing biased peer critiques, or even plagiarizing reviewed materials and using ideas that have been shared during peer-review processes. Peer reviewers must understand the tremendous professional responsibilities associated with having access to others' intellectual efforts or performance appraisal data. Siedlecki emphasizes the importance of just and fair treatment of the reviewed peer by the evaluator. There are often times when reviewers should recuse themselves from review activities if the peer is personally known or a competitor of some sort (e.g., for funding resources) (Siedlecki, 2016).

Peer Review: Abstracts and Manuscripts

Peer review is essential for high-quality scholarly work. It is usually conducted as a double-blind process. The reviewer is unfamiliar with the author of the submission, and the author receives feedback that is anonymous. Similar to the notion of double-blind research studies, the system protects the integrity of the decision making by divorcing the person from the quality of the work.

Double-blind peer review is incorporated into selection processes for most types of professional activities and venues (**BOX 3-5**). Many new advanced nurses find review procedures intimidating or confusing. Some would like to contribute as reviewers but do not know how to initiate this activity. Understanding the basic process is necessary

BOX 3-5 Select Peer-Review Activities

Manuscript review processes for journals
Podium abstracts for conference presentations
Poster abstracts
Dossier review by outside experts for tenure and promotion in university settings
Grant applications
Fellowship applications
Awards
Institutional Review Board research project submissions
Clinical ladder promotion processes
Root cause analyses

to actively contribute to nursing scholarship and to disseminate information that may be useful to the profession and to practice.

There is a need for expert nurses to serve as reviewers for nursing journals. Advanced nurses' expertise may be in education, research, administration, informatics, or clinical practice. Many journals have requests for reviewers posted on their home page. Some journals prefer publishing experience. Reviewers volunteer their services. Most are acknowledged through some type of simple gesture, such as an annual published list of reviewers in the journal, a certificate of acknowledgment, or a thank-you letter on journal stationery. Nurses should make certain to include reviewer activities on their curriculum vitae or résumé as a professional activity or professional service. Usually, reviewers serve a predesignated time commitment. Manuscripts are delivered to reviewers in an unscheduled, sometimes unpredictable, fashion, but there is usually a reasonable time period between manuscript review requests.

Manuscript reviews vary in format and process. Some reviews are submitted electronically, whereas other journals use hard-copy manuscripts with various options for review return. Reviewers are selected based on the manuscript topic and the reviewer's area of expertise. More than one reviewer is assigned to each manuscript.

Most journals provide verbatim feedback from reviewers to authors. Part of the peer-review process should be to provide constructive feedback in such a way that even when a manuscript is rejected, the author does not feel personally rejected or insulted. Most authors work very hard on manuscripts. This does not mean that all submissions are well written or even logical. Nonetheless, remember that the comments and criticisms written on the review page are going to be read by the author. If the review is too harsh or unkind, the writer may never submit another manuscript. Reviewers should be candid but should also be professional. Consider the review process as an opportunity to mentor and develop a colleague.

Advanced nurses may also elect to participate in peer-review processes for conferences. Most popular or highly regarded conferences are competitive. A call for abstracts is issued for both paper and poster submissions. Reviewers are needed to select those abstracts that are suitable for podium presentations versus those that are more appropriately shared in poster form. A percentage of abstract submissions will be rejected based on reviewers' critiques. The number of rejections will depend on the number of submissions. Reviewers play a key role in this process. Many organizations solicit abstract reviewers during conferences. This is a good way to serve an organization and get involved at an entry level in regional, national, or international conference planning.

▶ Succession Planning

Performance appraisals provide a unique opportunity to chat with staff about their talents, aspirations, and professional goals. These conversations create opportunities for succession planning, a critical workforce priority given the potential future nursing shortage resulting from nurse retirements over the next 5 years (Acree-Hamann, 2016). Talent recognition and management are vital obligations of advanced nurses. Recognizing aptitude for management, practice, teaching, or systems-thinking is one aspect of succession planning while nurturing these talents and encouraging nurses to continue to build these capacities requires a different set of activities. Advanced nurses need to consider how they can contribute to supporting leadership transitions across the many types of essential professional nursing services.

Succession planning is not unique to nursing and is often a priority within organizations as they consider how to recognize, recruit, retain, and develop talented employees. Nursing's aging workforce contributes to a particular sense of urgency regarding succession planning (Acree-Hamann, 2016; Griffith, 2012; Manning, Jones, Jones, & Fernandez, 2015). Health care peculiarities that complicate the challenges of building leadership capacity across educational and practice environments include system complexities, financial uncertainties, and rapidly evolving technologies and informatics requirements. Efforts have been undertaken to understand the unique needs of succession planning within the nursing profession (Fray & Sherman, 2017) and to implement interventions in response to institutional demands.

Published literature offers an array of succession planning programs that advanced nurses may want to consider. A Future Nursing Unit Managers program was designed to enhance the managerial and leadership talents of potential nursing unit managers (NUMs) (Manning et al., 2016) by incorporating succession planning principles identified in the published literature but often not linked to specific implementation strategies. This particular program was modeled around identified core principles, including organizational support, identification of skills and competencies necessary for the position and based on a map derived from the job description, talent detection, gap analysis of skills and competencies of program participants, and development opportunities (Manning et al., 2016). Program evaluation findings supported the value of the program. There were eight participants at the time of publication and half had moved into some type of NUM position following the program.

The University of North Carolina Medical Center, a Magnet™ designated academic medical center, addressed its goal of developing internal nurse leaders by establishing a Nursing Leadership Academy (Strickler, Bohling, Kneis, O'Connor, & Yee, 2016). Similar in some respects to the NUM program, the academy was designed to support succession efforts as nurse leaders were promoted. The goal was to establish a bench of potential leaders available for new opportunities as formal leaders. Academy efforts have resulted in numerous internal promotions while also reducing external recruitment expenses (Strickler et al., 2016).

The Veterans Health Administration (VHA) has also addressed the need for succession planning by using a different strategy, creation of a useful database to identify candidates for nursing leadership positions based on interest, willingness, and ability to accept such a position (Weiss & Drake, 2007). The database has access that is restricted to the nurse executive group and to those in the office of nursing services. A variety of position options are included in the database and career data are obtained from interested staff and approved by the appropriate nurse executive based on verification of leadership potential. The database is robust and data may be modified as needed (Weiss & Drake, 2007). Opening the database to the entire VHA system allows access to agencies outside of candidates' local areas and doing so ensures that each individual VHA health care enterprise has access to the talent within the larger organization.

Successful succession planning must take into account the varied needs, perspectives, and experiences of nursing professionals as influenced by age, culture, sex, gender, and other demographic characteristics. Generation Y nurses were born between 1980 and 2000 and are often labeled "millennials." Literature describes them as comfortable with diversity of all sorts, capable of working in teams, interested in work–life balance, and proficient with technologies.

Sherman (2015) points out that this generational cohort values flexible leaders that offer meaningful and frequent feedback. Performance feedback is very important to this generation and Generation Y nurses are often in paths for advancement early in their career trajectories (Sherman, 2015). Advanced nurses should consider how to guide and nurture this group of relatively new nurses, not only because of the flexibility, optimism, and confidence often characteristic of millennials, but also because of their potentially powerful and important contributions to the health care workforce. Their passion for environmental causes, technologies, equity, and diversity offer much-needed perspectives and attitudes to the nursing profession.

Seasoned nurses also have unique needs that should inform performance appraisal and succession planning. The aging nursing workforce is a real concern, and a global issue. The median age of RNs in the United States was 48 years in 2008 and 45.4 years in Canada creating a worrisome scenario of inadequate workforce numbers to provide care for aging populations (Armstrong-Stassen, Cameron, Rajacich, & Freeman, 2014). Published research findings support that nurse managers are unaware of the unique needs of seasoned nurses. Literature also reveals that experienced nurses fail to receive useful and supportive evaluative feedback (Armstrong-Stassen et al., 2014). This may be a challenge that advanced role nurses, as well as nursing teams, need to explore and address so as to assist in retaining the expertise of this valuable cohort.

Partnering performance appraisal and succession planning in a deliberate fashion offers opportunities for retaining and advancing nurses. Advanced nurses have an important role to play in both endeavors. There may be a need for advanced nurses to work with their particular professional organizations to increase conscious consideration of succession planning. Cursory reviews of CNL competencies (American Association of Colleges of Nursing [AACN], 2013), Adult-Gerontology CNS competencies (AACN, 2010a), Nurse Practitioner core competencies (National Organization of Nurse Practitioner Faculties [NONPF], 2017), and Adult-Gerontology Primary Care NP competencies (AACN, 2010b) reveal that these competencies do not address succession planning. Most do not address performance appraisal processes although there is mention of coaching and/or mentoring. Nurse Manager competencies (American Organization of Nurse Executives [AONE], 2015) explicitly address succession planning as a component of human resource leadership skills (p. 6). Staff evaluation and retention are also included (AONE, 2015). Because succession planning and performance appraisal are important to the entire nursing team, including the many diverse types of advanced nurses, it seems reasonable to advocate for greater collective attentiveness to both activities.

▶ Conclusion

Participating in performance appraisal processes and working with nurses to address deficiencies or build on strengths are challenging aspects of advanced nurses' responsibilities. Many supervisors cringe at the thought of giving honest feedback to employees, particularly if this feedback relates to performance deficiencies, disciplinary concerns, or the possibility of employment termination at the conclusion of a probationary period.

These are certainly stressful events; however, advanced nurses are wise to consider the benefits of the performance appraisal process. They may be able to offer the struggling employee a very real opportunity to improve performance. Advanced nurses, particularly those in roles that are not administrative line positions, are typically regarded by staff as nurse advocates, rather than perceived as potentially threatening. This rapport provides them with the means to make a difference in the professional life of a nurse and the work life of a nursing team.

Performance evaluation may also be best viewed as a continuous quality improvement activity that has the potential to truly change practice. Verbal coaching, written kudos, reminders of practice expectations, and gentle nudging are interventions that can foster strong relationships between nursing staff and advanced nurses. Continuous evaluative feedback may elicit higher levels of professional practice and improved patient care outcomes. From this perspective, the advanced nurse's role in performance appraisal has the potential to be empowering and uplifting. Concrete skills, logistical and legal responsibilities, and documentation habits need to be developed, but resources are available and should be used as the advanced nurse learns to contribute to an expert and fair appraisal process.

References

Acree-Hamann, C. (2016). A call to action: Succession planning needed. *Newborn & Infant Nursing Reviews, 16*, 161–163. doi:10.1053/j.nainr.2016.07.001

American Association of Colleges of Nursing. (2010a). Adult-gerontology clinical nurse specialist competencies. Retrieved January 17, 2018, from http://www.aacnnursing.org/Portals/42 /AcademicNursing/pdf/AdultGeroCNSCompetenc ies-2010.pdf?ver=2017-05-17-102046-357.

American Association of Colleges of Nursing. (2010b). Adult-gerontology primary care nurse practitioner competencies. Retrieved January 17, 2018, from http://www.aacnnursing.org /Portals/42/AcademicNursing/pdf/Adult-Gero-NP-Comp- 2010.pdf?ver=2017-05-17-102558-170.

American Association of Colleges of Nursing. (2013). Competencies and curricular expectations for Clinical Nurse Leaders™ education and practice. Retrieved January 17, 2018, from http://www .aacnnursing.org/Portals/42/CNL/CNL-Competencies-October- 2013.pdf?ver=2017-07-20-193433-107.

American Organization of Nurse Executives. (2015). AONE nurse manager competencies. Chicago, IL: Author. Retrieved January 17, 2018, from http://www.aone.org/resources/nurse-leader - competencies.shtml.

Armstrong-Stassen, M., Cameron, S., Rajacich, D., & Freeman, M. (2014). Do nurse managers know how to retain seasoned nurses? Perceptions of nurse managers and direct-care nurses of valued human resource practices. *Nursing Economics, 32*, 211–218.

Aslan, M., & Yildirim, A. (2017). Personality and job satisfaction among nurses: The mediating effect of contextual performance. *International Journal of Caring Sciences, 10*, 544–552.

Association of Registered Nurses of Newfoundland and Labrador. (2015). Continuing competence program framework. Retrieved January 17, 2018, from https://www.arnnl.ca/sites/default/files /documents/RD_CCP_Framework_Revised.pdf.

Briggs, L. A., Heath, J., & Kelley, J. (2005). Peer review for advanced practice nurses. What does it really mean? *AACN Clinical Issues, 16*(1), 3–15.

Chandra, A. (2006). Employee evaluation strategies for healthcare organizations—a general guide. *Hospital Topics, 84*(2), 34–38.

DelPo, A. (2005). *The performance appraisal handbook: Legal & practical rules for managers.* Berkeley, CA: Nolo.

DelPo, A., & Guerin, L. (2003). *Dealing with problem employees: A legal guide* (2nd ed.). Berkeley, CA: Nolo.

Dougherty, M. (2006). Editorial: The value of peer review. *Nursing Research, 55*(2), 73–74.

Fray, B., & Sherman, R. (2017). Best practices for nurse leaders: Succession planning. *Professional Case Management, 22*, 88–94.

Gbadamosi, G., & Ross, C. (2012). Perceived stress and performance appraisal discomfort: The moderating effects of core self-evaluations and gender. *Public Personnel Management, 41*(4), 637+. Retrieved January 16, 2018, from Academic OneFile, go.galegroup.com/ps/i.do?p=AONE&sw=w&u=drexel _main&v=2.1&id=GALE%7CA3 14347849&it=r&asid=18962ecfd474a93479c6b38f4840df28.

Griffith, M. B. (2012). Effective succession planning in nursing: A review of the literature. *Journal of Nursing Management, 20*, 900–911. doi:10.1111/j.1365-2834.2012.01418x

Hewko, S., & Cummings, G. (2016). Performance management in healthcare: A critical analysis. *Leadership in Health Services, 29,* 52–68. doi:10.1108/LHS-12.2014-0081

Jackson, E. (2012). Ten biggest mistakes bosses make in performance review. *Forbes.* Retrieved January 17, 2018, from https://www.forbes.com/sites/ericjackson/2012/01/09/ten-reasons -performance- reviews-are-done-terribly/#2d31cfcc5ee0.

Kellner, A., Townsend, K., Wilkinson, A., & Lawrence, S. (2016). Learning to manage: Development experiences of hospital frontline managers. *Human Resource Management Journal, 26*, 505–522. doi:10.1111/1748-8583.12119

Locke, E., & Latham, G. (2002). Building a practically useful theory of goal setting and task motivation: A 35-year odyssey. *American Psychologist, 57*(9), 705–717.

Mamchur, C., & Myrick, F. (2003). Preceptorship and interpersonal conflict: A multidisciplinary study. *Journal of Advanced Nursing, 43*(2), 188–196.

Manning, V., Jones, A., Jones, P., & Fernandez, R. (2015). Planning for a smooth transition. Evaluation of a succession planning program for prospective nurse unit managers. *Nursing Admin Quarterly, 39*, 58–68. doi:10.1097/NAQ.0000000000000072

Mantesso, J., Petrucka, P., & Bassendowski, S. (2008). Continuing professional competence: Peer feedback success from determination of nurse locus of control. *Journal of Continuing Education in Nursing, 39*(5), 200–205.

Mathews, D. (2000). Developing a perioperative peer performance appraisal system. *Association of PeriOperative Nurses, 72*(6), 1039–1042, 1044, 1046.

McAllister, M., & Osborne, Y. (1997). Peer review: A strategy to enhance cooperative student learning. *Nurse Educator, 22*(1), 40–44.

MCG Experts. (2017). Performance appraisal biases. *Management Study Guide.* Retrieved June 29, 2017, from http://managementstudyguide.com/performance-appraisal-bias.htm.

National Organization of Nurse Practitioner Faculties. (2017). Nurse practitioner core competencies content. Retrieved from http://c.ymcdn.com/sites/www.nonpf.org/resource/resmgr/competencies /2017_NPCor eComps_with_Curric.pdf.

Shaneberger, K. (2008). Managing your staff's performance. *OR Manager, 24*(6), 23–24.

Shepard, G. (2005). *How to make performance evaluations really work.* Hoboken, NJ: Wiley.

Sherman, R. (2015). Recruiting and retaining generation Y perioperative nurses. *AORN Journal, 101*, 138–143. doi:10.1016/j.aorn.2014.10.006

Siedlecki, S. (2016). The ethics of peer review: What to know before saying "yes." *Nursing Management, 47*(7), 44–48. doi:10.1097/01.NUMA.0000480762.22417.43

Siriwardena, A. N., & Gillam, S. (2014). Patient perspectives on quality. *Quality in Primary Care, 22*, 11–15.

Spiva, L., Jarrell, N., & Baio, P. (2014). The power of nursing peer review. *Journal of Nursing Administration, 44*, 586–590. doi:10.1097/NNA.0000000000000130

Strickler, J., Bohling, S., Kneis, C., O'Connor, M., & Yee, P. (2016). Developing nurse leaders from within. *Nursing, 46*(5), 49–51. doi:10.1097/01.NURSE.00000482261.78767.c2

Swift, S., Moore, D., Sharek, Z., & Gino, F. (2013). Inflated applicants: Attribution errors in performance evaluation by professionals. *PLoS ONE, 8*(7), e69258. doi: 10.1371/jounal.pone.0069258

Van Woerkom, M., & de Bruijn, M. (2016). Why performance appraisal does not lead to performance improvement: Excellent performance as a function of uniqueness instead of uniformity. *Industrial and Organizational Psychology, 9*, 275–281. doi: 10.1017/iop.2016.11

Vuorinen, R., Tarkka, M. T., & Meretoja, R. (2000). Peer evaluation in nurses' professional development: A pilot study to investigate the issues. *Journal of Clinical Nursing, 9*(2), 273–281.

Walters, G. (2000). A checklist for better understanding of the peer review process. *RN Update, 31*(4), 4–5.

Weiss, L. & Drake, A. (2007). Nursing leadership succession planning in Veterans Health Administration. Creating a useful database. *Nursing Administration Quarterly, 51*, 33–35.

Zemke, R. (1991). Do performance appraisals change performance? *Training, 28*(5), 35–39.

CHAPTER 4

Healthcare Business Essentials: A Primer for Advanced Nurses

Mary Beth Kingston, MSN, RN, NEA-BC and **Patti Rager Zuzelo**, EdD, RN, ACNS-BC, ANP-BC, CRNP, FAAN

N ursing administration is a specialty that requires a combination of business savvy and regulatory expertise with an understanding of clinical practice demands. Advanced nurses have a systems perspective and an understanding of modes of influence that provide valuable insight to the finance and business aspects of nursing.

Nurse executives require formal expertise in business and nursing administration, and nurses in all advanced roles require a grasp of health care business principles and a clear understanding of the health care system. This knowledge is necessary for rational, effective practice in multidisciplinary settings with outcomes emphases and tight fiscal constraints. Basic familiarity with health care and nursing "business" is critical for advanced nurses practicing in a variety of roles who are expected to develop new programs and improve clinical and operational processes. Basic business acumen is also useful for the advanced nurse who envisions future employment and advancement in nursing administration.

▶ The Context of Nursing Practice: An Overview of the U.S. Healthcare System

A variety of well-written resources are available on this subject. Shi and Singh (2015) provide an overview of the U.S. health care system that is concise and essential. Advanced nurses are advised to understand different types of managed care organizations

(MCOs), including health maintenance organizations (HMOs), preferred provider organizations (PPOs), exclusive provider organizations (EPO), and point of service (POS) plans. It is also helpful to appreciate the significant changes that are occurring as the health care system moves from volume-based to value-based reimbursement models, including programs driven by the Patient Protection and Affordable Care Act (ACA) and health care reform.

MCOs are part of a larger group referred to as third-party payors because they are connected to two other key parties of interest in health care, the patient and the provider (Shi & Singh, 2015). Other members of the third-party payor group include insurance companies, Blue Cross/Blue Shield, Medicare, and Medicaid. Each third-party payor pays differently, depending on its reimbursement method and contractual arrangement.

Full payment fee-for-service is a rare arrangement when compared with other forms of reimbursement. Fee-for-service refers to being paid for specific tests, procedures, or admissions, but the reimbursement does not typically cover the generated charges or, depending on the payor, even the cost of the service. Providers determine charges, bills are generated, and insurers pay. The higher the charges, the greater the net revenue. Diagnosis-related groups (DRGs) were an early strategy for curtailing the spiraling costs associated with fee-for-service arrangements.

Third-Party Payors

The *payor mix* of an institution is a critically important variable in the assumptions underlying institutional budgets. Advanced nurses need to have a general sense of the payor mix of their practice or service line. They must also understand the payor mix of the employing institution or network as this mix directly influences the amount and variability of revenue streams available for all types of services, including educational programs, equipment, and the affordability of staffing mix and nurse-to-patient ratios.

In terms of payor mix, private or commercial insurers tend to pay a higher percentage of charges than government programs (Medicare and Medicaid). Payor mix varies for many reasons, including the income level, age, and employment status of the population served in a hospital, clinic, or other health care setting. Reimbursement from payors can influence behavior (**TABLE 4-1**).

Managed Care Organizations

HMOs are the earliest forms of MCOs and continue as a popular arrangement. The goal of HMOs is to reduce costs while providing quality care. Care is coordinated through the primary care provider, who acts as a *gatekeeper* to services and who safeguards against unnecessary tests or treatments. Payor policies are often a barrier to advanced practice nurses (specifically nurse practitioners) serving in this gatekeeper role (Hain & Fleck, 2014). Though practices vary, private or commercial plans may not recognize advanced practice nurses as primary care providers, thereby limiting their scope of practice. Even in states with full practice authority, payors may opt to not pay the advanced practice nurse directly or reimburse at a lower rate (Yee, Boukous, Cross, & Samuel, 2013).

HMOs offer services to maintain or improve health status, recognizing that it is more cost effective to avoid illness than to treat illness. Preventive services such as

TABLE 4-1 Impact of Payor Type

Payor Type	Percentage	Impact
Private (commercial) ■ Fee-for-service ■ Managed care **Subtotal**	 39% 14% **53%**	Private or commercial payors are the largest category of payor with a high percentage of fee-for-service. The incentive is to increase volume to increase revenue—more tests and procedures.
Government ■ Medicare ■ Medicaid **Subtotal**	 30% 8% **38%**	Typically, these programs pay a lower percentage of charges than private payors, with Medicaid reimbursement usually lower than Medicare. As the age of the population increases, Medicare percentage will rise. This example is a relatively low government payor mix minimizing impact of political decisions that impact reimbursement.
Miscellaneous ■ Self-pay ■ Other **Subtotal**	 5% 4% **9%**	Others may include bad debt, charity care, and workers' compensation and does not pose a significant financial risk in this example.
Total	**100%**	

smoking cessation, weight management, physical fitness, and routine wellness visits are examples of services designed to reduce the risk of disease and to intervene early when illness occurs. HMOs usually pay providers a fee per person on a contracted basis. This fee is referred to as *capitation*. Enrollees are restricted to service providers, including hospitals, physicians, laboratories, and other diagnostic service facilities within the network. There are a variety of HMO models with differing physician arrangements (e.g., staff models with HMO-salaried providers, group models with contracted physicians within a group practice rather than employed physicians, network models with a variety of contracted medical groups, and the independent practice association [IPA] model, in which the IPA shares risk and assumes responsibility for utilization and quality management) (Shi & Singh, 2015).

PPOs offer enrollees more choices and increased control over their utilization of specialists. Enrollees can opt for out-of-network service providers, albeit at a higher cost, through preestablished copayments (Shi & Singh, 2015). PPOs are typically more expensive in terms of plan premium HMOs (Campbell, 2016) and do not use capitation arrangements. They usually work on a contractual arrangement with providers in a modified fee-for-service approach. PPOs are the dominant form of the employer health coverage market, and 58% of workers are covered with this type of plan with a mean family premium as high as $14,000 in 2010 (Kaiser Family Foundation, 2010).

EPOs are similar to PPOs, but enrollees cannot receive reimbursed care from a provider outside of network (Briscoe, 2015). This arrangement prioritizes cost savings, though EPO plans provide flexibility in terms of choice. There is not a requirement to choose a primary care provider, nor a need to have a referral for specialist care. However, the network of providers and hospitals is limited and if care is received outside of this network, it will not be covered unless it is an emergency. Knowing the panel of included providers and sites is therefore essential for enrollees. Limiting selection of providers and services is the key to reducing costs.

POS plans combine features of both HMOs and PPOs. Enrollees are typically required to select a primary care provider who makes referrals to specialists within the network when needed. Plans may vary, and there are usually no or minimal costs or deductibles for care provided by the primary care provider. As in a PPO model, individuals can receive care from providers out of the network but will be subject to greater out-of-pocket costs and copayments.

Private Health Insurance

Blue Cross/Blue Shield plans are nonprofit and cover hospital and physician services. In addition to Blue Cross and Blue Shield, other private health insurance plans may be purchased as an individual or family member or purchased as an employee participating in an employer-provided plan. Private health insurance is a program not provided for or administered by the government. Private health insurance plans are offered in a variety of forms, including MCOs, indemnity, or fee for service.

Public Health Insurance

The Centers for Medicare and Medicaid Services (CMS) are responsible for Medicare and Medicaid programs. CMS is organized within the U. S. Department of Health and Human Services (DHHS) and has a strategic plan that includes objectives related to regulatory, budgetary, and quality responsibilities for a variety of stakeholders (CMS, 2013) (**BOX 4-1**). Advanced nurses require a basic

---

BOX 4-1 CMS Mission, Vision, and Strategic Goals

Mission: As an effective steward of public funds, CMS is committed to strengthening and modernizing the nation's health care system to provide access to high quality care and improved health at lower cost.
Vision: A high quality health care system that ensures better care, access to coverage and improved health.

Strategic Goals:
- Better care and lower costs
- Prevention and population health
- Expanded health care coverage
- Enterprise excellence

Data from Centers for Medicare and Medicaid Services (2013).

understanding of CMS and its programs, given that many hospitals and health care practices are significantly influenced by regulations and reimbursements controlled by CMS.

Title 18 of the Social Security Amendment of 1965 provided for Parts A and B of Medicare, whereas Title 19 established the Medicaid program. Medicare provides publicly financed health insurance to elders, regardless of income. Some disabled people and individuals with end-stage kidney disease are also covered (Shi & Singh, 2015). Prescription benefits have been added via Part D benefits, and most people pay a monthly premium for this coverage. Medicare Parts A and B cover different types of benefits. In general, Part A covers hospitalization and short-term nursing home stays following hospitalization. Part B covers physicians' bills and other outpatient services. Elders pay part of the premium expense of Part B, whereas Social Security taxes pay for Part A (CMS, 2014).

Traditional Medicare does not typically cover all expenses, including copayments and deductibles. Enrollees may choose to purchase a supplemental insurance policy (Medigap, also known as Part C) that is sold by private insurance companies. Medicare will first pay the Medicare-approved portion of health care costs for services and then the Medigap contribution will be applied. Medicare does not provide coverage while traveling outside the United States and Medigap policies will often include this provision. Another option for elders is to enroll in a Medicare Advantage plans. Private insurance companies contract with Medicare to provide all Part A and Part B benefits. These plans include HMOs, PPOs, and prescription drug coverage (Cubanski et al., 2015).

Medicaid is a public health insurance program for individuals with low income. It is a combination of a federal and state program, subject to federal standards but administered by states. Individual states have flexibility to determine populations and services that are covered under the program. In 2017, Medicaid and the Children's Health Insurance Plan (CHIP) covered over 74 million low-income Americans, including infants and children, parents, pregnant women, people with disabilities of all ages, and elders with very low incomes. Approximately three quarters of nonelderly Medicaid recipients are from working families (Kaiser Family Foundation, 2017). The ACA increased the income eligibility for Medicaid, though not all states opted to participate in this expansion. Services covered by Medicaid vary by state, but a number of states have elected to cover optional services, including dental care and prescription drugs. While Medicare and Medicaid are government programs, health care services are provided by private entities.

Federal expenditures have dramatically increased since the inception of these programs. The United States spent $3.2 trillion on health care in 2015, an average of $9,990 per person. The health spending share of gross domestic product in 2015 was 17.8% (CMS, 2015). This per capita spending is more than twice the average of other developed countries; yet, the outcomes, specifically life expectancy and infant mortality, are no better and in some instances worse than those countries that spend less. Growth in health care spending is predicted to annually increase by 5.6% during the period 2016–2025 (CMS, 2015). As health care costs climb, federal, state, and local governments exert more stringent controls over reimbursements. Simultaneously, health care consumers and practitioners demand increasingly sophisticated and expensive technologies and services.

Health Care Reform

The high cost of health care in the United States has led to a number of legislative efforts to curb costs while maintaining and improving quality. One of the most significant is the ACA, which was signed into law in March 2010. There are many aspects and complexities to this law, but a few key provisions include the following:

- Expanding access to insurance coverage
- Increasing consumer insurance protections that emphasize prevention and wellness
- Improving health quality and system performance
- Promoting health workforce development
- Curbing the rise of health costs

While there has been debate about the success of the ACA, the number of uninsured Americans has decreased since its implementation. Health care costs have still continued to rise, though at a lesser rate than in prior years. Some insurers have opted out of the state exchanges, limiting choice and increasing copayments for service. There have been efforts to replace the ACA with other health care proposals that address rising costs, as well as access to and quality of care. ACA and related health care factors continue to be active and ongoing concerns within Congress.

Value-Based Care and Alternative Payment Models

The traditional fee-for-service model incentivizes strategies that increase the number and volume of services to increase revenue. This payment model does not reward providers and organizations based on health care outcomes. As a result of increasing health care costs and quality and safety concerns, government payers, health plan organizations, and employers are beginning to focus on value-based payment models aligning payments and penalties based on quality, costs, and outcome measures.

There are a variety of alternative (value-based) payment models. An alternative payment model (APM) is an approach that provides incentive payments to organizations or networks to provide care that is high quality and cost effective. APMs can be utilized with a population, specific clinical condition, or care episode.

In a *shared savings* model, organizations are paid fee-for-service, but if spending is below a preset target, they share in the savings as a bonus. *Shared risk* models are similar to shared savings, but organizations also pay a penalty if spending exceeds the target. In a *bundled payment* arrangement, organizations are paid for an episode of care rather than separate payments for hospital, physician, and outpatient care related to a specific condition (**EXEMPLAR 4-1**). One area that CMS has focused on is bundled payments for total joint replacement. These models promote achievement of quality outcomes as well as cost reduction.

Accountable Care Organizations

An accountable care organization (ACO) is a network of physicians, nurses, other health care providers, hospitals, and additional care delivery sites that work together to deliver high-quality coordinated care to their patients (CMS, 2017a). The ACA created Medicare shared savings programs (MSSPs) rewarding ACOs with financial

EXEMPLAR 4-1 Improving Quality and Efficiency to Maximize Bundled Payment Arrangements

Advanced nurses can play a significant role in identifying improvements in quality and efficiency in bundled payment arrangements. As part of a comprehensive joint management program, the nurse manager, clinical nurse specialist, and clinical nurse leader evaluated the postoperative care on an orthopedic unit. Their focus was on ambulation and pain management, as both play a significant role in recovery and costly inpatient length of stay. Compression devices are important, but inefficient in terms of early ambulation. The advanced nurses identified a compression device that could be used while ambulating, thus increasing patient mobility and reducing time spent in removing and reapplying devices. After a review of best practices in pain management and collaboration with physician colleagues, the advanced nurses implemented a pain protocol that essentially avoided the use of parenteral narcotics, utilizing oral medications and a cooling device on the knee. Education was provided preoperatively to support these measures. As a result, the hospital length of stay was reduced and the incidence of readmission decreased.

savings for providing cost-effective care and positive patient outcomes. Preventive services, wellness programs, elimination of unnecessary tests and procedures, and provision in the most appropriate and low-cost setting are cornerstones of the ACO approach. In the MSSP, financing remains fee-for-service but the incentive is only paid if the preset targets are achieved. CMS has continued to build on the ACO strategy, developing programs that can receive additional incentive payments by assuming greater financial risk.

Early results from the Medicare ACO MSSP programs are demonstrating mixed results (Baseman, Boccuti, Moon, Griffin, & Dutta, 2016). In 2014, the Medicare ACO programs generated savings of $411 million; however, after paying bonuses for the savings, the overall program resulted in a loss of $2.6 million to the Medicare trust fund. Performance on quality measures has been good or better than the traditional Medicare program (Baseman et al., 2016).

Population Health

Population health has been defined by Kindig and Stoddart (2003) as "the health outcomes of a group of individuals, including the distribution of such outcomes within the group (p. 381)." Alternative payment models may or may not be used in a population health model, but achieving desired quality and financial outcomes currently focuses on prevention, promotion of health behaviors, early intervention, and case management for those with significant health care issues. Data and predictive analytics are essential in determining individuals at risk for complications, hospital readmissions, and high cost care. Intensive care management is often utilized to coordinate complex care. Social factors that may impact health, including access to food and transportation, are often considered, though these services are rarely reimbursed. The goal is to improve outcomes and reduce costs by promoting health.

Value-Based Purchasing

CMS has initiated a hospital value-based purchasing (VBP) program that rewards acute care hospitals for the quality of care delivered by providing incentive payments. The payments are based on (1) the quality of care provided to Medicare patients, (2) patient experience, and (3) adherence to clinical practices and processes. This program was established as part of the ACA and rewards hospitals based on value and outcomes, rather than volume. Providing incentives or payment based on quality of care, cost effectiveness, and service is also utilized in ambulatory, home care, and long-term care settings. The move from volume to value provides advanced nurses with a unique opportunity to demonstrate the impact of nursing on clinical outcomes and the organization's bottom line.

Specific measures are identified and typically include outcomes in the following categories (CMS, 2017b):

- Mortality and complications
- Health care–associated infections
- Patient safety
- Patient experience
- Process
- Efficiency and cost reduction

Advanced nurses need to appreciate the changing and challenging context in which health care services are provided in the United States. A basic familiarity with various insurance models, differences between Medicare and Medicaid programs, the effect of payor mix on health care organizations' budgets, and the move from volume to value will assist the advanced nurse in understanding the challenges confronting health care organizations and society. The interplay between cost and reimbursement and quality outcomes has significant influence on the *bottom line* of health care organizations. Understanding these concepts is important for well-informed nursing practice. There is concern that advanced nurses may have inaccurate or inadequate understanding of CMS programs (Zuzelo et al., 2004) and that this knowledge deficit may impact care and disadvantage the public by artificially limiting the accessibility of advanced nurses to health care service recipients.

Although advanced nurses are not consistently involved in budget and business processes at organizational or network levels, they are often involved in these activities at the unit or department level or by service line. Advanced nurses participate in capital budget development through product evaluations and recommendations. Clinical nurses often ask nurses in advanced roles to explain budget processes, and it is not uncommon for program administrators to solicit the input of advanced nurses regarding basic operating and capital budget needs. Many nurses in various advanced roles have some budgetary responsibilities that range in scope and accountability. Understanding the pressures of health care organization financing is critical to the success of the organization-at-large and also to the individual programs and departments within the system. Upcoming sections explain key concepts of nursing and capital budgets and provide strategies and tools for product evaluation, particularly given the importance of selecting products that satisfy the needs of the organization at an acceptable price point.

▶ Budget Process Essentials

The degree of advanced nurses' involvement in the budget process varies depending on the organization and the advanced nurses' roles and job responsibilities. Advanced nurses' exclusion from the process can represent a missed opportunity for nursing administration. The experience and expertise of the advanced nurse, as well as the clinical or operational focus of the nurse's role, has the potential to add value to many facets of the budget process, including resource planning for new clinical programs, identification of quality-of-care issues, and comparison of equipment and clinical supply items. The advanced nurse must have knowledge of general processes and principles of budgeting, to have a positive impact on critical finance activities and decisions.

The budget is an annual process of identifying anticipated revenues and expenditures for an organization. It provides a framework to allocate resources that support ongoing operations and programs. Additionally, the budget serves as a monitoring and evaluation tool throughout the fiscal year (FY) (**BOX 4-2**). The FY is defined by each organization; it can correlate with the calendar year (January through December) but more often follows a July through June or October through September time frame.

Budgeting has often been described as an organization's best guess regarding future performance and expenses. However, the budget is based on a careful review of factors that might influence revenue and expenditures. The organization's strategic plan provides the framework for beginning the review process. The external environment, prior year performance, new programs, additional physician practices, and marketing initiatives are carefully reviewed. Additional sources of information include projected salary and price increase, regulatory changes, and estimations of charity care and bad debt.

The organization may start the budgeting process in a number of ways. In zero-based budgeting (ZBB), each budget request is justified every cycle regardless of prior history. Use of ZBB requires that managers justify why they should spend the organization's resources in the manner proposed. Each planned activity or project must include an analysis of cost, benefit, alternatives, and measures of performance. One major drawback to ZBB is the amount of time required to review and justify, at times, routine operational costs in great detail on an annual basis.

Historical or baseline budgeting begins with the organization's historical data and builds on the readily available past performance of its operations. Historical budgeting works well in organizations with predictable operations. This method of budgeting saves time and is less likely to result in an omission of a key event, trend, or expense. Alternatively, it may also result in inclusion of items that no longer have relevance.

BOX 4-2 Budget Functions

1. Identify anticipated revenues.
2. Identify planned expenditures.
3. Provide a framework for resource allocations.
4. Monitor spending.
5. Evaluate accuracy of allocation decisions.
6. Evaluate fiscal responsibility.

TABLE 4-2 Budget Approaches: Zero-Based Budget Versus Historical Budget			
Budget Type	**Description**	**Advantages**	**Disadvantages**
Zero-based budget	Start at zero. Justify each expense and revenue source.	1. Tight control over resources 2. Dollars allocated based on need rather than history	1. Time consuming 2. Justify routine, required expenses
Historical budget	Begin with previous budget. Build on past performances.	1. Works well in predictable situations 2. Saves time 3. Less likely to omit key events or trends	1. May budget for irrelevant items 2. May not scrutinize expenses as thoroughly

In practice, many health care organizations use a combination of methods, relying on historical or baseline data combined with assessment of trends. A ZBB approach is frequently used when proposing new programs and initiatives (**TABLE 4-2**).

Types of Budgets

There are several types of budgets: operating budgets, revenue budgets, expense budgets, and capital budgets.

Operating Budget

The operating budget is the financial plan for the organization's day-to-day activities. It details the immediate goals for revenues, volumes, and expenses. The operating budget is extremely detailed and is used for monitoring throughout the year. The revenue and expense budgets make up the operating budget.

Revenue Budget

The revenue budget is the projected income for the FY. The primary source of revenue in a health care organization is the delivery of health care services. Volume projections in each department drive the revenue budget. The definition of volume or *units of service* varies with the specific patient care area, but includes visits in the emergency department and clinic settings, patient days in the inpatient areas, procedures in the surgical suite, and numbers of tests in the laboratory.

Volume is a major factor in calculating anticipated revenue, but there are other primary considerations. Federal and state reimbursement changes and contractual relationships with payors have a significant effect on revenue projection. Assumptions are also made regarding the acuity level of patients, specifically the case mix index (CMI) that affects Medicare reimbursement. The CMI is a marker of the severity of a patient's illness and is tracked by Medicare.

In the inpatient areas, the length of stay (LOS) and number of patient days affects revenue projections from admissions. LOS varies by specialty area and is influenced by historical data and the organization's ability to move patients to the appropriate level of care at the right time. LOS is typically longer on an inpatient behavioral health or rehabilitation unit as compared to a general surgical patient care area. If an organization has the ability to move patients from an acute care area to a skilled or long-term nursing facility, then the LOS may be reduced.

The number of patient days is another key revenue budget metric. The number of budgeted admissions multiplied by the LOS results in total number of patient days (**BOX 4-3**). The number of patient days has a direct effect on patient revenue and expense. Many payors reimburse based on a case rate or diagnosis. In this instance, a prolonged LOS results in additional expense without corresponding revenue. If a payor pays a per diem rate, then an increased LOS might enhance revenue. Patient days are also an important metric in determining the nursing expense budget.

Expense Budget

The expense budget includes salaries, supplies, fees, purchased services, repairs, maintenance, consulting, education, insurance, depreciation, and other miscellaneous items. Health care expenses, particularly in nursing, are largely made up of salary expenses.

Salary Expenses. Salary expense can be divided into productive and nonproductive time. Productive time is time actually worked, and nonproductive time includes sick, holiday, vacation, orientation, and education hours. Productive hours include direct time or time spent in caregiving activities. Indirect hours include unit secretarial, nurse manager, and educator time.

Direct caregiver hours are usually classified as variable. These hours adjust to the patient care volume. Areas with minimum staffing requirements and those that have difficult-to-predict daily volume (e.g., emergency departments, labor and delivery services) cannot routinely flex direct care staff. Fixed hours are those required to run the unit regardless of fluctuating volume and census and include positions such as the unit secretary, housekeeper, and nurse manager.

Nonsalary Expenses. Supplies are second in importance to salary in the health care organization's budget. Supply expenses can also be categorized as fixed versus variable. Patient care supplies and forms usually fluctuate or vary with patient days. Expenses that are fixed include phone services and electricity. Many organizations have joined group purchasing programs to take advantage of reduced supply prices

---

BOX 4-3 Number of Patient Days with Example

Admissions × Length of Stay = Patient Days

20,000 annual admissions × 6 days LOS = 120,000 patient days

when purchased in quantity. Supply costs can often be a large component of the budget, particularly in surgical areas.

The Bottom Line. The bottom line or net income from operations is commonly measured as net patient revenues minus the total operating expenses (**BOX 4-4**). The organization's operating margin is the percentage of profit realized from the operations of its day-to-day business. Profit can be defined simply as the difference between net expenses and net revenue.

Capital Budget

The capital budget is developed separately from the operational budget and pertains to the organization's plan for investments in building or plant and major equipment. The capital budget is driven by the organization's strategic plan and is composed of two components: (1) equipment purchases, building plans, and plant maintenance that occur within the annual budget cycle; and (2) those that exceed 1 year in length. A defined dollar amount typically determines whether an item is defined as capital. The amount varies, but usually is at least $500 and may exceed $5,000. This has implications for the operating budget. For example, if the manager of a unit is purchasing equipment that falls under this threshold, the item will not be considered capital and will be reflected in the unit operating budget.

The annual capital budget begins with identification of equipment needs or building/renovation projects for the upcoming year. Patient care equipment needs may be unit based, program specific, or they may cut across clinical specialty lines. The initial list in nursing is often generated at the department level and should be developed by the nurse manager or director with significant input from advanced nurses and nursing staff. Examples of capital items are critical care monitoring equipment, dialysis machines, scales, hospital beds, and mattresses. Identification and communication of need are crucial steps, and the advanced nurse can play a major role in this area. Identifying and evaluating products as part of the capital budget process are important advanced nurse responsibilities, depending on the type of advanced nurse practice.

Communication with other departments is particularly important when developing the capital budget. Determining which department is responsible for capital purchases may be confusing. For example, stretchers are purchased by the transport service for general use, yet the emergency department, operating room, and radiology areas purchase stretchers for their specific areas.

Many capital requests from other departments affect nursing practice and patient care, particularly related to renovating existing patient care areas. Capital requests may require renovation, and this need must be noted early and identified as an associated cost (**FIGURE 4-1**). For example, if monitoring equipment is purchased and the current electrical outlets are inadequate or in difficult-to-reach locations, renovation needs must be taken into account and communicated to the facilities and maintenance director (**FIGURE 4-2**).

Company XYZ Capital Expenditure Request

Company:	XYZ		
Department:	1000-Admin		
Description:	Patient Ceiling Lift	Request Owner:	John Doe
Project ID:	123	Funding Owner:	Nursing
Project In Service Month:	July	Project In Service Year:	2020
Project Function:	↓ Medical / Medical / Non-Medical	Status:	↓ New / New / Replacement

Capital Expenditure Summary:

Install new patient ceiling lift to increase staff and patient safety.

Additional Considerations That Impact This Capital Request:

Facility personnel will need to assist with inspection and support.

Vendor:	Lifts, Inc.	Attach Quote:	

Importance to Department: (1 - 5)   1 - High Priority

FIGURE 4-1 Capital Expense Request.

Once items for a specific area are identified, the manager generally identifies the following information:

- A description of the item or equipment
- The number of items needed and whether this is a replacement or addition
- The date or quarter of the FY the purchase will take place
- Priority of each item

The manager typically works with the purchasing department to provide supporting documentation. The advanced nurse often plays a role in comparing different vendors' products and networking with others to learn about new technology and efficacy.

Company xyz Capital Expenditure Request

Capital Budget (over $5k each item)

	QTY	Amount		2020 Budget
Movable Equipment:				$ -
Fixed Equipment:	2	$ 2,000.00		$ 10,000.00
Buildings:				$ -
Land:				$ -
Software:				$ -
Improvements:				$ -
Freight:	2	$ 250.00		$ 500.00
Subtotal:				$ 10,500.00
Tax (if taxable):				$ 588.00
Total Capital Requested:				$ 11,088.00

Expense Budget (under $5k each item)

	2020 Budget
Minor Equipment:	$ 2,000.00
Installation:	
Storage:	
Training:	
Other:	
Subtotal:	$ 2,000.00
Tax (if taxable):	$ 112.00
Total Expense Requested Related to Capital Project:	$ 2,112.00

FIGURE 4-1 *(Continued)*

Building the Inpatient Nursing Budget

Nursing expenses are primarily based on salary or personnel budget. The foundation of the salary budget is the full-time equivalent (FTE) (**BOX 4-5**). It is important to note that the FTE is not a person, merely a time equivalent. Nursing job requirements for being considered a full-time employee vary widely, particularly with 12-hour shifts and increasing flexibility in scheduling. A nurse who works three 12-hour shifts per week is considered full time in many organizations, but the budget will reflect the position as a 0.9 FTE (**BOX 4-6**).

Company XYZ
Capital Request Form

SPACE, BUILDING & RENOVATION REQUEST

Capital Project # _____

To be completed by Department Head

DEPT. # _____   PROJECT DATE REQUESTED   _____

DEPARTMENT NAME _____ PHONE# _____

Campus Location   Building   Floor

1. Request for: _____ Renovation   _____ Relocation of Dept/   _____ Additional
                                    of Area   Equipment   Space*

                         _____ Reconfiguration _____ Installation of New   _____ Other
                                    of Area   Equipment

2. Description of Work:

3. Justification for
   Work.

Signature of Department Head: _____ Date _____

Signature of Vice President: _____ Date _____

To be completed by Director Facilities Management

4. Cost Estimate Breakdown   Projected Length of Project   _____
   A. Project can be accomplished:

      _____ With in-house labor and materials.
      _____ Through outside contracting.
      _____ Through a combination of in-house effort and contracting.
      _____ DOH Approval/Notification required
   B. Costs
      Material Costs: $ _____
      Contractor Costs: $ _____
      In-House Labor Costs $ _____
      I. S. Costs (cabling/terminations) $ _____
      Other Costs $ _____

      Total Project Estimate $ _____

Comments: _____

Signature of Vice President Facilities: _____ Date _____

Administrative Use Only

Ranking: _____   Approved _____   Denied _____   Deferred _____

Administrator Signature: _____   Date _____

PLEASE ATTACH DOCUMENTATION FOR EACH REQUEST TO THIS FORM!

March 24 2018

FIGURE 4-2 Space Renovation Form.

The number of FTEs required to provide care is determined in a number of ways. Nursing units begin with a standard and then match the standard to the projected volume. Inpatient units often utilize nursing hours per patient day (NHPPD) as the standard or metric, that is, the number of hours of care divided by the number of patient days (**TABLE 4-3**). The required nursing hours are based on a variety of factors, including the type of unit, acuity of the patient population, and patient outcomes.

Specialty areas that do not utilize NHPPD use other standards. In the emergency department, nursing hours per patient visit is the metric. In the operating room, the number of staff required is case dependent, but also determined by a standard FTE per room.

BOX 4-5 Full-Time Equivalent (FTE) Calculation

40 hours per week × 52 weeks/year = 2,080 hours or 1 FTE

BOX 4-6 Three 12-Hour Shifts/Week Employee

36 hours per week × 52 weeks/year = 1,872 hours
1,872 hours/2,080 hours = 0.9 FTE

TABLE 4-3 Sample Calculation of Required FTEs Based on a Standard NHPPD

Projected patients days	7,300 patient days (equates to an average daily census [ADC] of 20 patients) 7,300 patient days/364 days/year = 20 patients/day
NHPPD standards	10
Patient days × NHPPD standard	*Total number of direct care hours required*
7,300 patient days × 10 NHPPD	73,000 direct care hours
73,000 direct care hours/2,080 (1 FTE)	35.09 required FTEs

Establishing the number of direct care FTEs is not the final step in building a nursing budget. Not all of an FTE's 2,080 hours per year are productive or worked hours. Replacement time must be built in to provide coverage for nursing staff during non-productive time including vacations, holidays, and sick time usage.

How Is Benefit Time Determined?

Benefit time is calculated by subtracting the number of benefit hours from the total FTE time (**BOX 4-7**). In practice, there is individual variability with factors such as seniority playing a role in the amount of vacation time. Most organizations use an average to calculate time. It is important to recognize that on units with high percentages of senior staff, organizational averages may not be the best barometer for calculating benefit time.

Staffing Patterns and Ratios

A nursing budget can also be built by starting with a staffing pattern. Staffing patterns relate to NHPPD, but the budgeting process starts a bit differently depending

BOX 4-7 Benefit Time Calculations

Benefit Time

Vacation time = 4 weeks vacation annually or 160 hours

Sick time = average 6 days annually or 48 hours

Holiday time = 6 days annually or 48 hours

Personal time = 3 days annually or 24 hours

Educational time = 4 days annually or 32 hours

TOTAL = 312 hours

2,080 hours (1 FTE) – 312 hours of benefit time = **1,768 hours actually worked**

In this scenario, 312 hours, or 15% of total hours, will need to be replaced per FTE.

FTEs × 15% = total number of direct care FTEs required

BOX 4-8 Using Staffing Ratios to Budget FTEs

Assumptions

Unit census = 20 patients

Nurse-to-patient ratio = 1:4

Number of required staff = 5

Three 8-hour shifts = 15 staff

Replacement factor 15% (see Box 4-7): 15 staff × 0.15 replacement factor = 2.25 FTEs

Total number of required staff:

15 FTEs + 2.25 FTEs = 17.25 FTEs

on the metric. Recently, nurse–patient ratios have been a topic of debate and discussion. For example, California has a legislated 1:5 nurse (RN)–patient ratio on medical-surgical units, and the number of FTEs is based on this metric (**BOX 4-8**). When using a staffing pattern to build the budget, LPN and assistive staff would be added to the matrix.

Again, indirect salaries need to be added, including medical clerks, nurse manager, clinical nurse specialist, and any other support staff that are in the nursing budget. A replacement factor must be built in for the medical clerks, but is not included for the nurse manager or clinical nurse specialist.

Once FTEs are determined, the type of hours or who will be filling the FTEs is a key decision. The following areas must be considered:

- Skill mix (percentage may already be determined by standard or history)
- Special programs, such as weekend rates/shift differentials
- Use of supplemental staff

Skill Mix

Skill mix refers to the proportion of licensed to nonlicensed caregivers in a patient care delivery model. Some organizations use an RN/LPN to nursing assistant/technician ratio and others use an RN to LPN/nursing assistant technician ratio. Ideally, the skill mix should be determined by carefully examining the patient population being served and identifying skills and tasks required to provide care. In practice, many factors affect skill mix determinations.

Available RN supply affects skill mix. During times of RN shortage, skill mix percentages often decrease due to inability to fill positions. Skill mix can also affect cost. Higher skill mix equals higher salary dollars. When developing the budget, the manager most often follows the historical trend for skill mix, unless a justification for change is submitted. The advanced nurse can assist in identifying whether a change in skill mix is required based on the assessed needs of the patient population being served.

Typically, the historical pattern for skill mix varies based on the patient population and level of care. Critical care units tend to have a very high RN mix, and long-term care facilities have a lower RN mix. Nursing research has begun to focus on the impact of skill mix on patient outcomes.

Frith, Anderson, Tseng, and Fong (2012) identified an inverse relationship with RN mix and medication errors. A decrease in medication errors was demonstrated as the proportion of RNs increased. However, findings did not generate specific staffing recommendations. Aiken and colleagues (2017) explored nursing skill mix in European hospital settings using a cross section of data from patient discharges, hospital characteristics, and nurse and patient surveys. Data analysis revealed that a richer nurse skill mix was associated with lower odds of mortality, lower odds of low patient hospital ratings, and lower odds of poor quality reports, poor safety grades and other poor outcomes after adjusting for patient and hospital factors (Aiken et al., 2017). Findings support that for every 10% reduction in the proportion of professional nurses there is an associated 11% increase in the odds of death. In this hospital sample, consider that there was an average of six caregivers for every 25 patients, four of whom were professional nurses. Substituting one nurse assistant for a professional nurse for every 25 patients would be associated with a 21% increase in the odds of dying (Aiken et al., 2017). Nurses in all types of advanced roles can track outcome data on individual units and identify associations between outcomes and staffing to determine whether changes are required.

Incentives and Differentials

Organizations differ on how specific program incentives and differentials are captured. If shift differential or weekend program salary rates are not incorporated into the budget, then the unit will be over budget during the year, even though the hours of care remain constant.

The manager is responsible to identify the percentage of staff working hours requiring pay above the base salary rate. During times of nursing shortages, incentive programs such as sign-on bonuses, additional differentials for night shift, and retention bonuses proliferate. Targeted incentives can be beneficial during unanticipated volume increases or nursing shortages, but can be difficult to administer and maintain.

Sign-on bonuses for new hires often create resentment among long-term staff. Sunsetting or ending very rich programs can feel like a pay reduction or takeaway to staff. The advanced nurse is instrumental in identifying workplace issues that promote retention and a satisfying work environment. Carefully reviewing past history and judicious use of supplemental staff are strategies that can reduce the need for incentives. If programs are in place or anticipated during the year, they must be included during the budgeting process.

Supplemental Staff

Workload increases, staff vacancies due to resignations or leaves of absence, or increases in required staff numbers related to new programs lead to supplemental staffing strategies. Supplemental staff can include internal nursing pools, temporary staff provided by an external agency, increased hours for part-time staff, and overtime. With the exception of part-time staff increasing hours to full-time status, these options increase salary costs due to the higher associated hourly rate.

Supplemental staff salaries are frequently the cause of a major variance in the nursing budget. It is crucial that the nurse manager realistically project supplemental staff needs and closely monitor these costs. Obviously, filling vacant positions reduces the need for supplemental staffing.

Using *per diem* pool staff has become a major strategy for many organizations. Per diem staff usually have a minimum requirement of hours, no or reduced benefits, and a significantly higher hourly rate. In units with high vacancy rates, an interesting shift may occur. Nurses who have benefits through their spouses/partners or do not need benefits coverage may choose to shift from full-time positions to per diem. They receive a higher hourly rate, often work up to full time, and have a reduced holiday and weekend commitment. In this case, the manager depends on the per diem staff for regular hours and does not have the flexibility of the per diem pool to cover high-volume needs or replacement for leaves and sick calls.

With a fairly consistent average daily census, a wise strategy is to hire full- and part-time staff into budgeted positions utilizing per diem staff for flexibility. An exception is in units with a widely fluctuating census, such as in neonatal intensive care units. In this type of unit, allotting a percentage of FTEs to per diem or pool staff is an important strategy for efficient resource management. When the census increases, per diem staff can increase their hours. If a decrease in census is sudden and prolonged, the number of full-time staff required to use nonproductive time may be minimized.

Additional sources of premium pay are overtime and temporary staffing. Overtime can be incidental, short times to complete work, or additional shifts. A number of organizations do not budget overtime, but inevitably a late sick call will result in the request for a staff member to stay, even if it is for a short time. Historical data are important in budgeting overtime; however, scheduling practices can often play a role. Prescheduling overtime or schedules that consistently create an overtime situation, such as scheduling staff for four 12-hour shifts within a week, are often reasons for an overage or increase in overtime pay.

Temporary or agency help also provides a degree of flexibility, particularly during times of sustained volume. For example, if an organization has historical data that identify an increase in the average daily census of 20 patients during the month of January, utilizing temporary staff might be a viable strategy.

Temporary supplemental staffing agencies can provide local individuals on a day-to-day basis, provide a "block" agreement for a longer time frame, or provide a consistent individual for a specific time period. Again, the hourly rate is significantly higher than the average staff nurse salary and can have a negative impact on the bottom line.

Predictive Analytics

There are a number of software and staffing and scheduling tools that can assist in predicting staffing needs based on demand, typically based on historical data. Greater accuracy in matching supply to demand assists in identifying the core staffing needed at a given point in time. It may also reduce the time that scheduled nurses are unexpectedly not needed for a particular shift, which can be a major source of dissatisfaction if occurring frequently.

The Demand for Close Observation

Many organizations wrestle with the need for close observation, also known as one-to-one or sitter care. The advanced nurse can play a major role in establishing sitter criteria and working with staff to identify appropriateness of one-to-one observation. This type of monitoring is clearly required for suicidal patients and in specific clinical situations. Sitters are frequently utilized to prevent falls, inadvertent tube removals, elopement, and wandering. With the focus on restraint-free environments, the use of sitters has increased. It is important to review past usage history and assess the needs of the anticipated patient population during the budget process. Working with physicians and other members of the health care team to identify appropriate alternatives to one-to-one care is a key strategy.

Video or remote monitoring has demonstrated promising results in reducing costs associated with the need for *one-to-one* observations while achieving desired safety outcomes (Burtson & Vento, 2015). A centralized monitoring system allows one or more trained individuals to observe a number of patients concurrently and then alerting the nurse if there appears to be an imminent risk of fall or elopement. Key to the success of this intervention is identification of appropriate patients and effective communication systems (**EXEMPLAR 4-2**).

 EXEMPLAR 4-2 Remote Video Monitoring to Protect Patients from Harm

A general medical unit in an academic teaching hospital often cares for patients with dementia who require close observation for wandering and fall prevention. At any given time, this unit often has five patients that require this level of supervision. The additional staffing requirements would be 5 nursing assistants or other designated sitters per shift or an additional 15 in a 24-hour time frame. This requirement places a significant burden on the unit staffing model as nursing assistants may need to be reassigned from their responsibilities to augment sitter staffing needs.

The hospital recently implemented a remote video program. The advanced nurse, a clinical nurse specialist, evaluated all patients requiring sitters against criteria for participation in the remote video program option. Four patients met the criteria. The remote monitoring program supports one trained individual who monitors multiple patients. In this scenario, staffing needs were reduced to two sitters per shift. One sitter stayed on the unit with the patient who did not meet video monitoring criteria and one sitter remotely watched four patients. The 24-hour staffing requirements were reduced from 15 sitters to 6 sitters, resulting in a less burdensome impact on unit staffing and decreased labor costs while maintaining required safety precautions.

Justification Considerations for Nursing Staffing

It is important to note that although NHPPD and staffing patterns can be used to build the nursing budget, these figures are calculated averages. Staffing inpatient care areas on a daily basis must take into account the population of patients and the roles and responsibilities of the care providers.

The American Nurses Association (ANA, 2012) recognizes that appropriate nurse staffing is integral to achieving safe, quality outcomes. It asserts that ascertaining appropriate staffing requires dynamic decision making that incorporates consideration of many variables. Cost effectiveness is an important consideration and the reimbursement structure should not affect nurse staffing patterns or level of delivered care. Select core components include but are not limited to the following:

■ Quality, cost-effective health care relies on appropriate nurse staffing.

■ "All settings should have well-developed staffing guidelines with measurable nurse sensitive outcomes specific to that setting and healthcare consumer population that are used as evidence to guide daily staffing" (ANA, 2012, p. 6).

■ Registered nurses are full partners collaboratively working with other interdisciplinary health care professionals.

■ Registered nurses, including direct care nurses, must have a meaningful voice and active role in staffing decisions to ensure they have the time necessary to meet patient needs and complete nursing duties.

■ Staffing need determinations must be based on analysis of data, including patient characteristics, the care environment, and staff characteristics (skill set, mix, professional characteristics, and previous staffing patterns that have demonstrated effectiveness on outcomes of importance).

■ "Appropriate nurse staffing should be based on allocating the appropriate number of competent practitioners to a care situation; pursuing quality of care indices; meeting consumer-centered and organizational outcomes; meeting federal and state laws and regulations; and attending to a safe, quality work environment" (ANA, 2012, p. 6).

These principles demonstrate the complexity of the various factors that must be considered when determining appropriate nursing staffing.

Often the NHPPD is budgeted based on the prior year, and nursing leadership needs to make the case for an adjustment or increase. In recent years, there has been a concerted effort to benchmark nursing staffing data. Participation in national benchmarking initiatives, such as the National Database of Nursing Quality Indicators (NDNQI), has been increasing.

The NDNQI compares an organization's actual nursing care hours by specialty to the median of other participating hospitals on a quarterly basis. Nursing hours as reported by the NDNQI are the direct care provider hours and do not include indirect time. Nurse-sensitive quality indicators, such as the development of nosocomial pressure ulcers and fall rates, are also benchmarked in the NDNQI database. Data comparisons, including patient care outcomes and nurse-sensitive quality data, can provide a powerful tool when preparing budget justification for changes in nursing hours of care.

A number of investigators have studied the relationship between nurse staffing and patient outcomes. Aiken, Clarke, Sloane, Sochalski, and Silber (2002) noted that in hospitals with high patient–nurse ratios, surgical patients experience higher risk-adjusted 30-day mortality and failure-to-rescue rates than hospitals with lower ratios. In a more recent international study in nine countries, Aiken and colleagues (2014) found that an increase in nurses' workload increases the likelihood of inpatient hospital mortality. Similar findings were demonstrated in a study of surgical patients in Pennsylvania that suggested differences in nurse–patient ratios have an impact on postoperative mortality with lower ratios resulting in fewer deaths (Shekelle, 2013). The body of nursing research examining nurse staffing and outcomes is building, and the advanced nurse can play a role in continuing to examine this relationship.

Variance Reporting

Budget monitoring during the year usually occurs on a monthly basis. Actual revenue and expense reports are compared to the budget figures. Identifying a variance is the first step, but analysis is essential to make needed adjustments. Factors that contribute to a positive or negative variance are numerous and multifactorial and cannot always be controlled. A report describing the reason for a discrepancy is consistently required for a variance of 5% or more.

FTEs, actual dollars spent, and revenues vary with patient volume, but NHPPD and other standards remain constant. Supplemental staffing costing premium pay is a common area of negative variance in nursing. A unit could be well within the budgeted NHPPD or other standard, but have a negative dollar variance due to higher hourly rates.

Another metric that is used is the nursing costs per patient day. Cost per patient day encompasses the total salary and supply costs for a specific unit and divides it by the number of patient days. The higher salaries of supplemental staff or unusual supply usage are reflected in the total cost. A unit or department may end the month or even the year within budget, but not have flexed appropriately to the units of services. It is also possible in a variable budget context to be over budget and justify this variance as due to volume increases. Cost per patient day is an important metric that often demonstrates failure or success in adjusting staff and associated expenses to volume fluctuations.

Additional reasons for negative volume variances (*over* the budget) include unusually high sick calls, use of nonproductive time for vacation, unanticipated leaves of absence, high patient acuity, and supply costs for specific patient populations (e.g., gowns and gloves). Righting course may be necessary, but not at the expense of providing the agreed-upon standard (NHPPD, hours per visit) of care.

Nursing Budget Considerations in a Value-Based Environment

Nursing's impact has not always been quantifiable in the fee-for-service world. As nursing moves toward payment for outcomes and, in some instances, penalties for not achieving those outcomes, the profession has an opportunity to connect the impact of its practice to the bottom line of an organization. Advanced nurses can play a role in identifying staffing factors such as turnover, inadequate resources, and high use of agency staff that might impact the achievement of clinical outcomes. Another consideration is the importance of cross-continuum care and communication. In an era of population health, nurses need to think beyond the care delivered in the inpatient setting. Utilizing nurses' full capabilities in the inpatient, ambulatory, clinic, and home care settings becomes essential when the focus is on maintaining the health of a specific group of patients. Budgetary impact might include the need for additional assistive personnel, additional time for communication to nurses in other settings, and a renewed focus on coordination of complex care.

Preparing for the Capital Budget: Product Evaluation

Although advanced nurses may not be the architects of the hospital or nursing budgets, their clinical and operational expertise has the potential to inform many budget projections and decisions. Advanced nurses are especially needed as contributors to the capital budget process, particularly to lead or participate in product and equipment identification and evaluation. They influence the quality of the care environment and efficiency of the work environment by assisting in the provision of cost-effective, quality devices and products that improve care processes and positively affect outcomes.

Nurses in advanced roles are often involved in evaluating and selecting products and medical devices that are used in a variety of clinical settings. There is little in the literature to guide advanced nurses through this decision-making process. A review of published nursing literature reveals that perioperative nurses are at the forefront of product and device selection and management. Perioperative nurses and nurses in other specialized settings and departments are high-volume end users of hospital products. Given the emphasis on interprofessional collaboration and team-based decision making, it makes sense that such multidisciplinary input should be used for medical device and product evaluation activities.

There are more products than ever from which to choose. In 1992, Berkowitz, Diamond, and Montagnolo observed that in the early 1980s, there were more than 6,000 distinct types of medical devices and an estimated 750,000 brands, models, and sizes produced by approximately 12,000 manufacturers worldwide. The number and varieties have increased over the past 25 years, particularly when considered within the context of the technological and computerization explosion that has occurred in health care during this same period of time.

Selecting the right product and most appropriate technology or device requires effort. Fiscal resources are limited, so product and device decisions must be good. Most hospitals' capital equipment budgets are smaller than the amount of total requests, so competition for dollars is fierce between equally worthy projects. The goals of product evaluation include selecting products and devices that (1) meet specific performance criteria, (2) are safe for both patients and staff, (3) encourage positive patient outcomes, and (4) are cost effective for all stakeholders (Halvorson & Chinnes, 2007).

Opportunities to Explore Devices and Products: Trade Shows

Trade shows and conferences are good venues for exploring new products. The American Association of Critical Care Nurses' (AACN) National Teaching Institute (NTI) & Critical Care Exposition has the largest trade show for critical care nurses, advanced practice nurses, and nurses who care for critically ill patients (AACN, 2018). The Association of peri-Operative Registered Nurses (AORN) Global Surgical Conference and Expo includes a large exhibit hall filled with new products, technologies, and services. Other specialty organizations also work to provide opportunities for conference attendees and product experts to meet, mingle, and network over patient care needs, customizable products, software platforms, and other latest and greatest devices. Advanced nurses should make certain to visit vendors and keep current with new product opportunities. Vendors usually have business contact cards, flyers, white papers, and samples that can be brought back to the work setting for group consideration. Although some products and devices may initially appear cost prohibitive, careful analysis may reveal that new equipment could reduce expenditures related to high-ticket patient care concerns such as LOS, complications, nurse injuries, and patient safety enhancements.

Product Evaluation and Medical Device Competencies and Considerations

Malloch (2000) suggested that advanced nurses making purchasing decisions need three new competencies specific to product evaluation: end-user accountability, evidence-based product selection, and nursing commercial competence. End-user accountability relates to achieving specific results. Evidence-based product selection means that advanced nurses need to collect important end-user clinical information from staff members who preview the product or equipment. Nursing commercial competence is balancing clinical intent with economic impact. Malloch (2000) emphasized that advanced nurses need to consider the real value of different choices by analyzing alternatives and their consequences.

Advanced nurses and staff may be inclined to think of price as the most important purchase consideration. Certainly, given constrained resources, product and device costs are important considerations. Contino (2001) identified that there are two ways to consider costs when purchasing equipment. These include the payback period, defined as the number of years required to recover the original investment, or the internal rate of return, calculated to determine whether the generated revenue will cover the purchase cost. Advanced nurses should understand that there are other components affecting supply costs besides price, including but not limited to (1) environmental impacts such as disposability and recycling options, (2) technological congruity with other systems currently in use in the practice setting and expenses associated with connecting or revising, (3) options for communication with the electronic health record system, (4) satisfying regulation requirements including Health Insurance Portability and Accountability Act (HIPAA) and other privacy concerns, (5) infection control considerations, and (6) ease of repair, maintenance, and diagnostic surveillance options. Vendor reputation and supports should also be considered (Plonien & Donovan, 2015).

AORN updated guidelines for evaluating and selecting products used in perioperative settings in 2010 (Stanton, 2017). A newly renamed and updated AORN publication, *Guideline for Medical Device and Product Evaluation,* will be published in the *Guidelines for Perioperative Practice* in 2018, to provide evidence-based guidance to perioperative team members as they design and implement a process for evaluating U.S. Food and Drug Administration (FDA)–approved medical devices and products used in the perioperative care setting (Stanton, 2017). Advanced nurses should consider similar, evidence-based guidelines for other practice areas, or building on the efforts of the AORN, as a reasonable way to ensure consistency, fairness, and quality in decision making.

Opportunities for Staff Engagement

Nurses in advanced roles should consider establishing an interprofessional team for product selection and medical device evaluation processes. As an added bonus to the spirit of teamwork that may be generated by the collaboration, evaluation projects offer staff opportunities to learn the research process by devising small-scale studies that are practical and interesting. Pelter and Stephens (2008) designed an experimental study to compare first-attempt success rates, patient comfort, and insertion time between urinary catheterizations using a new device designed to facilitate urethral catheterization and catheterization procedures without the new device. Consenting patients were randomly assigned to one of the groups. The nurses conducting the urethral catheterization procedure also received informed consent. Two-tailed student t-tests and chi-square tests were used for statistical analysis. A small sample size limited the generalizability of the results; however, study findings did suggest that while the device had little influence on the dependent variables, findings indicated that nurses are challenged by urethral catheterization and some find that this is a difficult procedure to master.

This study (Pelter & Stephens, 2008) provides a simple but elegant example of an opportunity to engage staff in research while evaluating devices in the clinical setting. The basic setup of this particular project may be applied to a variety of product evaluation opportunities. For example, nurses could brainstorm outcomes or dependent variables of interest related to hygiene products, dressings, airway-securing devices, or any number of other devices, products, or systems and then use basic experimental or quasi-experimental designs to answer relevant questions. Research questions may relate to comparing different products as part of the purchase decision, determining whether a product is successfully addressing a particular clinical concern or looking at already established products to ascertain if implementation processes require improvement.

Opportunities Through Group Purchasing Arrangements

Plonien and Donovan (2015) comment that many agencies participate in group purchasing organization (GPO) agreements that provide cost savings through negotiation of large purchase orders. Such GPO arrangements also promote standardization. However, there are times when physicians have preferences for similar products that come from vendors other than those in the GPO. Physician product preferences are often distinct from product or device costs and these desires set the stage for conflict. Plonien and Donovan (2015) strongly advise including surgeons on intraprofessional purchasing committees. They also describe two methods to influence purchasing behaviors rather than using an autocratic approach. One method is the formulary model, where limits are placed on the variety of manufacturers and products. Another option is the payment-cap model, which uses price caps for particular item categories (Plonien & Donovan, 2015, p. 428).

Value Analysis

Products that do not add value to the practice environment should be avoided (Plonien & Donovan, 2015). To determine value, advanced nurses should incorporate evidence and performance improvement priorities. Efficient resource utilization is paramount and making certain that a new item has additive benefits to the unit or department's established arsenal of products and devices connects to performance improvement (Plonien & Donovan, 2015).

Theft Concerns

Over 25 years ago, Lyons (1992) reminded nurses that theft opportunities and preventions should be a consideration in product evaluation. Theft persists as a relevant concern that contributes to serious financial loss. Barlow (n.d.) comments that medical equipment may be sold online. Excluding embezzling and other crimes, small item theft is also a worry because it makes a difference to the bottom line. When providers, staff, patients, and families steal chargeable, consumable supplies, there is an associated cost. High-frequency pilfering involves many items that might be best included in room rates or some sort of per diem supply cost applied per patient day (**BOX 4-9**).

It may be wise for advanced nurses to consider the possibility of item attractiveness and thievery when considering products and devices. Some equipment requires chargeable housing that is not easily stolen. Other devices are simply not appealing to would-be thieves due to their limited practicality outside the health care setting. If a new product or device has a high theft appeal, advanced nurses may need to consider the additional expenses associated with storing the equipment or product and tracking its use.

BOX 4-9 Select Items Frequently Stolen from Hospitals

Items
Thermometers
Fans
Toilet paper
Telephones
Tissue
Linens
Gowns
Incontinence products
Baby towels
Office supplies
Baby formula
Bandages
Baby gowns and outfits
Scrubs
Towels
Bath blankets
Energy saver light bulbs
Baby blankets
Bed exit systems
Dopplers
Digital thermometers

Safety Concerns

Nurses in advanced roles should consider searching for reports of adverse events (AEs) involving medical devices as a step in product evaluation. The FDA maintains a publicly available medical device reporting Manufacturer and User Facility Device Experience (MAUDE) database (FDA, 2017a). MAUDE data consist of reports submitted by mandatory reporters, manufacturers, importers, and device user facilities, as well as reports from voluntary reporters such as health care professionals, patients, and consumers (FDA, 2017a).

The online database provides access to information on medical devices that may have malfunctioned or caused serious injury or death. MAUDE may be searched for reports that have been submitted over the previous 10 years. MAUDE is not intended to suggest cause-and-effect factors and it does not represent all known safety data for a particular device (FDA, 2017a).

Advanced nurses may not be aware of the rich data made available through the FDA's Center for Devices and Radiological Health (CDRH). This center provides information about regulatory decisions and associated rationales, descriptions of regulatory processes, and data to support CDRH activities. MAUDE is a CDRH database. There is also a recalls database, medical devise databases, and other searchable databases (FDA, 2017b). The available information has tremendous implications for advanced nurse practicing across all types of clinical and operational settings, regardless of specialty or population.

One study using the MAUDE database analyzed reports of da Vinci robotic surgical system instrument failures to analyze possible root causes of failures and trends that might be useful to know (Friedman, Lendvay, & Hannaford, 2013). Instrument failures (N = 565) were discerned via the reports and although there were likely other failures that were not reported, the retrieved data illustrated the importance of devising standard failure reporting policies in practice settings so that failure rates and device concerns can be improved. Advanced nurses should consider the implications of this database for practice improvements and policy development and include such information during device inservicing and education programs.

The What-If and More-Is-Better Syndromes of Materials Management

It is important to remember that there is usually more than one way to perform a procedure or more than one product to accomplish a job. The best product, defined in any number of ways, is not always needed. An average product may work just as well and may suit the needs of the organization quite satisfactorily. The problem is that advanced nurses may equate average with cheap. Lyons (1992) directs material managers to assist advanced nurses in understanding that quality can be defined as meeting the requirement or the need. Average products may be the better choice.

Lyons (1992) emphasizes that need must be separated from want. The *what-if* syndrome tends to encourage practitioners to think of every possible scenario, no matter how unlikely, and then to look for equipment or products that can address these unlikely situations (**EXEMPLAR 4-3**). This type of thinking drives up projected costs that may lead to rejection of the proposed capital budget expenditure.

EXEMPLAR 4-3 The *What-If Syndrome* of Product and Device Purchasing

Several medical intensive care unit (MICU) nurses attended a regional critical care conference. During the conference's trade show, the nurses came across a new automatic blood pressure cuff system. This system was very appealing for a number of reasons; in particular, it had a safety feature for cuff size and placement that the nurses believed would help to ensure the accuracy of MICU vital signs assessment.

The conference attendees brought information back to their colleagues. The nurses were enthusiastic about the product, as there had been recent problems with assessment inaccuracies related to incorrect cuff fit and placement that had compromised patient assessment data and potentially affected care. The nurses evaluated the project per the recommended checkpoints and concluded that the equipment should be submitted for review during the capital budget request period. As the nurses developed their proposal, they discussed the number of automatic cuffs that would be required on the unit. Some nurses believed that each room required this new system. Others were concerned that "extras" were required because equipment "always walks." Each estimated figure cost more due to the increasing numbers of requested cuffs. The advanced nurse was consulted for assistance with the capital budget request.

The advanced nurse began the consultation process by reviewing the nurses' rationale for requesting this particular blood pressure monitoring system. Other brands of automatic cuffs were available and were considerably less expensive. The advanced nurse asked the staff to identify the "typical" types of patients who required such sophisticated technology. The advanced nurse encouraged the staff to think in terms of "must have" rather than "nice to have." The nurses believed that patients with small upper arm circumferences and patients with above-average arm circumferences required these cuffs, in other words, patients who were outliers specific to arm circumference size. The advanced nurse worked with the staff to isolate the approximate number of MICU patients who met these criteria on an average shift. The nurses agreed that approximately two patients per shift were difficult to fit with the standard automatic blood pressure system, leading to accuracy concerns. After further guided discussion, the staff identified a simple strategy for confining the equipment on the unit to prevent loss. The nurses also developed guidelines for staff to consider when deciding whether to use manual, standard automatic, or specialized automatic blood pressure cuffs.

The staff decided to requisition the budget for two of the new, specialized automatic blood pressure cuffs. They realized that their opportunity for expenditure approval was better with a tight proposal that clearly avoided the "more-is-better" syndrome. Although there was no guarantee that the equipment request would be approved, the nurses felt confident that if the request was denied, it would be denied due to funding limitations or competing priorities rather than due to an unrealistic needs assessment.

The *more-is-better* syndrome encourages the belief that if one is good, two must be better (Lyons, 1992). Nurses in advanced roles must assist staff in identifying exactly what is needed in terms of the number of products or the frequency of equipment use. Determining an accurate measure of "need" is important for calculating direct and indirect costs. Need does not have to pertain to number of units. It may also apply to the features of technological products (**EXEMPLAR 4-4**).

EXEMPLAR 4-4 The *More-Is-Better Syndrome* of Product and Device Purchasing

The surgical trauma unit's nurses and physicians were interested in replacing the unit's cardiac monitors. The biomedical engineering department agreed that it was time to replace the aging system. The staff contacted several reputable vendors and began to explore monitor options.

As the group was introduced to increasingly sophisticated equipment options, the nurses and physicians began to acquire the *more-is-better* syndrome. They were surprised and impressed with the various technological advances and were amenable to the sales representatives' premise that their patients deserved the best. The monitors were capable of powerful analyses, and the data collection and alarming options were impressive. After a few months of investigation, the group began to think about fiscal and clinical practice realities and asked a critical care advanced nurse to offer an unbiased opinion.

The advanced nurse preliminarily collected historical data from the staff and physicians to explore the capabilities of the current monitoring system and to contrast these opportunities with the functions that were actually used on a regular basis. The interprofessional group was surprised to learn that the old monitoring system was not used to peak efficiency. Certain capabilities, including ST-segment monitoring and historical trending data, were rarely used for nursing assessment or medical management, despite the perceived importance of the functions. The advanced nurse emphasized to the group that if monitoring capabilities were identified in policies and procedures as essential to quality of care and a required part of routine assessment, the nurses and physicians were potentially inviting risk or compromising care by failing to follow the established protocols that they had developed!

The advanced nurse began the group process by meeting with the physicians and nurses to determine what monitoring functions were critical to patient care. The advanced nurse emphasized that unless equipment features are consistently used, they may become more of a care liability than benefit. Staff was asked to prioritize equipment functions. Physicians were involved in discussions specific to detailing the information that they really would use for patient care management. Nurse educators were asked to review the equipment options from the perspective of teaching and learning.

The advanced nurse compiled this information and developed a list of desired monitoring capabilities that would be valued and consistently utilized by nursing and medical staff. This list was reviewed by the prospective users and validated for accuracy. Vendors were asked to respond to this list. Equipment was selected based on the match between price and capabilities. This experience revealed to practitioners that more is not always better. There is no value in paying for equipment capabilities that are not desirable or are underutilized. Liabilities may increase if monitoring capabilities are available but not used by staff in the intended way. Educational needs should be considered as well. If orientation and in-service demands are too complex or rigorous, the likelihood of staff using the equipment correctly is reduced. The advanced nurse cautioned the group that neither more nor less is better. Rather, it is wisest to get exactly what is needed at an affordable price.

Nurses in advanced roles should be actively engaged in product and device identification, selection, and evaluation. Product and device possibilities should be considered methodically with a clear idea to the intent and need underlying the review process (**TABLE 4-4**). Deliberate review processes may be enhanced by using a product evaluation tool that can be used to solicit feedback from nurses and other involved health care professionals (**TABLE 4-5**).

TABLE 4-4 Product and Device Evaluation Checkpoints

Product/Device Consideration	Suggestions
1. Review and verify manufacturer claims for accuracy.	Advanced nurses should ensure that manufacturer claims are accurate. Products may not perform as promised during clinical use. Review the fine print of claims and make certain that these attestations are accurate when products are actually put to the test in clinical situations.
2. Compare available products or devices.	Advanced nurses should compare products during clinical use. Select a few competing products or devices and compare them.
3. Consider ease of use and maintenance.	Consider how easy the product or device is to use. This consideration includes ease of cleaning and storing.
4. Pay attention to ergonomics and product size and weight.	Advanced nurses should pay attention to the influence the product has on body mechanics. If a product requires repetitive movements, muscle straining, or periods of prolonged standing, solicit input from staff and other health care professionals as to the potential for injury, particularly given the aging nursing workforce.
5. Evaluate the complexity and readability of the manufacturer's product instructions.	Review the written instructions for clarity, readability, and accuracy. Advanced nurses should explore whether troubleshooting information is available in print and/or Web forms. It may be reasonable to ascertain whether a 24-hour contact is accessible for troubleshooting, particularly if a product or device is new to the setting.
6. Consider safety features and prioritize features that are absolutely essential.	Advanced nurses should encourage staff to think about what could go wrong and ways in which the device might be misused. It's important to make certain that critical safety features cannot be turned off. Some devices may have delay switches that reset after a period of time to avoid the need to deliberately reset safety features once discontinued.

(continues)

TABLE 4-4 Product and Device Evaluation Checkpoints *(continued)*

Product/Device Consideration	Suggestions
7. Estimate anticipated training costs.	Advanced nurses should calculate the training costs associated with assuring competent use of new devices and equipment. Some products are quite sophisticated and may require hours of training. Others may warrant competency assessments. Explore whether vendor-packaged training materials, including computer or Web-based instruction, are available.
8. Determine ease of repair.	Many devices and products are sophisticated by design and require experts for repairs or maintenance activities. If the institution cannot afford the cost of backup equipment or cannot justify the expense of developing in-house repair expertise, it may be difficult for staff to work without equipment when it malfunctions. Consider expenses associated with repair, replacement, and/or extended warranties.
9. Determine security issues.	Consider if this product or device requires protections from theft. Is this a product or device that is likely to be appealing to would-be thieves? Can the product be used outside of the health care facility? Is there a secondary market or home use for this item? If thievery is a concern, consider strategies for securing the product, restricting its access, or monitoring its use.
10. Determine environmental impact.	Advanced nurses should investigate the costs associated with cleaning or disposing of the product. Environmental impacts are important not only in terms of the chemicals or processes necessary for cleaning but also the biodegradability and bulk of items when no longer useful. Are parts recyclable?
11. Provide device safety reports.	Review MAUDE databases for information about reported safety concerns that may be relevant to the devices that are under consideration.

TABLE 4-5 Product/Device Evaluation Tool Example

Characteristic	Evaluation 1 = Unacceptable 2 = Poor 3 = Adequate 4 = Good 5 = Highly beneficial	Rank Importance of This Characteristic to the Purchase Decision 1–20	Comments: Follow-up Needs (with Assigned Responsibility)
1. Simplicity of use: • Size of print on buttons • Manipulability of equipment • Weight • Height (Does it fit in the patient room?) • Portability • Amount of space required for storage			
2. Instructions: • Readability of written instructions • Availability of additional instructional materials (e.g., DVD, laminated information cards, signs, computer-based instruction) • Vendor-provided education programs • Step-by-step guidelines for competency development			

(continues)

TABLE 4-5 Product/Device Evaluation Tool Example *(continued)*

Characteristic	Evaluation 1 = Unacceptable 2 = Poor 3 = Adequate 4 = Good 5 = Highly beneficial	Rank Importance of This Characteristic to the Purchase Decision 1–20	Comments: Follow-up Needs (with Assigned Responsibility)
3. Safety features: • Alarm featured • Battery life and indicators • Default settings • Most common errors and failures with related safeguards • Reset buttons • Expiration dates (on products) • Associated allergens • Risk to staff			
4. Amount of time needed to initially learn how to use the equipment: • Preliminary in-service time • Predicted frequency of use and impact on nurse competence • List of users and associated education needs			

5. Repair services:
   - In-house repair versus contracted repair
   - Guaranteed turnaround time for repairs
   - Replacement policy
   - Weekend/after business hours/holiday support
   - Repair expense
   - Availability of replacement parts

6. Shared dependency on other departments:
   - Components stored and managed off nursing unit?
   - Materials management training
   - Consistent coding and identification of parts between nursing and other departments
     - Distribution and clear designation of "who-does-what and when"
     - Off-hours responsibilities for each department

7. Ergonomics:
   - Repetitive motions
   - Impact on standing/sitting
   - Potential for staff injury

8. Required dexterity for safe use

(continues)

TABLE 4-5 Product/Device Evaluation Tool Example *(continued)*

Characteristic	Evaluation 1 = Unacceptable 2 = Poor 3 = Adequate 4 = Good 5 = Highly beneficial	Rank Importance of This Characteristic to the Purchase Decision 1–20	Comments: Follow-up Needs (with Assigned Responsibility)
9. Environmental impact: · Discard versus clean, sterilize · Recyclable, if discarded · Product ingredients · Efficiency of product packaging and impact on trash volume · Ozone discharge, air quality effects, scents, chemical usage · Is product manufactured in eco-friendly industry/packaging center?			
10. Expense: · Purchase cost · Maintenance cost · Miscellaneous cost			
11. Security: · Theft prevention · Tracking location · Physical security options (e.g., locks, mounting)			

(continues)

12.	Potential impact on patient care outcomes of concern					
13.	Patient perspective: · Alarm noise · Transportability for mobile patients · Patient safety					
14.	Impact of misuse: · Worst-case scenario when equipment fails · Opportunities for incorrect use					
15.	What patient care problems does this product fix?					
16.	Product capabilities that are useful in this clinical setting as compared to capabilities not useful/required					
17.	Gaps in processes within and/or between departments that this product may create					
18.	Gaps in processes within and/or between departments that this product may solve					
19.	Clinical and nonclinical stakeholders: · Who is potentially affected by this purchase decision?					

TABLE 4-5 Product/Device Evaluation Tool Example

(continued)

Characteristic	Evaluation 1 = Unacceptable 2 = Poor 3 = Adequate 4 = Good 5 = Highly beneficial	Rank Importance of This Characteristic to the Purchase Decision 1–20	Comments: Follow-up Needs (with Assigned Responsibility)
20. Time required from securing the product (start) to finishing with the product (end) (nursing time utilized by this product per usage)			
21. Technology: • Possibility of interference with existing systems in use? • Wireless connectivity? Automatic updates? • Integration with electronic health record or other computerized systems/software platforms?			
22. References or commentary from nonbiased users			

▶ Conclusion

Health care resources are limited, and advanced nurses are obliged to participate in activities that promote the highest quality of care using the dollars that are available. Understanding the budget process, engaging in conversations and data collection activities that inform the budget, teaching and coaching staff to develop a better sense of the fiscal realities of care, and contributing to capital budgets through product and device evaluations are responsibilities of nurses in advanced roles. Many teaching moments related to health care administration processes are experienced by advanced nurses as they work closely with nurses at the point of care. Having a good understanding of the business basics of nursing is an excellent way to contribute to the managerial functions of the institution, functions that are critical to the overall success of the organization.

References

Aiken, L. H., Clarke, S. P., Sloane, D. M., Sochalski, J., & Silber, J. H. (2002). Hospital nurse staffing and patient mortality, nurse burnout, and job dissatisfaction. *Journal of the American Medical Association, 288*, 1987–1993.

Aiken, L. H., Sloane, D. M., Bruyneel, L., Van den Heede, K., Griffiths, P., Busse, R., . . . Sermeus, W. (2014). Nurse staffing and education and hospital mortality in nine European countries: A retrospective observational study. *The Lancet, 383*, 1824–1830.

Aiken, L. H., Sloane, D., Griffiths, P., Rafferty, A. M., Bruyneel, L., McHugh, M., . . . Sermeus. W, RN4CAST Consortium. (2017). Nursing skill mix in European hospitals: Cross-sectional study of the association with mortality, patient ratings, and quality of care. *BMJ Quality & Safety, 26*, 559-568. Retrieved April 25, 2018, from http://qualitysafety.bmj.com/content/26/7/559

American Association of Critical Care Nurses. (2018). National Teaching Institute 2018. Exhibitor information. Retrieved January 6, 2018, from https://www.aacn.org/conferences-and-events/nti/exhibitors.

American Nurses Association. (2012). *Principles for nurse staffing* (2nd ed.). Retrieved January 6, 2017, from http://nursingworld.org/MainMenuCategories/ThePracticeofProfessionalNursing/Nursing Standards/ANAPrinciples/ANAsPrinciplesofNurseStaffing.pdf.

Barlow, R. D. (n.d.). Preventing theft a loss cause. Devices, dollars and supplies disappearances lead to dismal fiscal results. Retrieved January 6, 2018, from http://www.hcsbureau.com/articles-details.html?id=103.

Baseman, S., Boccuti, C., Moon, M., Griffin, S., & Dutta, T. (2016). *Payment and delivery system reform in Medicare: A primer on medical homes, accountable care organizations, and bundled payments.* Menlo Park, CA: Kaiser Family Foundation. Retrieved January 7, 2018, from http://files.kff.org/attachment/Report-Payment-and-Delivery-System-Reform-in-Medicare.pdf.

Berkowitz, D., Diamond, J., & Montagnolo, A. (1992). Maximizing purchase decision factors other than price. *Hospital Material Management Quarterly, 13*(4), 27–31.

Briscoe, B. (2015). Beyond the numbers. Understanding health plan types: What's in a name? Retrieved January 7, 2018, from https://www.bls.gov/opub/btn/volume-4/understanding_health_plan_types.htm.

Burtson, P. L., & Vento, L. (2015). Sitter reduction through mobile video monitoring: A nurse-driven sitter protocol and administrative oversight. *Journal of Nursing Administration, 45*(7/8), 363–369.

Campbell, T. (December 15, 2016). Which plans are cheaper: HMOs or PPOs? Retrieved January 7, 2018, from https://www.fool.com/investing/2016/12/15/which-plans-are- cheaper-hmos-or-ppos.aspx.

Centers for Medicare and Medicaid Services. (2013). CMS strategy: The road forward 2013-2017. January 7, 2018, from https://www.nadona.org/wp-content/uploads/2016/05/CMS-Strategy.pdf.

Centers for Medicare and Medicaid Services. (2014). Medicare program. General information. Retrieved October 4, 2017, from http://www.cms.hhs.gov/MedicareGenInfo/.

Centers for Medicare and Medicaid Services. (2015). National health expenditure projections 2016–2025. Retrieved January 7, 2018, from https://www.cms.gov/Research-Statistics-Data-and-Systems/Statistics-Trends-and-Reports/NationalHealthExpendData/Downloads/proj2016.pdf

Centers for Medicare and Medicaid Services. (2017a). Accountable care organizations. Retrieved October 20, 2017, from https://www.cms.gov/Medicare/Medicare-Fee-for-Service-Payment/ACO/.

Centers for Medicare and Medicaid Services. (2017b). Hospital value-based purchasing. Retrieved January 7, 2018, from https://www.cms.gov/Outreach-and-Education/Medicare-Learning -Network-MLN/MLNProducts/downloads/Hospital_VBPurchasing_Fact_Sheet_ICN907664.pdf

Contino, D. (2001). Proposing the "capital" in capital budgets. *Nursing Management, 32*, 10, 13.

Cubanski, J., Swoope, C., Boccuti, C., Jacobson, G., Casillas, G., Griffin, S., & Neuman, T., Kaiser Family Foundation's Program on Medicare Policy. (2015). A primer on Medicare: Key facts about the Medicare program and the people it covers. Retrieved January 7, 2018, from http://files.kff.org/attachment /report-a-primer-on-medicare-key-facts-about-the-medicare-program-and-the-people-it-covers.

Friedman, D. C., Lendvay, T. S., & Hannaford, B. (2013). Instrument failures for the da Vinci Surgical System: A Food and Drug Administration MAUDE Database study. *Surgical Endoscopy, 27*, 1503–1508. doi:10.1007/s00464-012-2659-8

Frith, K., Anderson, E., Tseng, F., & Fong, E. (2012). Nurse staffing is an important strategy to prevent medication errors in community hospitals. *Nursing Economics, 30*(5), 288–294.

Hain, D., & Fleck, L. (2014). Barriers to nurse practitioner practice that impact healthcare redesign. *OJIN: The Online Journal of Issues in Nursing, 19*(2).

Halvorson, C., & Chinnes, L. (2007). Collaborative leadership in product evaluation. *AORN Journal, 85*(2), 334–352.

Kaiser Family Foundation. (2010). Family health premiums rise 3 percent to $13,770 in 2010, but workers' share jumps 14 percent as firms shift cost burden. Retrieved January 7, 2018, from https://www.kff.org/health-costs/press-release/family-health-premiums-rise-3-percent-to-13770 -in-2010-but-workers-share-jumps-14-percent-as-firms-shift-cost-burden/

Kaiser Family Foundation. (2017). Medicaid pocket primer. Retrieved October 10, 2017, from https:// www.kff.org/medicaid/fact-sheet/medicaid-pocket-primer/.

Kindig, D., & Stoddart, G. (2003). What is population health? *American Journal of Public Health, 93*(3), 380–383.

Lyons, D. (1992). Making the purchase decision: Factors other than price. *Hospital Materiel Management Quarterly, 13*(4), 55–62.

Malloch, K. (2000). Purchasing pointers. Wise buys. *Nursing Management, 31*(5), 30.

Pelter, M., & Stephens, K. (2008). Evaluation of a device to facilitate female urethral catheterization. *Medical-Surgical Nursing, 17*, 19–25.

Plonien, C., & Donovan, L. (2015). Continuing education. OR leadership: Product evaluation and cost containment. *AORN Journal, 102*, 426–432. http://dx.doi.org/10.1016/j.aorn.2015.07.007

Shekelle, P. G. (2013). Nurse patient ratios as a patient safety strategy: A systematic review. *Annals of Internal Medicine, 158*, 404–409. Retrieved January 7, 2018, from http://annals.org/aim /fullarticle/1656445/nurse-patient-ratios-patient-safety-strategy- systematic-review.

Shi, L., & Singh, D. (2015). *Essentials of the U.S. health care system* (4th ed). Burlington, MA: Jones and Bartlett Learning.

Stanton, C. (2017). Guideline first look. Guideline for medical device and product evaluation. *Periop Briefing, 106*(5), 7–9. http://dx.doi.org/10.1016/S0001-2092(17)30955-9.

U.S. Food and Drug Administration. (2017a). MAUDE. Manufacturer and user facility device experience. Retrieved January 6, 2018, from https://www.accessdata.fda.gov/scripts/cdrh/cfdocs/cfMAUDE /search.CFM

U.S. Food and Drug Administration. (2017b). CDRH transparency. Retrieved January 6, 2018, from https://www.fda.gov/aboutfda/centersoffices/officeofmedicalproductsandtobacco/cdrh /cdrhtransparency/default.htm

Yee, T., Boukus, E., Cross, D., & Samuel, D. (2013). Primary care workforce shortages: Nurse practitioner scope-of-practice laws and payment policies. National Institute for Health Care Reform (NIHCR) Research Brief No. 13. Retrieved January 7, 2018, from http://nihcr.org/analysis /improving-care-delivery/prevention-improving-health/pcp-workforce-nps/

Zuzelo, P., Fallon, R., Lang, A., Lang, C., McGovern, K., . . . Mount, L. (2004). Clinical nurse specialists' knowledge specific to Medicare structures and processes. *Clinical Nurse Specialist, 18*, 207–217.

CHAPTER 5

Confronting Workplace Violence: Creating and Sustaining a Healthy Place to Work

Patti Rager Zuzelo, EdD, RN, ACNS-BC, ANP-BC, CRNP, FAAN

A healthy work environment is essential for quality patient care. Environments that are highly stressed, morally uninhabitable (Peter, Macfarlane, & O'Brien-Pallas, 2004), demoralizing, and abusive are associated with high registered nurse (RN) turnover rates (Hayes et al., 2006; Way & MacNeil, 2006) and an increased number of errors (American Association of Critical-Care Nurses [AACN], 2016). Many factors encourage a sick organizational dynamic. These factors include but are not limited to opportunities and triggers for both physical and verbal assaults, heavy workloads with long hours, power differentials, and poor, ineffective work relationships.

Advanced nurses have opportunities to positively influence these concerns by working to reduce opportunities for workplace violence (WPV) of all types, establishing positive communication processes, developing interprofessional communication opportunities, and enhancing efforts to address workload concerns. Nurses in advanced roles need to contribute to WPV reduction efforts by collecting data that can be used to determine whether policies, procedures, and planned interventions designed to reduce WPV are effective. They also need to consider both research and evidence-based practice initiatives to counter the gamut of violence in all its forms. This chapter offers information, strategies, and resource suggestions that will be useful to nurse leaders working toward healthy work environments through creative and comprehensive violence-reduction strategies.

▶ Workplace Violence

As society becomes more violent, WPV, also known as occupational violence (Shea, Sheehan, Donohue, Cooper, & De Cieri, 2017), becomes more commonplace. Workplace shootings accounted for 405 fatal injuries in 2010 and comprised 78% of all workplace homicides (Bureau of Labor Statistics [BLS], 2015). WPV is recognized as an occupational hazard for health care providers, including nurses. BLS compiles data concerning workforce statistics and organizes these data by occupational sectors and supersectors. The Health Care and Social Assistance sector, comprised by establishments that provide health care and social assistance for individuals (BLS, 2017a), is included in the education and health services supersector (BLS, 2017a).

BLS tracks work-related fatalities, injuries, and illnesses and defines "work-related" as when a work environment event or exposure caused or contributed to the resulting condition or significantly worsened a preexisting condition (BLS, 2017b). There were 123 work-related fatalities attributed to the health care and social assistance sector in 2015; a fairly consistent number over 4 years of data collection and ranging from 121 to 123 fatalities (BLS, 2017b). Nonfatal occupational injuries and illnesses resulting from violence and other injuries caused by persons or animals for those working in health care and social assistance roles in private, state, and local government totaled 14 events (BLS, 2016a). The victims of nonfatal WPV in 2014 were predominately female (67%) and approximately two-thirds worked in the health care and social service industry. Nearly one-quarter of victims needed 31 days or more of recovery time away from work while 20% required 3–5 days of work release time (National Institute for Occupational Safety and Health [NIOSH], 2017a).

In response to the impact of WPV on health care and social services employees, several labor unions, AFL-CIO, American Federation of Teachers, Communications Workers of America, International Brotherhood of Teamsters, Service Employees International Union, and United Steelworkers petitioned the Secretary of Labor with the claim that the Occupational Safety and Health Administration (OSHA) efforts to protect these health and social services workers are inadequate and the unions used BLS data to support their position. Subsequent to this petition, National Nurses United sent a separate petition. Both petitions included proposals for training programs, record keeping, and a prevention plan (Safety + Health, 2016).

ECRI Institute, formerly known as the Emergency Care Research Institute, is a nonprofit organization focused on applying scientific research to improve patient care outcomes (ECRI, 2017a). This organization, as well as others, makes the case that violent events are underreported in the health care setting (ECRI, 2017b). Given that nurses, in particular, underreport for many reasons including the belief that violence is an expected part of nurses' work and a fear of retaliation, sobering BLS data and NIOSH reports present advanced nurses with an open challenge to create evidence-based strategies to eliminate WPV and ensure that nurses have a safe place within which to provide excellent care.

The violence problem is serious and insidious yet remains inconsistently regulated. Some states require employers to administer WPV programs, including California, Connecticut, Illinois, Minnesota, New Jersey, and Oregon. New York requires public employers to run such programs. Washington does not require WPV programs but does require WPV incident reporting (American Nurses Association [ANA], 2017a). Approximately 42 states have regulations providing penalties for assault charges and specifically including nurses in the language of the law. There are some states that have setting-specific regulations related to violence against personnel; settings include emergency departments (EDs), mental health/psychiatric facilities, or public health.

Contributing to the legal morass are laws that approach WPV in health care from a different perspective. In addition to penalizing those who assault nurses, Ohio authorizes hospitals to post warnings about violent behaviors; Hawaii passed a resolution encouraging employers to develop and implement conduct standards and policies to reduce workplace bullying (ANA, 2017a). Trotto (2014) points out that this state-level push is directed toward reducing violence risk for those working in the health care professions. These laws are often modifications of existing codes to include nurses and/or first responders designed to charge perpetrators of violence with felonies in response to assaulting or committing battery against designated personnel.

The ANA (2017b) provides a model bill for states, entitled "The Violence Prevention in Health Care Facilities Act." This bill is developed in recommended language that includes background facts that lend support to the need for such a bill. One critical point is the assertion that it is realistic to decrease and allay the impact of violence (ANA, 2017b). The model bill provides definitions of covered health care facility, health care worker, and violence or violent act. Recommended provisions include the establishment of a violence prevention program and a violence prevention committee that include nurses with direct care responsibilities. Other committee members need to have some sort of expertise or experience in violence prevention. The model bill charges covered health care facilities with responsibility for education, training, record keeping, and establishing a postincident response system. The proposed bill asserts that the covered agency shall not retaliate against any health care worker for reporting occasions of violence (ANA, 2017b).

Compounding the contextual complexities of violence in health care, WPV is inconsistently defined, and differences between violence and aggression are not established (Rippon, 2000); and there is a dearth of intervention studies (McPhaul & Lipscomb, 2004) examining the effectiveness of implemented programs, policies, and procedures designed to reduce the incidence or severity of violent behaviors. Some scholars suggest that the conceptualization of WPV needs to be reconsidered to a more holistic and comprehensive conceptualization that does not rely on the notion of a paid workplace (Van De Griend & Messias, 2014). A concern with a narrow WPV understanding that connects work to income is that this perspective excludes consideration of the many types of unpaid work that women perform. The violence that occurs in these unpaid situations is certainly experienced within a *work* context.

Van De Griend and Messias (2014) assert that the current definition is andocentric and excludes much of the work that women do in places that are not formal workplaces. This is an important concern that warrants attention and consideration, particularly given the nursing profession's undeniable connection to traditionally labeled "women's work"; however, for purposes of this chapter and its particular attention on the paid health care setting environment, WPV will be traditionally considered while still noting that there is much work to be done within the broader context of violent events or risk of violence in places in which work of any sort is done.

The health care culture is resistant to recognizing that nurses are at risk and demonstrates complacency related to accepting the idea that violence is simply part of the job of nursing. Despite the increasing attention paid by health care professionals to the topic and experience of violence, there is little evidence that systems of care are successfully intervening to reduce occasions of violence and to assure nurses that they are safe at work. There is a good bit of published literature examining the stories of violence and sharing the details of WPV and its intended and unintended consequences but not the necessary science aimed to fix the problem.

Advanced nurses are uniquely positioned to address all types of WPV and to promote healthy work environments. There is a broad spectrum of violent behaviors in health care, including violence directed horizontally or vertically between health care providers or violence focused on nurses from patients, families, and visitors. Bullying behaviors, including between students and nurse educators and between new and established employees also require remedy. Cyberbullying is increasingly problematic and can be quite damaging to the individuals against whom the attacks are directed. Advanced nurses need to also consider opportunities for eliminating social media bullying, including threatening, uncivil email correspondence.

Background Information

The NIOSH is a research agency of the Centers for Disease Control and Prevention (CDC) in the U.S. Department of Health and Human Services (DHHS) (NIOSH, 2016). Its mandate is to "develop new knowledge in the field of occupational safety and health and to transfer that knowledge into practice" (NIOSH, 2018). It is easy to confuse NIOSH with OSHA (Occupational Safety and Health Administration), but they are different. OSHA is a regulatory agency in the U.S. Department of Labor that is responsible for ensuring the safety and health of American workers.

NIOSH and OSHA are excellent government resources for advanced nurses intrigued by the science of WPV and interested in possible risk-reduction strategies. Both agencies host websites that offer continuing education opportunities; multimedia resources; and other downloadable materials, including scientific reports. A particularly good resource is the online course for nurses addressing WPV offered by NIOSH (2017b) (https://www.cdc.gov/niosh/docs/2017-114/). Since NIOSH and OSHA are government agencies, materials are free and permissions for use are not required.

Definitions of Workplace Violence

There are many definitions of WPV and varying types of violence ranging from offensive language to homicide. WPV may also be referred to by its synonym, occupational violence. NIOSH (2017c) defines WPV as "the act or threat of violence, ranging from verbal abuse to physical assaults directed toward persons at work or on duty" WPV includes any act or threat of physical violence, harassment, intimidation, or other threatening behavior occurring at the workplace (OSHA, n.d.[a]) and psychological violence, abuse, mobbing or bullying, racial harassment, and sexual harassment. Cyber-based or Web-based bullying related to work encounters or relationships is another form of WPV.

Advanced nurses need to keep in mind that although bullying and uncivil behaviors are often acknowledged in nursing literature as forms of violence, these potentially damaging behaviors are not tracked as data indicators of WPV. Although bullying, harassment, and incivility do affect retention, patient safety, and professional engagement and may escalate to episodic or sustained injury that leads to missed days of work or other measurable outcomes, these behaviors are not included in WPV datasets and may be best remedied using different strategies and interventions than those used to reduce occupational violence associated with assault and/or fatalities.

The Pervasiveness of Violence: Who Is Hurt?

The U.S. Department of Justice delivered a 2011 report on WPV that compiled and examined data from 1993 to 2009. This report included data from the National Crime Victimization Survey (NCVS) and the BLS Census of Fatal Occupational Injuries (Harrell, 2011). Key points of this summary analysis include the following: (1) Law enforcement employees experienced the highest proportion of WPV followed by those in retail sales, but approximately 10% of WPV victims worked in medical occupations. The rate of WPV per 1,000 employed nurses from 2005 to 2009 was 8.1; physicians' rate was 10.1 and the rate for professionals working in mental health was 17 per 1,000 employees. (2) The percentage of WPV experienced in the total medical occupation category from 2005 to 2009 was 10.2% and the percentage for the total mental health occupation category, including professional, custodial care, and others, was 3.9%. (3) From 2005 through 2009, strangers committed the greatest proportion of WPV acts with approximately 53% of events against males and 41% against females. The proportions of males and females were roughly the same when examining victims of intimate partner violence in the workplace. (4) Current or former coworkers committed 16% of WPV against males and approximately 14% against females. Of note, patients were more likely to direct violence in the workplace against females than males (Harrell, 2011).

One particularly interesting finding revealed by the data analysis was the relationship of alcohol or drugs to WPV. Nurses often attribute violence in the ED to the influence of alcohol or drugs; however, approximately 40% of WPV did not involve an offender under the influence of alcohol or drugs as compared to 22% of nonworkplace-related violence. The report also noted that drug/alcohol use of about 36% of the offenders in WPV events and 41% in non–WPV events were not known (Harrell, 2011).

Violent behaviors include interactions that occur between coworkers, supervisors, patients, families, visitors, and others (McPhaul & Lipscomb, 2004). Research findings suggest that nonphysical violence is highly associated with physical violence and should be seriously addressed as part of comprehensive WPV prevention plans (Lanza, Zeiss, & Rierdan, 2006).

An Organizing Framework for WPV: Violence Typologies

Established typologies are helpful organizing frameworks and provide a context for developing interventions and researching the effectiveness of these interventions. Capozzoli and McVey (1996) developed a typology over two decades ago that organizes occasions of violence based on where it originates and where it occurs. This WPV categorization describes three types:

Type 1: Violence originates in the workplace and occurs in the workplace.

Type 2: Violence originates in the workplace and occurs outside the workplace.

Type 3: Violence originates outside the workplace but occurs in the workplace.

An example of Type 1 violence is when a hospital worker perceives that he or she has been victimized by an arbitrary evaluation that has led to a suspension. The employee comes to the work setting looking for retribution and directs this hostility toward the manager or to anyone else in the hospital. Type 2 violence is exemplified by the nurse who has a disagreement with the nightshift charge nurse. The nurse learns the charge nurse's home address and spray-paints his automobile. Property destruction is considered a violent act, although many people might first think of murder or physical assault as examples for this type of violence. Type 3 violence may be illustrated by the shooting death of a nurse in the parking lot of the hospital by an estranged spouse.

Capozzoli and McVey's (1996) violence typology differs in structure from the categorization offered by the Federal Bureau of Investigation (FBI) National Center for the Analysis of Violent Crime (NCAVC), Critical Incidence Response Group (CIRG). The FBI taxonomy identifies four broad categories of WPV that focus on perpetrator and victim characteristics within the broad context of the workplace (Rugala, Isaacs, & NCAVC, 2003). The FBI typology is used by NIOSH (2006) (**TABLE 5-1**).

TABLE 5-1   FBI Violence Typology with Nursing Practice Examples

Violence Type	FBI Definition (Rugala et al., 2003)	Exemplar
Type 1 (criminal intent)	Violent acts by criminals who have no other connection with the workplace, but enter to commit robbery or another crime.	Nurses working in the intensive care unit return to their locker room at the conclusion of their shift to find that the lockers have been forcibly opened. Credit cards, cash, and electronic devices have been stolen. Hospital security and police suspect that outside thieves entered the facility pretending to be visitors.
Type 2 (customer/client)	Violence directed at employees by customers, clients, patients, students, inmates, or any others for whom an organization provides services.	An emergency department nurse is pushed by an angry family member because of a delay in receiving laboratory results.
Type 3 (worker-on-worker)	Violence against coworkers, supervisors, or managers by a present or former employee.	A nursing assistant (NA) is suspended from work as a result of a serious and witnessed patient care incident that compromised safety. The NA waited in the parking lot until the nurse witness finished the shift and accosted the nurse.
Type 4 (personal relationship)	Violence committed in the workplace by someone who doesn't work there, but has a personal relationship with an employee—an abusive spouse or domestic partner.	A physician's spouse enters the patient care unit to confront the physician about domestic issues. The discussion escalates into verbal abuse and threats of physical battery.

Data from Rugala, E. A., & Isaacs, A. R. (Eds.). (2003).

Violence Resulting from Criminal Intent (Type 1)

Type 1 (criminal intent) violence preventive strategies include physical security measures including bright lighting, alarms, lock placements, cameras, and equipment designed to reduce outside accessibility (Rugala et al., 2003). These strategies are unique to this type of violence because the perpetrator has no connection to the workplace unlike the other violence categories. Type I violence accounts for about 80% of workplace homicides often because the criminal is carrying a weapon. For the most part, this type of violence is directly related to vulnerabilities associated with job characteristics (e.g., taxi drivers or late-night retail clerks). Victims often work in isolation and, sometimes, in dangerous locations. Accessibility to cash amplifies the risks (Rugala et al., 2003).

While nurses are not often working in these sorts of circumstances, they do conclude shifts at times of night and early morning that may contribute to lonely walks to parking garages or to public transportation sites. Health care employees also are often required to go to isolated areas of hospital facilities by themselves to complete certain tasks or retrieve necessary care-related items. Nurses and other health professionals work in increasingly diverse types of health care facilities and each work setting and its associated environment likely has its own opportunities for criminally motivated violence.

High Frequency Categories of Nurse-Targeted WPV

The majority of threats and assaults against care providers come from patients, families, and visitors (McPhaul & Lipscomb, 2004; NIOSH, 2006; Rugala et al., 2003) and are reflective of Type 2 WPV. This is a particularly high-frequency category of WPV as related to health care provision, particularly in settings recognized as risky for occasions of violence. Nursing home settings, psychiatric/behavioral health facilities, and EDs provide opportunities for close contact with patients and families under circumstances that can be stressful and fast paced for all concerned. Additionally, care demands are often high and patient/family expectations may be unmet contributing to a pressure-cooker environment that may trigger violent interactions.

Types 3 and 4 violence may have associated clues or warning signs prior to an act of WPV. Observed behaviors that evoke an intervention, even if this response is in the form of reporting the concerning comportment or action, are welcome and should be encouraged by advanced nurses. With warning, preventive measures can be taken prior to escalated aggression including assault, battery, or homicide.

Although the Capozzoli and McVey (1996) and FBI (Rugala et al., 2003) typologies differ, both are useful to law enforcement, policymakers, and advanced nurses and administrators because they organize a complex phenomenon, WPV, into manageable and meaningful categories. Categorization facilitates pattern recognition when attempting to research the effectiveness of interventions based on type of violence. The typologies offer opportunities for considering a variety of preventive strategies that may target different aspects of WPV. These approaches potentially work synergistically to protect nurses and other employees and providers practicing in diverse health care settings.

Legal and Regulatory Requirements—Healthy and Safe Work Environments

Employers are legally and morally obliged to promote a safe work environment that is free from violence in all its forms. Advanced nurses need to be well aware that hospital employment is hazardous work that requires a robust arsenal of preventive strategies to create a healthy and secure work environment. OSHA (n.d.[b]) has regulated through Section 5(a)(1) of the Occupational Safety and Health Act of 1970 (OSH Act of 1970) that employers have a duty to provide each worker both "employment and a place of employment which are free from recognized hazards that are causing or likely to cause death or serious physical harm" to the employees (OSH Act of 1970, Sec. 5. Duties). There are also OSHA-approved state plans that are supplemental to the federal OSHA program. Twenty-six states, Puerto Rico, and the U.S. Virgin Islands have these plans in place. There are also nine states that require certain types of health care facilities to have WPV prevention programs in place. Enforcing these state regulations is the responsibility of state-designated authorities rather than OSHA. The OSH Act, Section 11(c), also provides protections to employees who exercise the rights granted to them under the act (OSHA, n.d.[b]). These protected rights fall under the domain of the Whistleblower Protection Programs (OSHA, 2017).

In addition to federal regulations as enforced by OSHA, The Joint Commission (TJC), an independent accreditation body for health care organizations, has responded to WPV concerns in health care settings given the adverse impact that violence, including bullying, has on patient care outcomes. TJC issued a directive in 2009 that mandated a hospital response to disruptive behaviors perpetrated by employees, including physicians (Johnson, Boutain, Tsai, & de Castro, 2015). TJC has since crafted several standards related to WPV. These standards relate to a variety of organizational types including hospitals, nursing homes, behavioral health facilities, and others. Standards relevant to WPV include Environment of Care, Emergency Management, Leadership, and Performance Improvement. Much of the systemwide focus on WPV reduction includes partnership between patient safety and worker safety programs within the context of a culture of safety that includes high reliability principles and a just culture (OSHA, n.d.[c]).

TJC offers a variety of reports that provide executive-style summaries of timely concerns while offering insights, recommendations, and resources to those advanced nurses who are seeking guidance in the select subject domain. One example is an edition of *Quick Safety: An Advisory on Safety and Quality Issues* that addresses WPV and provides an overview of prevention strategies to reduce WPV risk factors. Resources with hyperlinks are provided and these resources include a variety of cutting-edge agencies including CDC and the National Research and Training Center (TJC, Division of Health Care Improvement, 2014). Nurses in advanced roles may find these briefs useful as staff education tools while also having utility for guiding working groups focused on violence reduction.

Causative Factors of Violence

Approximately one-third of violent events in the general public are caused by personality conflicts and related stressors (Capozzoli & McVey, 1996). Published literature supports that the health care sector experiences violent behaviors across all types of settings (NIOSH, 2002a; Trossman, 2006) but most frequently from patients, visitors, and patients' family members in EDs and psychiatric facilities (Edward, Ousey, Warelow, & Lui, 2014; McPhaul & Lipscomb, 2004; NIOSH, 2002b; Shea et al., 2017). Health care workers are frequently assaulted by patients, particularly those with dementia or schizophrenia (Denenberg & Braverman, 1999; McGill, 2006).

Ascertaining an accurate count of the frequency and types of violent incidences in health care settings on a national level is not currently possible, as there is no database or mandatory reporting mechanism in place. However, the number of states requiring WPV reports from hospitals is increasing. One such example is the California Division of Occupational Safety and Health (Cal/OSHA) mandatory WPV reporting system. This statewide online reporting program pertains to general acute care hospitals, psychiatric hospitals, and special hospitals and follows requirements of Senate Bill 1299 including a public report issued annually by January detailing the total number of reported incidents, names of reporting hospital facilities, outcomes of related investigations, any citations issued against a hospital, and a plan for violence prevention (Cal/OSHA, 2017). Not too many years ago, hospitals rarely volunteered information about the occasions of violence occurring in their facilities; rather, violence was considered the cost of doing business (Love & Morrison, 2003). Reporting programs provide an optimistic opportunity to collect and use real data to create effective violence-reduction programs.

Although the circumstances and context of WPV varies, it is not uncommon for health care workers to unintentionally aggravate stressful situations (Duxbury & Whittington, 2005; Hollinworth, Clark, Harland, Johnson, & Partington, 2005). When work environments are stressed and highly charged, nurses, physicians, or other health care workers may escalate aggressive behaviors by responding rudely, callously, or impatiently to patients, families, or coworkers. Duxbury and Whittington (2005) found that patients from inpatient mental health units perceived poor communication to be a significant precursor to aggressive behaviors.

Findings from a study that explored nurses and behavioral health associates' (BHAs) responses to violent inpatient interactions that occurred on a behavior health unit suggest that nurses and care associates recognized that there are often opportunities for improving communication and for enhancing professional behaviors (Zuzelo, Curran, & Zeserman, 2012). Findings revealed that behavioral health unit nursing staff appreciated the value of empathy and de-escalation techniques but also acknowledged that dealing with the emotional and physical aftermath of violence directed at them from patients is difficult. They described that feeling violated, angry, and scared are common reactions that affect the nurse-patient dynamic during future encounters, particularly if the interaction feels risky (Zuzelo et al., 2012). These sorts of patient care encounters support that one of the most common types of WPV occurs when the verbalization or behavior of another employee, a patient, or a visitor is perceived as threatening (Clements, DeRanieri, Clark, Manno, & Kuhn, 2005; Edward et al., 2014).

Nurses interact with patients or family members who are under the influence of drugs or alcohol and these interactions require a level of finesse and communication expertise that may be in short supply when staffing levels are inadequate and staff is fatigued. Significant and chronic staff shortages, high acuities, and more violence-prone patients, including elders with dementia and patients with substance abuse or metabolic issues, increase the likelihood of violent encounters (McPhaul & Lipscomb, 2004).

Besides personality conflicts, violence perpetrated by employees is often related to a threat to job, threat to person, and extended working hours (Capozzoli & McVey, 1996). Job threats trigger employee worries about meeting basic needs for survival. Many employees live check by check without the means to afford housing, food, or family expenses during a period of unemployment. Although most people solve their needs using socially acceptable methods, when an employee believes that these acceptable methods are ineffective, he or she may resort to unacceptable tactics. Even people who are usually balanced and reasonable may reach a breaking point (Capozzoli & McVey, 1996).

When employees perceive that they have been victims of unfair or capricious treatment, they may respond violently. Capozzoli and McVey (1996) noted that in most cases of employee or ex-employee violence, the event was preceded by an event or sequential events in which the individual perceived that he or she was treated unfairly by superiors. Extended working hours can also be stressful and may trigger helplessness. If other employees do not mind the extra hours, the stressed employee may also feel isolated and ostracized, worsening the potential for violent behavior (Capozzoli & McVey, 1996).

Conceptual Frameworks for Understanding Violence

Conceptual frameworks have been developed to explain the theoretical underpinnings of WPV and each theory offers a different way to consider the WPV phenomenon. The Haddon Matrix, developed by William Haddon, Jr. (1968), approximately five decades ago, connects public health domains to WPV (Runyan, 1998; Safety Lit, n.d.). The matrix includes such factors as host, agent, disease, and phases; and primary, secondary, and tertiary to explore and assess the many factors associated with injuries and their severities (Safety Lit, n.d.). The host is the victim, whereas the agent or vehicle is a combination of the perpetrator, weapon, and force of the assault. The environment is split into the physical and social environment. The matrix is a tool that is useful when selecting strategies for injury prevention measures.

The matrix is constructed with four columns and three rows combining the concepts of pre-event, event, and post-event phases (rows) to the factors (columns). The factors, host, agent/vehicle, physical environment, and social environment interact with each other. Injuries are usually the result of sequential events rather than a discrete moment in time (Runyan, 1998; Safety Lit, n.d.).

A helpful example of the Haddon Matrix is when a patient fall is the culmination of a pain experience requiring narcotic analgesia with a call bell out of reach and side rails in the up position. The patient, or host, may have urinary urgency and impulsivity concerns related to a previous stroke. The floor may be slippery, and the patient may be barefoot. The patient's room may be situated far from the nurses' station. In addition, other patients' family members may have heard the patient yell for help prior to climbing out of bed and falling but did not know how to alert staff and were uncomfortable going into the patient's room. These factors, if more fully developed on a Haddon Matrix, would provide insight into interventions that would fit into each cell, thereby generating a variety of strategies for addressing this particular problem.

A second theory, the Broken Windows Theory (Kelling & Wilson, 1982), is a popular criminal justice theory that has had significant influence on law enforcement and local activism (McPhaul & Lipscomb, 2004) and may have applicability to medical environments (Zhou et al., 2017). The theory asserts that when low-level crime is tolerated or ignored, the environment becomes increasingly conducive to more serious crime. In other words, environments with broken windows, stripped vehicles, and graffiti-clad buildings will have more serious crime than a neighborhood with clean walls, well-maintained yards, and no visible debris or destruction.

Advanced nurses need to know that there has been some controversy surrounding police programs purportedly based on the Broken Windows Theory and its presumed connection to high-arrest programs. In 2015, Kelling defended the theory and asserted that it was being used in ways contrary to its meaning. Kelling reinforced that the theory is about reducing the level of disorder in public spaces.

The Broken Windows Theory may not be uniquely relevant to health care, but perhaps it offers insight into the possible influence of environment on patient and family behaviors. For example, a dirty, trash-strewn waiting room area without windows and no magazines or toys may be more highly associated with hostility as compared to a waiting area that is clean, fresh-smelling, with a television, current magazines, newspapers, and various comfort supplies. This example is hypothetical but does have commonsense appeal.

Another example of the relevance of the Broken Windows Theory is offered by Zhou et al. (2017) in their examination of factors that contributed to hospital WPV as informed by hospital administrators and patients. Zhou et al. postulated that the medical environment consists of a hardware environment and a social environment and suggested that recognizing a **first** broken window can be an opportunity for administrators to respond and repair the broken entity so that an orderly environment is restored. The purpose of the study was to use the theory to reduce opportunities for violence by establishing strategies to eliminate hospital WPV triggers that corresponded to six factors: medical staff, patient-related, hospital environment, policy and institutional, social psychological, and objective events (Zhou et al., 2017). Study methods and findings offer interesting use of the Broken Windows Theory and point out opportunities to frame WPV within a theoretical construct that offers advanced nurses intriguing possibilities for viewing WPV through a unique lens.

Injury epidemiology, occupational psychology, and criminal justice offer strategies for understanding generalized society violence and more circumscribed occasions of violence, including those occurring in health care settings. An additional perspective described in nursing literature relates to violence as a response to oppression (Hedin, 1986; Hutchinson, Vickers, Jackson, & Wilkes, 2005; Roberts, 1983, 2000, 2015). Horizontal WPV, lateral violence, or bullying is a significant concern in nursing, although it is not a phenomenon unique to the nursing profession (Hutchinson, Vickers, Jackson, & Wilkes, 2006). It has been suggested that bullying requires examination beyond the confines of oppressed group behavior theory to include broader environmental and organizational perspectives (Hutchinson et al., 2006; Hutchinson, Wilkes, Vickers, & Jackson, 2008). Roberts (2015) suggests that purposeful leadership and nursing empowerment are two essential components to bullying reduction efforts. These efforts need to include resources available to encourage culture shifts and intervening to influence the power dynamics that contribute to lateral violence (Roberts, 2015).

Setting the Stage for Understanding Hospital Violence

"WPV is one of the most complex and dangerous occupational hazards facing nurses working in today's healthcare environment" (McPhaul & Lipscomb, 2004, p. 1). This danger reflects the risk of violent behavior victimization within society at large but may also be related to hesitancy and uncertainty within the health care system. Hospitals are concerned with patient satisfaction and recognize that health care consumers feel a sense of entitlement in terms of the quality of service.

Patient satisfaction is an important health care outcome measure. The Hospital Consumer Assessment of Healthcare Providers and Systems (HCAHPS) survey is the first national, standardized survey of patients' perspectives of hospital care. Results are publicly reported (HCAHPS, 2018). Since July 2007, hospitals subject to the Inpatient Prospective Payment System (IPPS) of the Centers for Medicare and Medicaid Services (CMS) have been required to fully participate in HCAHPS to receive full annual payment (HCAHPS, 2017). The Patient Protection and Affordable Care Act of 2010 (also known as Obamacare) included HCAHPS performance as a component of the calculation of hospital payment received through the Hospital Value-Based Purchasing program (HCAHPS, 2017).

Most advanced nurses recognize the significance of patient satisfaction on participants' responses to the HCAHPS survey, officially titled, *CAHPS® Hospital Survey*. It may be challenging for advanced nurses and other health care system leaders to underscore the importance of treating staff with respect and using nonviolent methods of communication while simultaneously emphasizing the institution's friendliness, approachability, and interest in meeting individual "customer" needs. It is also probable that hospital employees and administrators may be less likely to redirect and, if needed, reprimand families and patients who exhibit and verbalize unsafe behaviors or violence toward staff. In addition, because the culture of health care settings is to promote empathy and understanding, agencies may unintentionally create an environment in which there may be acceptance of unacceptable behavior (Rew & Ferns, 2005).

In response to violence perpetrated by the public against the United Kingdom (UK) National Health Service (NHS) staff, the health service established the Campaign to Stop Violence Against Staff Working in the NHS: NHS Zero Tolerance Zone (NHS, 1999). At the time of the campaign start, NHS health care workers were four times more likely to experience WPV than the general public. Estimates suggested that health care workers were approximately 26 times more likely to be seriously injured than members of the general public (Rew & Ferns, 2005). The Zero Tolerance Campaign focused on reinforcing to the public that violence against NHS health care workers is unacceptable while assuring staff that violent and intimidating behavior will not be tolerated.

WPV continues to be a concern across the NHS with a persistently low level of reporting. Some fear that care providers, including physicians, may perceive WPV as inevitable (BBC News, 2008). Published resources support that verbal and physical abuse of NHS staff persist (Health and Safety Executive, n.d.; NHS Wales, 2013); however, health care agencies are persistently advancing this issue with the public and with health and social care employees. Regulations reinforce that WPV perpetuated by the public—specifically, patients and family members—will not be tolerated and is in fact illegal. A flyer written by a medical practice in England provides one example of an educational handout that details the Zero Tolerance policy and procedures of its medical practice (Hope Farm Medical Centre, 2016).

The NHS structure provides opportunity for a single voice message about WPV and the health care system's stance on zero tolerance. Complexities of the U.S. health care system and the lack of singular focus within a care system model that encourages competition among provider entities may contribute to barriers in WPV reduction efforts. Perhaps advanced nurses need to consider strategies to build coalitions and partnerships that commit to providing public education about zero tolerance toward violence and employee harm. Nurses in all sorts of roles need to work with interprofessional colleagues to make certain that violence is not tolerated as just part of the expected daily work of health care providers.

Types of Violence in Health Care Settings

Health care settings around the globe are at risk for a variety of violent behaviors. Violence may be manifested as verbal abuse, sexual harassment, racial harassment, bullying, property damage, threats, murder, physical assault, and cyberbullying. Spector, Zhou, and Che (2014) conducted an integrative review of WPV perpetrated against nurses in the Anglo, Asian, European, and Middle Eastern regions and found that approximately 31.8% of nurses were exposed to physical violence, 62.8% to nonphysical violence, 47.6% to bullying, and 17.9% to sexual harassment during the year prior to data collection. In the United States, national data are not collected on verbal threats or assaults; BLS only reports on injuries severe enough to require time away from work. A direct result of inadequate or absent data collection specific to occasions of violence is the lack of clear descriptive statistics concerning the frequency of verbal and physical violence (Clements et al., 2005) and an accurate understanding of the measure of injuries resulting from violence (Love & Morrison, 2003).

Lateral or horizontal violence frequently occurs in health care agencies. Lateral violence is a form of bullying, nurse to nurse, and is usually directed toward nursing staff perceived as less powerful. Newly graduated nurses and younger nurses are particularly vulnerable to this form of violence (Edward et al., 2014; Roberts, 2015; Zhou et al., 2017). Hutchinson et al. (2008) define bullying as referring to a variety of hidden behaviors that are difficult to substantiate: "Perpetrators aim to harm their target through a relentless barrage of behaviours that may escalate over time and include being harassed, tormented, ignored, sabotaged, put down, insulted, ganged-up on, humiliated, and daily work life made difficult" (p. 21). Examples of lateral violence include nonverbal expressions of disdain or skepticism, rude or belittling comments, sabotaging another nurse by withholding relevant information, scapegoating or blaming, passive aggressive communication, and gossiping (Griffin, 2004). Bullying is tolerated because many nurses experienced it as a rite of passage and regard it as normal. Newly licensed nurses are one such group vulnerable to lateral violence during their early practice (Blando, Ridenour, Hartley, & Casteel, 2014; Goldberg, 2006; Griffin, 2004). This type of violence may be considered an undesirable form of hazing as graduate nurses are initiated into the ranks of professional nurses (**EXEMPLAR 5-1**).

EXEMPLAR 5-1 Horizontal Violence: Confronting a Saboteur of New Nurse Success

Oleksandr Bondar, RN, BSN, is a recently graduated professional nurse who was hired directly into a busy 12-bed medical intensive care unit (MICU). He was initially very enthusiastic about the employment opportunity, although a bit concerned about the demanding expectations that he recognized would be particularly challenging given his lack of MICU experience and his novice RN status. At the time of his job offer, the MICU nurse manager assured him that he would be well supported by an expert and professional nursing staff and a carefully constructed, individualized orientation program. Oleksandr had done quite well in his baccalaureate program and was considered a top-performing student. He had previously worked as an emergency medical technician and also had a military background. During his previous work

(continues)

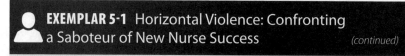

EXEMPLAR 5-1 Horizontal Violence: Confronting a Saboteur of New Nurse Success   *(continued)*

experiences, he demonstrated mature thinking and an optimistic, friendly presence that typically led to positive performance evaluations and leadership opportunities.

Oleksandr's orientation experience started in the classroom and he excelled in both simulated and computerized activities. After 4 weeks of intense academic preparation, he was assigned to work with Melanie Schrift, RN, a highly experienced critical care nurse with a reputation for a no-nonsense approach to practice and an occasionally formidable personality that some found to be intimidating.

During the first few shifts of the clinical preceptorship experience, Oleksandr shadowed Melanie. She explained to him that she was legally responsible for the quality of his care and she needed to be confident that he would not "screw up." He worked diligently to meet her expectations and to acquire an understanding of MICU processes. Melanie increasingly focused on his assessment skills and his knowledge of pathophysiology. She would often quiz him in front of other staff members and, occasionally, in front of patients. The questions were challenging and if he answered incorrectly or with less detail than she required, Melanie would correct him and chastise him in front of observers. These behaviors increased in frequency over the subsequent shifts and, eventually, Melanie incorporated nonverbal expressions of dissatisfaction or irritability that included deep sighs, eye rolling, and sarcastic comments about him to other staff members.

Oleksandr grew increasingly frustrated and felt disempowered. He recognized that his confidence was shaken by these experiences. Accustomed to hard work yielding successful outcomes, he was somewhat taken aback by Melanie's aggressiveness. He began to consider her interactions with him as demonstrations of bullying. Oleksandr was concerned about the effect of this bullying on his status within the staff group and potentially on patients and families as they witnessed passive-aggressive "coaching" at the bedside. He recognized that job opportunities were reasonably plentiful and that he could likely find a different job; however, he determined that it was important for him to address the situation and do what he could to stop the bullying behaviors directed at him. He was also committed to preventing similarly uncivil experiences for other new MICU hires.

Oleksandr devised a personal action plan that included the following activities:

1. Discuss the situation with the nurse manager and the nurse educator. Present his perspectives, concerns, and specific examples with a request for acknowledgement of his viewpoints and verbalization of support.
2. Utilize literature-supported strategies for directly confronting the bullying behaviors demonstrated by Melanie at the time of occurrences.
3. If bullying persists, directly speak with Melanie about his concerns in the company of a third party to ensure that mutual understanding was achieved with a satisfactory action plan.

Oleksandr followed through on his plan as devised. The nurse manager expressed concern for him and a keen interest in retaining him on the staff while assuring him of readily available support. She acknowledged that his preceptor could be "rough" but also shared that Melanie had demonstrated excellent supervisory and coaching skills during previous preceptorship experiences. The manager encouraged Oleksandr to implement his plan and to alert her if managerial input was required. She made clear to Oleksandr that bullying of any sort would not be tolerated and if the situation did not improve or if it worsened, an immediate response to support him would be evoked.

EXEMPLAR 5-1 Horizontal Violence: Confronting a Saboteur of New Nurse Success *(continued)*

The nurse educator concurred and provided him with her cell phone number to facilitate a rapid response to problems, if needed.

Oleksandr then considered recommendations offered by the literature and discussed during one of his undergraduate leadership courses. He considered that some nurses might justify behaviors characterized as rigorous or "tough love" (Leong & Crossman, 2016, p. 1357) as acceptable to encourage resilience; however, tough love or rigor may also be euphemisms for horizontal or workplace violence and these behaviors should be categorized as violent and immediately terminated. He reflected on the value of direct and clear communication between nurses and the confrontation avoidance tendencies that many nurses display in the workplace.

Oleksandr reviewed published literature that he had explored while in school, including *Crucial Conversations* (Patterson & Grenny, 2011) and *Crucial Accountability* (Patterson, Grenny, McMillan, & Switzler, 2012). He also read about cognitive rehearsal (Bowllan, 2015) and began practicing responses to the verbal and nonverbal messages that were frequently offered by Melanie and working on scripting a response to eye-rolling, public chastisement, and aggressive posturing during question and answer sessions. Oleksandr discussed these techniques with colleagues external to the workplace, shared his rehearsed responses with the nurse manager and the nurse educator responsible for his orientation program, and role-played with his friends from school. After a few days, Oleksandr felt prepared to confront the behaviors.

During each bullying encounter with Melanie, including condescension, nonverbal aggressions, or unwarranted criticisms and sarcastic comments, Oleksandr directly and calmly countered with a statement that compelled acknowledgement. One such example occurred at the end of the shift when Oleksandr was providing report to the incoming staff. Melanie interrupted and rolled her eyes. Oleksandr countered, "I see that you rolled your eyes in response to my report. I may have missed an important point. Please share your concern and I will address it." Another situation arose at the bedside of a newly admitted patient. When Melanie began to quiz Oleksandr using rapid-fire speech and aggressive body language, Oleksandr responded by noting, "Mr. Smith is in need of getting comfortable. Let's have this conversation outside the room once we have tended to his care priorities." Each time that Oleksandr directly responded to the disrespectful comment or behavior, Melanie appeared unsettled and stopped.

After a few confrontations, each handled calmly and respectfully, Melanie's behavior shifted and Oleksandr's confidence increased; he felt a sense of renewed accomplishment and confidence. His nurse manager met with him and commended him for his response to the event. She also noted that although the bullying had improved, she would need to discuss the behavior with Melanie to make clear that the bullying had been observed and would not be tolerated, particularly if she was interested in future opportunities to precept new hires.

Approximately 6 months later, Oleksandr successfully completed his orientation requirements and his probationary period. He and Melanie had developed a stable professional relationship. Oleksandr was asked to provide his department with an overview of his orientation experience and he determined that one aspect of this presentation would be horizontal violence or bullying. Oleksandr was particularly interested in contrasting a rigorous approach to orientation versus an approach akin to bullying. His perspectives were well received and discussion opportunities included feedback from the more-senior staff specific to the overwhelming responsibilities

(continues)

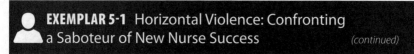

EXEMPLAR 5-1 Horizontal Violence: Confronting a Saboteur of New Nurse Success   *(continued)*

of supervising while managing an assignment, feeling uncertain about the best approaches to coaching a new nurse, and a distaste for orientation evaluation processes. The staff determined that it needed to explore opportunities to develop programs and policies around the following priorities:

1. Evaluation strategies that support the new nurse while also responding to the need to accurately determine whether the orientee is competent in nursing care priorities.
2. Recognition of bullying behaviors and individual/team responsibilities to halt such behaviors, particularly when witnessed.
3. Strategies that support robust and rigorous learning experiences within a context of kindness and caring.
4. Direct, clear, and honest communication techniques.
5. Skillful dialogue techniques to use when important conversations or critical confrontations need to occur.
6. Opportunities to nurture new nurses in ways that enhance team and confidence building.
7. Consistently applied policies to support a zero tolerance approach to workplace violence, particularly between staff and team members but also including patients and visitors.

When students or newly licensed nurses are victims of bullying behaviors, they may view such interactions as the norm in nursing and perpetuate the violent behaviors as they, in turn, progress to work with new nurses or students (Longo & Sherman, 2007). As with other types of violence, if institutions do not proactively protect staff through zero tolerance policies, lateral violence goes unrecognized and unpunished, allowing it to perpetuate. Advanced nurses need to keep in mind, however, that antibullying policies do not necessarily provide victims with sufficient protection against bullying and they do not assure victims that there will be expert guidance available to them from human resource staff about the best ways to manage bullying events (Cowan, 2011).

Violent verbal outbursts, aggressiveness, inappropriate criticisms, and publicly humiliating tirades are not atypical behaviors in health care organizations. Verbal abuse is common in the operating suite (Buback, 2004; Chipps, Stelmaschuk, Albert, Bernhard, & Holloman, 2013) and is largely unprovoked and unexpected when directed at a nurse or other operating room employee from a surgeon. Nonphysical violence is normative in health care settings, and those employees who experience nonverbal violence are more than seven times more likely to experience physical violence (Lanza et al., 2006). A systematic review of nursing and workplace aggression found that the highest incidence of collegial aggression occurred from physician to nurse, although nurse-to-nurse aggression was also as high as 32% within clinical areas (Edward et al., 2014).

Upward vertical bullying occurs when staff members antagonize and continually challenge people in legitimate positions of authority (Goldberg, 2006), including new nurse managers or others new to formal advanced roles. It is also not uncommon for nurses to bully new residents or medical students or for physicians to abuse nurses with such regularity and aggressiveness that nurses are fearful to telephone or page with legitimate patient care concerns. Pharmacists also experience bullying and abuse, particularly from prescribers of all types, including physicians (Institute for Safe Medication Practices [ISMP], 2004a, 2004b).

Risk Factors for Violent Behaviors

Nurses and other health care providers work directly and intimately with unpredictable or explosive people thereby increasing exposure to violence risk. Patients may demonstrate unpredictability as a result of their medical condition such as brain injury (Pryor, 2005), psychiatric illness (Nachreiner et al., 2007; Zuzelo et al., 2012), or dementia. Diagnoses most often associated with violent behaviors include schizophrenia, bipolar manic illness, and comorbid substance abuse (Amoo & Fatoye, 2010). Some perpetrators exhibit explosiveness due to alcohol or drug use. Nursing work often requires one-on-one time with patients and family members. There are times when being alone increases vulnerability to violence, particularly when patients or family are impulsive, angry, and frustrated (**BOX 5-1**).

Family members and visitors may present to health care facilities in angry or impaired states. Too few staff and staff members working alone either during direct care interventions or simply as a result of a decreased personnel pool compound the risk for violence (McPhaul & Lipscomb, 2004). Long wait times (Pich, Hazelton, Sundin, & Kable, 2011), anxiety, and miscommunications; or lack of communications can also trigger violence. These risks for violence relate to Type II, customer/client violence (McPhaul & Lipscomb, 2004), personality conflicts, or any of the three types of violence described by Capozzoli and McVey (1996).

Other risk factors for victimization do not directly relate to patient care but are connected to types of health care–related enterprises or characteristics of individual nurses. Nursing educators are experiencing an increasing number of assaults by angry and violent students, particularly perpetrated by students who are failing or performing poorly (Love & Morrison, 2003). These violent episodes have the potential to spill into clinical education settings. In addition to setting, there are data suggesting

---

BOX 5-1 Examples of Opportunities for Nurse Assault

1. Transporting a patient to a department for a necessary test during off-business hours with an on-call employee opening the department
2. Traveling in an elevator confined with a confused, combative, or angry patient
3. Transporting a deceased patient to the morgue, if the morgue is in a low-travel area
4. Providing patient care in a room with doors closed and equipment or furniture blocking easy exit
5. Sharing information with angry family members regarding a highly stressful patient care event
6. Traveling to and from the parking facilities, particularly if it is later or earlier than the common shift end and start times
7. Picking up medications or supplies during off-peak hours in distant, poorly monitored areas of the building

that nurses with a history of victimization are more vulnerable to WPV (Anderson, 2002a, 2002b; Edward et al., 2014), and risk of violence varies by nurse license type (Nachreiner et al., 2007).

Larger societal influences directly affect the risk for violence in health care settings. Stress, substance abuse, economic pressures, and life's uncertainties contribute to the likelihood of violence. During the first half of 2016, violent crime increased by 5.3% inclusive of murder, rape, robbery, aggravated assault, property crime, and burglary (FBI, n.d.[a]). In the United States in 2015, the population based on U.S. Census Bureau estimates was 321,418,920 people and of this group, 1,197,704 were victims of violent crime and 15,696 were homicide victims (FBI, n.d.[b]). Domestic violence is commonplace, manifested by high rates of spousal, child, and elder abuse. Individuals living in a violent home learn that violence is a normal coping mechanism. Over time, achieving a feeling of normalcy by behaving violently becomes a positive reinforcement (Capozzoli & McVey, 1996). Individuals who are accustomed to using violence to solve problems and who use anger as an early response to stress pose particular problems in hospitals when confronted with uncertainty, delays, confusion, grief, and perceived power inequities.

There were 8,318,500 people employed in the BLS Major Group of 29-0000 Healthcare Practitioners and Technical Occupations in 2016 (BLS, 2016b) and an additional 4,043,480 individuals working in the BLS Major Group of 31-0000 Healthcare Support Occupations (BLS, 2016c). Community and Social Service Occupations, BLS Major Group of 21-0000 and comprised of counselors, therapists, social workers, health educators, and others had 2,019,250 employees (BLS, 2016d) yielding a combined total of over 14 million people working in some sort of health care–related capacity in the United States in 2016. This is a staggering number of citizens employed in settings related to health care provision. As hospitals struggle to provide care within an environment of fiscal shortages and resource competition, and health care delivery systems respond to market and reimbursement uncertainties, there are times when workforce reductions occur. Layoffs and terminations are highly stressful events and may trigger violent outbursts. Hospitals are not immune from personnel problems that may or may not be related to downsizing. Suspensions and other forms of disciplinary actions may also lead to violence.

In summary, many factors contribute to WPV and place nurses at risk. Typical interactions with patients, family, and visitors are potentially dangerous depending on the context of the interaction, the stress levels of the individuals involved, and the personal attributes and behavior patterns of each. Nursing is a "people business" and, as such, is risky. This risk is compounded by inadequate, inconsistent, or nonexistent policies and procedures regarding WPV. Assaults, particularly verbal, occur between health care workers of all types, including physicians, nurses, ancillary staff, and multidisciplinary team members. An apathetic response to WPV in hospital settings contributes to the acceptability of lateral and vertical violence.

Hospitals are microcosms of society and, as such, encounter similar problems as society-at-large. Larger economic forces on local, regional, and national levels, reimbursement challenges, and resource shortages create circumstances addressed through labor downsizing, layoffs, and terminations. These few examples suggest that WPV is a multifaceted event with the potential to increase in frequency and scope. Advanced nurses need to have an understanding of WPV in all its forms so that responsive systems can be designed that intervene in effective, efficient, and meaningful ways.

The Challenges of Establishing Violence Reporting Systems

Defining characteristics of violent behaviors are frequently assumed to be clear and well established. Some types of violence initially appear to be rather simple to describe and commonly understood; bullying or lateral violence may be a more abstract concern than more tangible types of violence such as physical assault. Johnson et al. (2015) caution that there is a lack of conceptual clarity that can make it difficult for managers to identify, label, and discipline perpetrators of workplace bullying. Critical discourse analysis of language used in workplace bullying policies of health care organizations and regulatory agencies reveals that workplace bullying is not discussed as an occupational health issue despite the adverse health outcomes experienced by bullying victims and witnesses (Johnson et al., 2015). Frequently used terms in policy documents included *disruptive behavior, harassment,* and *bullying.* Rarely were documents referenced to external sources. Findings support that varying words are used to describe unwelcome workplace dealings and these words are often not defined in meaningful and consistent fashion (Johnson et al., 2015; Roberts, 2015).

Johnson et al. (2015) found that there are often multiple workplace documents addressing bullying and other behaviors associated with violence, and documents within the same organization often differed in their definitions and descriptions. An additional problem is that many of the health organizations' documents were influenced by TJC, as mentioned, an organization primarily focusing on patient safety rather than worker safety, rather than relying on work efforts of agencies responsible for workplace concerns (Johnson et al., 2015).

Perhaps related to the individuality of health care organizations' policies and the associated definitional deficiencies, violence reporting rates are low (Edward et al., 2014), even though WPV is increasingly recognized as problematic and important. Rationales for low reporting rates vary. Explanations offered specific to NHS staff include nurses' belief that they are "too busy" to take time out for reporting and also nurses' belief that some violent situations are not worth reporting, including unintentional aggression manifested by confused or disoriented patients and verbal abuse from elderly or pain-ridden patients (Ferns & Chojnacka, 2005).

A systematic review by Edward et al. (2014) of the literature pertaining to WPV reveals several barriers to reporting, including:

1. Absent or murky policies and procedures pertaining to violence reporting
2. Poor or missing management support for the victim
3. Previous experiences of nurses who did report without an administrative response, who elect to not report subsequent events
4. Fear of retribution

Other WPV underreporting influences include ingrained perceptions of violence as normative in the caregiving environment (Pich et al., 2010) and a legal system that often discourages nurses from pursuing charges against perpetrators (Wolf, Delao, & Perhats, 2014).

The empathetic and caring nature of nursing care may also countermand a responsibility to report violence of any type. When patients react poorly to a diagnosis, for example, and lash out at the nurse, this behavior tends to be legitimized as a stress response. The threats of irate family members or verbal assaults of patient visitors are often rationalized as being a reaction to anxiety or an inappropriate response to a legitimate problem (e.g., a lengthy wait in the holding area of the ED or an unanswered call bell).

Contributing to the inclination to not report may be that when nurses recognize systems problems but feel unable to correct them, they are more likely to excuse inexcusable behaviors. Reporting such behaviors and getting the patient, family, or visitor "in trouble" may seem an injustice. Ferns and Chojnacka (2005) suggested that nurses need to begin putting themselves first rather than prioritizing the patients in an effort to change the status quo perspective that violence is an inherent part of the work of nurses.

Advanced nurses need to contemplate whether nurses are socialized to expect violence from physicians, managers, or those in roles perceived as powerful (Ferns & Chojnacka, 2005). Certainly the literature supports the premise that nurses in advanced roles, including formal administrative positions, are not perceived as advocates for staff specific to WPV (Edward et al., 2014; Wolf et al., 2014). When violent events occur, nursing work must continue. Patients require care and attention, services need to be provided, and schedules must be followed. As a result, it may be that nurses are accustomed to carrying on regardless of violent exchanges, whether physical, emotional, or psychological assaults. There is little time to step back and step out from work and actually contemplate the impact of the event. An interesting aspect of this socialization is that nurses who experience occupational burnout are more likely to abuse other nurses (Rowe & Sherlock, 2005), and nurses who regularly experience verbal abuse may be more likely to experience burnout, thus perpetuating the cycle of violence.

Addressing the underreporting of violent incidences is a critical concern that must be corrected as an early step in violence prevention. Available data are incomplete, and the effectiveness of interventions cannot be fully researched without an accurate representation of the baseline characteristics and frequencies of violent events. A first step to collecting data is to develop consistent operational definitions of injuries and defining characteristics of violent event types that can be monitored using institutional and, eventually, national databases.

The Lingering Effects of Violence

Victims of violent behaviors have diverse responses to the events. Victims may internalize their feelings regarding verbal assault events or minimize the event (Antai-Otong, 2001) with initial reactions including anger, humiliation, shock, or surprise (Buback, 2004). Acute stress reactions are likely to follow traumatic encounters involving actual or threatened death, physical harm, or other threats to the physicality of self or others (Antai-Otong, 2001). Victims of lateral violence, particularly newly licensed nurses, often react to the violence by seeking other employment, particularly within the first 6 months (Griffin, 2004).

Findings from a content analysis of data acquired via focus groups comprised of nurses and BHAs revealed that participants had varied emotional responses to assault behaviors perpetrated by patients toward staff (Zuzelo et al., 2012). Nurses and BHAs who were victims of WPV on behavioral health units described themselves as worrying about preventing further episodes so that they could avoid repeat victimization (Zuzelo et al., 2012). Staff was conscious of personal responses to violence and appreciated that an angry nurse response to violence could have a ripple effect during interactions with other patients. Participants occasionally resented the perpetrators. They worried about the safety of the care environment. Each occasion of WPV reminded staff members of their vulnerability to serious injury, which evoked feelings of fright. The nurses and BHAs felt violated by violent patients (Zuzelo et al., 2012).

Needham, Abderhalden, Halfens, Fischer, and Dassen (2005) explored the nonsomatic effects of patient aggression on nurses by conducting a literature review spanning publications printed from 1983 to 2003. Edward et al. (2014) reviewed similar literature extending through 2013. Findings from both reviews indicated that nurses experienced anxiety or fear post WPV events. A minority experienced posttraumatic stress disorder (PTSD) or some symptoms of it (Needham et al., 2005). There were a variety of cognitive effects including victims feeling disrespected, unappreciated, violated, humiliated, compromised, or robbed of rights. Some shared feelings of guilt and shame, whereas others became more callous toward patients and were doubtful of their personal security and competency (Needham et al., 2005). Published literature also revealed nurses' losing confidence, missing work, and avoiding the workplace in response to WPV (Edward et al., 2014).

A specific form of violence that may trigger nonsomatic effects in nurses is verbal abuse. Rowe and Sherlock (2005) investigated stress and verbal abuse in nursing using survey methodology. Respondents (N = 213) completed an adapted survey that incorporated the Verbal Abuse Scale and the Verbal Abuse Survey. The sample included RNs and LPNs employed at a Philadelphia teaching hospital with Level I trauma designation. The response rate was 69%. Interestingly, the respondents had been verbally abused by a diverse group of people including patients (79%), other nurses (75%), attending physicians (74%), patients' family members (68%), resident doctors (37%), interns (24%), and others (19%). The most frequent source of verbal abuse reported by these nurse respondents was nurses (27%) followed by patients' families, doctors, patients, residents, others, and interns. Staff nurses were the most frequent nursing source of abuse, responsible for 80% of the events, followed by nurse managers at 20%. Although most of the respondents were able to handle the anger, judging, criticizing, and condescension that were most often encountered as the abusing tactic, many did report response patterns of silence, passivity, calling out sick after the encounter, and having negative feelings about the workplace and the job (Rowe & Sherlock, 2005).

Roberts (2015) reviewed the published literature pertaining to lateral violence in nursing that has been produced over the past 30 years. Similar to the findings of Rowe and Sherlock (2005), Roberts found that bullying leads to reduced job satisfaction, enhanced stress, depression, anxiety, and intent to leave the practice setting. The desire to leave the employment setting is frequently attributed to lateral violence or bullying in the workplace.

Advanced nurses recognize that not all violent events are nonphysical. Homicides, although uncommon, do occur. The *Workplace Violence, 1993–2009 Special Report* compiled and published by the U.S. Department of Justice, Office of Justice Programs, Bureau of Justice Statistics (2011) reveals that nurses have an 8.1 rate of WPV per 1,000 employed persons. Mental health workers, professional, custodial, and other occupations have markedly higher rates of WPV. If an employee is injured as a result of a workplace injury, including WPV, workers' compensation insurance usually covers the expense (OSHA, n.d.[d]). For those organizations that are self-insured, the financial implications are staggering.

OSHA (n.d.[d]) notes that nurses and other caregivers are driven by injuries and stress to leave the profession. Advanced nurses must keep in mind that it is expensive to replace a nurse: approximately $27,000 to $103,000. When this sum is considered within the context of treatment expenses and lost wages, each and every nurse's WPV-related physical or nonphysical injury is fiscally costly. When nurses make decisions to leave the employment setting as a result of lateral violence or bullying, replacement costs are high. Additionally, advanced nurses may want to consider the expense associated with a nursing department or unit reputation as unsafe, unfriendly, and not collegial. The key takeaway message is that the expense of violence is high, not only in terms of human suffering but also in economic costs.

▶ Strategies for Violence Reduction

A comprehensive view of WPV encourages appreciation of its multifaceted nature and justifies the repeatedly published calls to establish robust and highly utilized reporting mechanisms, national databases, policy changes, institutional programming, and multidisciplinary task forces. Advanced nurses of all types and across all roles are uniquely suited to participate in these activities given their advanced educational preparation, leadership skills, and, likely, willingness to dig in and contribute to the hard work involved in creating, managing, and evaluating WPV systems.

There are resources available to advanced nurses and other health care leaders interested in effecting change in the phenomenon of violent workplaces. Formal study of threat assessment and WPV curtailment did not begin until the late 1980s with more obvious efforts in the 1990s that have persisted and increased. As a result, this field of study is relatively new, particularly as it relates to health care systems, and much of the work related to nursing has been descriptive. Nonetheless, there is some beginning evidence and certainly a good bit of descriptive data that may be used to inform potential intervention studies.

Establishing a Policy of Nonviolence

It is probably wise to begin with suggestions related to policy environment specific to WPV. Policy is not generally emphasized as a vehicle for change within programs of nursing education. Policy shapes what nurses do (Malone, 2005), and although not all nurses can be policy experts, it is important for advanced nurses to understand that policy environment provides the context and boundaries in which nursing is practiced. Malone (2005) offers a working framework for assessing the policy environment. Although published over a decade ago, this framework is useful for evaluating the policy environment specific to WPV and the deficiencies and strengths of such an environment.

Malone (2005) asserted that policy is a process rather than a static point and puts forth four distinctive policy characteristics that advanced nurses should consider:

1. A policy is always general.
2. A policy establishes a norm of behavior. Policies formalize decision making about what course of action is good or better than alternative actions.
3. Policy has scale and is intended to apply to different levels of a social organization.

4. There is always someone who makes policy decisions. The advanced nurse must figure out who this individual is within the health care system as part of assessing the policy environment of the system.

Ten questions drive the policy environment assessment (Malone, 2005). The questions provide a useful organizing framework when assessing the policy environment specific to WPV. Each question should be considered carefully to identify gaps and opportunities and to develop an appropriate plan for WPV reduction that encompasses policy change rather than simply rule approval, a less-substantive change. Policy requires "ongoing implementation activities, monitoring, and evaluation" (Malone, 2005, p. 137). The questions have been addressed based on the information provided in this chapter. Policy framework questions should be applied to the advanced nurse's practice setting. Answers may vary depending on the characteristics and circumstances of the institution under consideration.

What Is the Problem?

The problem of note is the occurrence of violent behaviors in hospitals and other health care settings directed toward all types of care providers, including nurses. Behavior categories include verbal and physical assaults, threats, and occasions of lateral or horizontal violence. To provide a more accurate definition of the *what* of this problem, it is necessary to define violence and to determine how to apply this definition when it is related to patient physical or mental illness. Is violent behavior, when part of a medical condition, a policy problem or a medical management problem? One example is aggressive behaviors manifested by elderly patients with dementia and consisting of hitting, scratching, pinching, or screaming at nurses. These behaviors are violent and undesirable. They may be reflective of inadequate medical management or ineffective nursing interventions. They also put nurses at risk for injury and contribute to an unsafe work environment.

Using the FBI model (Rugala et al., 2003), it may be reasonable to view all violent behaviors as unacceptable and reportable. In the example of the elderly patient with dementia attempting to strike a nurse while verbally abusing staff, the behaviors would be reported, but management of the situation would rely on medical and nursing interventions. This situation is different than a violent threat of harm directed toward a nurse from an ED visitor who is under the influence of alcohol. Both behaviors would be reportable, although the interventions triggered by each would be markedly different.

The policy problem includes the lack of national reporting mechanisms and the often confusing and unclear definitions and reporting methods used by individual institutions. The lack of robust data collection systems creates deficient benchmarking processes, incomparable intervention studies, and inconsistent trending. One contributing factor to this problem may be hospitals' current emphasis on patient satisfaction and service. Perhaps the current emphasis on servicing patient and family needs contributes to a sense of entitlement that encourages the belief of patients, visitors, and families that they may act in ways that are socially unacceptable but are forgiven in the hospital setting due to the stressful effects of illness, anxiety, and pain. This perspective minimizes the value of staff and negates the importance of civility and respect in all forms of human interaction. It also encourages staff to avoid reporting violent incidences.

An additional problem is that while many health care professionals report experiences as victims of violence, there is scant published literature addressing the various ways that nurses and other providers potentially contribute to hostile interactions. Negative staff interactions characterized by hostile or aggressive responses to patient, family, or visitor encounters do contribute to an escalation of anger and negative inpatient cultures (Duxbury & Whittington, 2005). Violence-enhancing reactions may relate to personal tendencies to address emotionally heightened encounters with aggression (Anderson, 2002a). There may also be a need for nurses to learn and practice communication techniques designed to establish therapeutic rapport with patients in the early phase of a potentially volatile situation (Casella, 2015). Active violence prevention on the part of providers by using verbal and nonverbal communication techniques is an important component of any WPV initiative in health care.

Nurses experiencing burnout may be more vulnerable to aggression (Winstanley & Whittington, 2002), and nurses with unresolved issues of childhood abuses may have an increased susceptibility to violence, particularly during their early years of professional practice (Anderson, 2002a). Advanced nurses need to consider that staff involved in perpetrating violence, including lateral WPV, may be disinclined to identify themselves as abusers and may require opportunities for candid dialogue and introspection following occasions of nonphysical or physical violence.

Where Is the Process?

The process of garnering attention for policy issues related to WPV is not simple given the many competing demands for resources within the health care system. Keep in mind that the generalized administrative ambivalence to violence directed toward nurses and other employees demonstrates that WPV recognition and reduction efforts are not often organizational priorities. WPV is a wicked problem that is not readily solved and any proactive approach runs the risk of creating problems and issues for the institution and its leadership. It is preferable to draw attention to this workplace issue before a dramatically violent event unfolds. Violence should be addressed proactively rather than reactively.

The insidious nature of lateral or horizontal violence and incivility in the workplace has far-reaching implications in terms of human and economic costs. The NHS campaign of the United Kingdom offers ideas for advanced nurses employed in a variety of roles within the U.S. health care system. As mentioned, a major thrust of the NHS Zero Tolerance Zone Campaign is educating the public that violence against NHS staff is unacceptable. The American public may require similar reminders.

Nurses need to be reminded that their safety is important. OSHA requires employers to take steps to ensure a safe and healthful workplace for employees (Capozzoli & McVey, 1996). Consistent with OSHA's stance, the ANA (2015) released its position paper, "Incivility, Bullying, and Workplace Violence." ANA supports zero tolerance for violence. The AACN (2004) has a "Zero Tolerance for Abuse" public policy that recognizes the relationship between abusive work environments and nurse turnover. AACN (2016) also has done significant work on healthy work environments based on its recognition of the indissoluble relationship among work environment, nursing practice, and patient care outcomes.

Advanced nurses must keep in mind that politics do affect policy. Effecting political change requires coalition-building activities and activism. Establishing WPV as a political priority means that nurse leaders need to galvanize rank-and-file nurses to apply pressure on government officials and the public remembering that there are many worthwhile political issues demanding resources and recognition. It may be a struggle to move the issue of WPV into the forefront of policy making.

How Many Are Affected?

When a problem affects only a few people, it is difficult to get the problem addressed through policies. In the case of WPV, many health care workers are affected. There is a need to mobilize this large number of nurses and other health care providers to give weight to the significance of the problem. WPV is an international concern. The International Council of Nurses (ICN) prioritized violence in 2001 by partnering with the World Health Organization (WHO), the International Labour Organization, and Public Services International to develop an effective worldwide antiviolence campaign (ICN, 2007).

ICN has held several international conferences on "Violence in the Health Sector" and it persists in championing issues related to nurses and violence. ICN (2017) recently issued a statement that addressed a recent arrest of a nurse who was correctly carrying out her duty. ICN made clear in its statement that nurses have a right to work in a "safe environment, free from violence." WHO is also very engaged in addressing the concerns of nurses and other health care providers as they struggle with WPV risks. WHO (2016) led a study of midwives (N = 2,400) from 93 countries that describes poor working conditions, including harassment, lack of security, and fear of violence. WHO (2015) also reported that health care workers responding to the Ebola virus disease (EVD) experience many occupational hazards, including violence. These select examples demonstrate that WPV is a serious, worldwide concern for health care workers, including nurses. Care providers put themselves at risk in the practice environment to provide essential services to those in need. While some risks are not violence related, certainly eliminating WPV as one of the potential hazards of the job is a societal obligation, in addition to an employer responsibility.

What Possible Solutions Could Be Proposed?

Before committing to any single solution, advanced nurses should consider alternatives and the likely advantages of a multipronged approach to the WPV concern. Nurses in advanced roles should reflect on whether possible solutions are politically palatable, practical, or achievable. It is important to select interventions that are acceptable to hospital staff (McPhaul & Lipscomb, 2004). For example, metal detectors in the ED may be the most desirable strategy for eliminating weapons threats but may present insurmountable manpower and budgetary challenges in small hospital facilities. Restricted access to the ED setting by reducing the number of entrances or locking the doors during low- or high-activity periods may be less expensive and actually solve the concurrent problem of too many people in crowded, tense circumstances waiting for access to inpatient areas.

An ED shooting event during which a police officer was slain by a criminal suspect illustrates that both suburban and urban care settings have risk for WPV and offers some real-world considerations for promoting safety in EDs. After the tragedy, medical center staff reevaluated hospital security and made improvements after consulting with law enforcement officials (Roman, 2007). Improvements included keeping criminal suspects separate from other ED patients, building a public safety room for the use of police officers taking suspects to the ED for testing, modifying entryways into the ED, bolting furniture to the floor in the sparsely furnished public safety room, and improving communication processes within the hospital. These interventions have led to effective improvements evaluated following a subsequent event of ED violence (Roman, 2007).

Advanced nurses may want to work with colleagues and use evidence-based tools for proactive identification of patients at risk for perpetrating violence. Kling et al. (2006) described the use of a violence risk assessment tool in an acute care hospital as a strategy for identifying potentially violent or aggressive patients. Nurse leaders may find it useful to consider options for identifying patients that may have a propensity for violence so that staff can implement strategies designed to deescalate aggression during care encounters.

What Are the Ethical Arguments Involved?

Distribution of resources (justice), privacy, nonmaleficence (do not cause harm), autonomy, veracity, and fidelity are key ethical principles requiring consideration when examining strategies for reducing WPV. It is just to allocate scarce resources to protect nurses and patients from violence, although these security expenditures may be chosen over competing and worthy budgetary demands. Patient and employee privacy must be maintained and protected to ensure that rights are not compromised. Autonomy relates to independent decision making based on honest information. Hospitals may need to consider both publicly acknowledging rates of violence and installing programs designed to curtail or eliminate assaults or threats in any form. Fidelity refers to promises and keeping vows. Certainly health care facilities are morally obliged to provide a safe environment for workers and patients.

At What Level Is the Problem Most Effectively Addressed?

WPV must be addressed on a variety of levels including policy making at federal and state levels. All states should have legislation that recognizes health care worker assault as a felony. Violence must be recognized as unacceptable, and the public needs to be informed that health care facilities are not required to tolerate violent behaviors. Consumer education should clearly notify patients, families, and visitors that violent behavior of any type will be reported and addressed, including law enforcement notification when assault or threats of assault are forthcoming during interactions with employees.

Health care agencies need to prioritize worker safety. To effectively address safety needs, hospitals and other facility types must establish safety systems with performance tracking that informs and measures employee safety improvement programs. The Joint Commission (2016) advises that many of the same standards and principles that have improved patient safety are applicable to worker safety. OSHA and TJC have partnered to provide information, guidance, and training resources related to employee health and safety. These materials may be accessed at www.jcrinc.com/about-jcr/osha-alliance-resources (TJC, 2016). One resource, "OSHA and Worker Safety: Assault Halt," provides access information to a compendium of OSHA resources available via the portal Worker Safety in Hospitals (TJC, 2016). The intent of the OSHA and TJC alliance is to provide health care systems with the tools needed to implement comprehensive WPV programs.

Hospitals need to establish policies regarding lateral and vertical violence as well as policies and procedures concerning safety improvements in patient transport and security systems. Health care facilities should also consider broader programs that include institutional threat assessment (Turner & Gelles, 2003), signage, and flexible staffing levels to avoid nurses practicing in isolation without rapid access to emergency support. Antiviolence exercises, including active shooter drills, should be considered to support workplace readiness and response training. Hospitals are vulnerable to this type of violence, and risk naiveté should be corrected.

At the unit level, educational programs and staff training exercises may increase awareness of WPV and provide staff with the skills necessary to avoid escalating patient and family aggression, particularly since there is considerable evidence that some nurses may poorly handle aggressive encounters with patients (Duxbury & Whittington, 2005; Edward, et al., 2014; McGill, 2006), visitors, and colleagues, and also contribute to episodes of horizontal WPV (Longo & Sherman, 2007). Recognizing that health care providers and workers can find themselves in verbal power struggles with patients that are not productive, frustrating, and potentially risky, one agency encourages employees to recognize this type of situation when it occurs and "tap in" by telling the involved worker that he or she has a phone call that requires immediate attention or some sort of similar intervention (Relias, 2016). This "tap in" intervention assists the first employee with gracefully exiting and allows for a change in the communication dynamic with the patient. This example illustrates the importance of employee training, including those practicing at the sharp point of care.

Who Is in a Position to Make Policy Decisions?

Within health care systems, it can be challenging to determine where the "buck stops" in terms of policy making. Identifying a persuasive and powerful administrative champion is critical for success. A zero tolerance for violence policy as a method of risk management is appealing for a number of reasons including institutional protection from lawsuits and negative publicity. Advanced nurses should evaluate the health care facility's executive level to ascertain who might be in a position to either implement policy decisions or influence key individuals who are directly able to determine policy.

Health care system administrators are compelled by TJC to address concerns related to safety and security risks, including how agencies will coordinate security activities with community agencies. Preparing for the possibility of an active shooter falls within the domain of this emergency operations standard (OSHA, n.d.[a]). Advanced nurses should consider opportunities to parlay their understanding of accreditation standards and regulatory requirements into a strong and reasonable case for consideration by administrators with policymaking responsibilities.

What Are the Obstacles to Policy Intervention?

Nurses are good problem solvers but often address issues indirectly rather than directly. Nurses' reluctance to report violent or threatening behaviors elicited from patients, families, colleagues, and other employees is an obstacle to developing and implementing effective nonviolence policies. Nurses may also be reluctant to confront perpetrators who may be dissatisfied with the suggestion that their behaviors need to be curtailed or modified. Advanced nurses need to have opportunities to build their anti-WPV skillset and since this topic is often not given required attention in graduate programs of studies or in workplace educational programs, nurses in advanced roles may feel unprepared to respond to policy inadequacies. Given that the number of doctoral prepared nurses is increasing, particularly those with doctor of nursing practice (DNP) degrees, it is likely that advanced nurses will increasingly find the peer support and expertise needed to effectively address WPV policy deficiencies.

What Resources Are Available?

Advanced nurses need to consider informational, advocacy, and economic resources (Malone, 2005). Nurses are positively viewed by the public with 84% of respondents to Gallup's annual survey of professions' ethical standards and honesty placing nurses in the top position (Gallup News, 2017). Nurses have high social capital but may need to more effectively use this social capital to the profession's advantage. Similar to the work of the NHS, public campaigns by the media and public service messages may be useful in directing attention to WPV in health care settings. Nursing organizations at the international, national, regional, and local levels may be useful allies.

Scholarly resources describing horizontal WPV including bullying and incivility are increasingly available through refereed publications. Developing a valid instrument for measuring workplace bullying would provide a potential mechanism for better understanding the WPV experience (Hutchinson et al., 2008). Quantifying the bullying phenomenon may provide advanced nurses with the means to measure the effect of programs designed to reduce workplace bullying in nursing.

Griffin and Clark (2014) offer cognitive rehearsal as an intervention against incivility and horizontal violence. This is an evidence-based strategy that was utilized in 2004 with graduate nurses as an intervention to respond to lateral violence experienced in nursing. A review of the published literature between 2004 and 2010 reveals that cognitive rehearsal offers value as a tool that enables nurses to shield themselves from oppressive and hostile behaviors. Griffin and Clark (2014) identified key points from the literature review, including building working definitions for incivility, bullying, and workplace mobbing; evidence that supports the use of cognitive rehearsal; and a common language to respond to incivility that empowers nurses to influence uncivil encounters by redirecting the focus on the priority concern of safe and high-quality patient care delivery.

More research is needed to establish evidence-based interventions for reducing WPV in high-risk areas, including the ED. Gillespie, Gates, Kowalenko, Bresler, and Succop (2014) designed a quasi-experimental, repeated measures design that collected survey data from ED employees pre and post a packaged intervention developed with multidisciplinary input specific to WPV that included an educational intervention, environmental changes, and policies and procedures. Effectiveness of the planned intervention was not demonstrated although there was a significant decrease in the number of violent events at two of the intervention sites. Likely more important than the results of this single study is the effort that was applied to addressing ED WPV via a well-designed research study that incorporated many voices. Advanced nurses should consider supporting these sorts of efforts and engaging when possible.

There are several commercial, contracted WPV training programs available for health care workers. Arbury, Zankowksi, Lipscomb, and Hodgson (2017) analyzed selected elements of 12 available programs. Each program differed in its approach and content. Arbury et al. (2017) noted that the most important content gap was inattentiveness to the unique needs of each facility related to risk assessment and policies. As mentioned, it is imperative for advanced nurses to address the potential risks associated with violence of all sorts, including homicidal violence perpetrated using guns and other weapons. The gap in facility-specific risk assessment and policies for risk deterrence, risk management, or responses to active shooters or hostage events is concerning. Arbury et al. (2017) provide an extensive list of criteria used to review the available training programs. Nurses in advanced roles may want to use these published criteria when considering programs that might be useful for unit, department, or systemwide WPV training.

NIOSH offers a web-based training program for nurses. The Occupational Violence program, entitled "Workplace Violence Prevention for Nurses," is a free, interactive course to help health care workers understand WPV (NIOSH, 2017; https://www.cdc.gov/niosh/topics/violence/training_nurses.html). Continuing education units are available upon course completion. Course objectives include (1) to identify institutional, environmental, and policy risk factors for WPV; (2) to recognize behavioral warning signs of violence in individuals; (3) to employ communication and teamwork skills to prevent and manage violence; (4) to identify appropriate resources to support injured health care workers; and (5) to take steps to implement a comprehensive WPV prevention program. The course has no prerequisites and there are 13 modules that take about 15 minutes each to finish.

How Can Advanced Nurses Get Involved?

Nurses in advanced roles should consider learning advocacy skills and developing an understanding of the political process. Becoming well informed is essential. Advanced nurses need to join lobbying efforts and initiate grassroots efforts to bring WPV topics to the forefront of public health discussion. Advanced nurses and those with whom they practice must commit to nonviolence in the workplace and model this behavior for their professional counterparts.

Whether addressing horizontal violence with newly licensed graduates or verbal assaults from colleagues, affecting changes in violence reporting policies and procedures related to patients and families, or forming and participating in multidisciplinary security task forces, nurses have the potential to positively influence the frequency and type of violent behaviors manifested in the work environment. Other strategies for eliminating health care violence include addressing personnel problems and establishing violence response teams.

Address Personnel Problems

Capozzoli and McVey (1996) offer suggestions for managing personnel problems with a focus on preventing WPV. Falcone (2017) suggests strategies for providing progressive disciplinary actions that may reduce the risk of a violent response. These recommendations may be viewed as preemployment, employment, and postemployment strategies. Advanced nurses may find themselves involved both peripherally and directly in personnel events, depending on the type of employee and associated job responsibilities.

Preemployment Strategies. Background checks of job applicants should be conducted to the full extent allowed by the law. It is important to ascertain the credibility of the applicant's work history, degrees, military record, and licensing. Negligent hiring suits are becoming more common, and employers are losing because they have performed inadequate background checks (Capozzoli & McVey, 1996). It may be reasonable to include personality testing and drug screening with preemployment testing, but institutions must bear in mind that personality tests must be administered by skilled professionals, and the Americans with Disabilities Act protects people with recognized disabilities. In addition, the preemployment interview is an important screening activity. There are times when advanced nurses lead or contribute to applicant interviews. Expertise in conducting interviews is an important advanced skill.

During Employment Strategies. Employee performance problems must be addressed in a timely fashion using accurate documentation. The institution's disciplinary process should be used, and employees should be afforded the protection and dignity of due process, as outlined in employee handbooks. Advanced nurses with managerial responsibilities should be trained in conflict resolution. If there is serious concern of violence from the employee in response to the disciplinary process, it is advisable to make certain that undercover security is available in close proximity. If such services are not available at the agency, the advanced nurse should discuss for-hire security services to ensure workplace safety (Falcone, 2017).

Postemployment Strategies. When the progressive disciplinary process ends and the employee is terminated, Capozzoli and McVey (1996) warn that terminated employees cannot be expected to act rationally. All termination paperwork should be ready at the time of the final interview. Immediately following this meeting, the employee should gather personal effects and collect the last paycheck. It is important to collect keys, identification badges, and any other items to avoid creating a need for the employee to return to the work setting. Security services should be readily available. Falcone (2017) shares that most WPV events occur on Mondays after a terminated employee has had the weekend to contemplate and stew over perceived wrongs. For this reason, Falcone (2017) recommends that disciplinary events take place early in the work-week so that the terminated employee has access to work services for questions and information. This consideration is also the rationale for scheduling progressive discipline and termination events early in the workday rather than at the end of a shift (Falcone, 2017).

Violence Response Teams

From a broader perspective, health care facilities should *anticipate* occasions of violence. There should be a crisis management plan for violent events, and security procedures should be developed and disseminated. It is helpful to hold security drills to ensure that employees know where panic buttons, alarms, and security phones are located and to make certain that employees recognize red flag behaviors and respond appropriately. The U.S. Department of Homeland Security (DHS, 2017) provides resources to assist workplaces in preparing and responding to an active shooter incident (**FIGURE 5-1**).

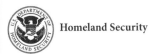 Homeland Security   Active Shooter Preparedness Program

Active shooter incidents, in many cases, have no pattern or method to the selection of victims, which results in an unpredictable and evolving situation. In the midst of the chaos, anyone can play an integral role in mitigating the impacts of an active shooter incident. The Department of Homeland Security (DHS) provides a variety of no-cost resources to the public and private sector to enhance preparedness and response to an active shooter incident. The goal of the Department is to ensure awareness of actions that can be taken before, during, and after an incident.

Active Shooter Preparedness Program
DHS maintains a comprehensive set of resources and in-person and online trainings that focus on behavioral indicators, potential attack methods, how to develop emergency action plans, and the actions that may be taken during an incident.

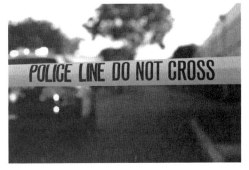

Active Shooter Online Training
This one-hour online course (IS-907 Active Shooter: What You Can Do) provides an introductory lesson on the actions that may be taken when confronted by an active shooter, as well as indicators of workplace violence and how to manage the consequences of an incident. To access this course, please visit the Federal Emergency Management Agency (FEMA) Emergency Management Institute online training website at http://www.training.fema.gov/is/crslist.aspx and type Active Shooter in the search bar.

Active Shooter Preparedness Workshop Series
These scenario-based workshops feature facilitated discussions to inform participants on the best practices associated with preparing for and responding to an active shooter incident. Through a dynamic exchange of information, these workshops provide participants an understanding of how to plan and aid in the development of an initial draft of an emergency action plan for their organizations. For more information on these workshops, please contact the Active Shooter Preparedness Program at ASworkshop@hq.dhs.gov.

Active Shooter Online Resources
There are additional resources available online to inform individuals on how to prepare for active shooter incidents. These resources range from booklets and pocket guides, to a 90-minute webinar that explains the importance of developing an emergency action plan and the need to train employees on how to respond to an incident. To access these resources, please visit http://www.dhs.gov/activeshooter.

Contact Information
For general information regarding the Active Shooter Preparedness Program, please email ASworkshop@hq.dhs.gov.

FIGURE 5-1 DHS (2016). Active Shooter Preparedness Program

DHS (2017). Active Shooter Preparedness Program. Retrieved from https://www.dhs.gov/sites/default/files/publications/dhs-active-shooter-preparedness-program-fact-sheet-01-16-508.pdf

Advanced nurses need to think about the "what-ifs" surrounding potential WPV events. Hostage taking, gun violence, assault, and homicide are only a few of the more dramatic occasions of WPV. Consider whether staff on all shifts would know how to manage particularly dangerous episodes of violence (e.g., a gun-wielding family member, an employee's domestic violence dispute that presents as an enraged and violent significant other arriving at the workplace, a knife-carrying patient who holds a staff member hostage). These events may seem unlikely; however, current events suggest otherwise and advanced nurses need to prepare for the possibility of such events, no matter how seemingly unlikely.

Critical incident stress debriefing should be considered a key component of WPV recovery efforts. The goal of critical incident stress debriefing is to promote a sense of psychological closure with regard to the concerning event. It is structured to assist the employee in making sense of the violence. Part of the challenge of working with nurses who have experienced violence at work is their tendency to dismiss the event as a normal occurrence in health care.

Debriefing in some form should routinely occur within 24–72 hours after violent events in a safe, blame-free environment (Clements et al., 2005). Debriefing activities should be voluntary. Nurses should contemplate developing debriefing programs to assist nursing staff with the psychological, emotional, and physical responses to WPV. Event debriefing assists staff with addressing their feelings and responses post violence (Zuzelo et al., 2012). Some nurses might also benefit from employee assistance programs. Advanced nurses should encourage staff to take full advantage of these programs and should refer employees to the employee assistance staff as needed. Programs need to be evaluated to determine effectiveness and modified accordingly.

▶ Conclusion

Advanced nurses have a critical role to play in ensuring that health care environments are healthy for both patients and employees. An environment is healthy when verbal and physical abuse of any kind is not tolerated, regardless of the social stature of the offender or the nature of the relationship in question. Incidences of WPV are increasingly frequent. The more typical violent behaviors may be limited to social bullying or terroristic email threats; however, these types of assaults have a significant cost in terms of nurse turnover rates and medical errors.

Hospitals and other types of health care agencies are historically open systems. Visitors enter at will with cursory security checks. Rarely is identification required, particularly during daylight hours. Opportunities for extreme violence, including hostage taking, physical assault, or homicide, are significant. Although national terrorism events have evoked significant changes in some aspects of society, most health care organizations have not yet attended to these issues in substantive or consistent ways.

Advanced nurses are in an ideal position to initiate WPV-focused discussions and development sessions. They should participate in interprofessional activities aimed at reducing the potential for violence and responding to occasions of actual violence with effective action that minimizes the likelihood of harm. Advanced nurses have expertise in varied areas with potentially wide nets for capturing the attention of a broad swath of key policy makers. Having a clear understanding of the magnitude of WPV concerns in health care and developing familiarity with the available resources already accessible for employee education provides an excellent starting point. Advanced nurses are charged with nurturing a workplace culture that has no tolerance for violence while also recognizing that agencies have realistic risks of violence and there must be operational response plans that are familiar to staff should violence occur.

References

American Association of Critical Care Nurses. (2004). Zero tolerance for abuse. Retrieved January 18, 2018, from http://studylib.net/doc/8822614/zero-tolerance-for-abuse---american-association-of-critical.

American Association of Critical-Care Nurses. (2016). AACN standards for establishing and sustaining healthy work environments. A journey to excellence (2nd ed.). Executive summary. Retrieved November 6, 2017, from https://www.aacn.org/~/media/aacn-website/nursing-excellence/healthy-work-environment/execsum.pdf?la=en.

American Nurses Association. (2015). Position statement on incivility, bullying, and workplace violence. Retrieved January 18, 2018, from http://nursingworld.org/DocumentVault/Position-Statements/Practice/Position-Statement-on-Incivility-Bullying-and-Workplace-Violence.pdf.

American Nurses Association. (2017a). Workplace violence. Retrieved October 21, 2017, from http://www.nursingworld.org/workplaceviolence.

American Nurses Association. (2017b). Model "state" bill. The Violence Prevention in Health Care Facilities Act. Retrieved October 21, 2017, from http://www.nursingworld.org/MainMenuCategories/Policy-Advocacy/State/Legislative-Agenda-Reports/State-WorkplaceViolence/ModelWorkplaceViolenceBill.pdf.

Amoo, G., & Fatoye, F. O. (2010). Aggressive behavior and mental illness: A study of inpatients at Aro Neuropsychiatric Hospital, Abeokuta. *Nigerian Journal of Clinical Practice, 13,* 351–355.

Anderson, C. (2002a). WPV: Are some nurses more vulnerable? *Issues in Mental Health Nursing, 23*(35), 351–366.

Anderson, C. (2002b). Future victim? *Nursing Management, 33*(3), 26–32.

Antai-Otong, D. (2001). Critical incident stress debriefing: A health promotion model for WPV. *Perspectives in Psychiatric Care, 37*(4), 125–132, 139.

Arbury, S., Zankowski, D., Lipscomb, J., & Hodgson, M. (2017). Workplace violence training programs for health care workers. An analysis of program elements. *Workplace Health & Safety, 65,* 266–272.

BBC News. (2008). Doctors not reporting assaults. *BBC News.* Retrieved June 6, 2008, from http://news.bbc.co.uk/go/pr/fr/-/2/hi/health/7178777.stm.

Blando, J., Ridenour, M., Hartley, D., & Casteel, C. (2015). Barriers to effective implementation of programs for the prevention of workplace violence in hospitals. *Online Journal of Issues in Nursing, 20*(1). Retrieved January 18, 2018, from http://www.nursingworld.org/MainMenuCategories/ANAMarketplace/ANAPeriodicals/OJIN/TableofContents/Vol-20-2015/No1-Jan-2015/Articles-Previous-Topics/Barriers-to-Programs-for-the-Prevention-of-Workplace-Violence.html.

Bowllan, N. M. (2015). Nursing students' experience of bullying: Prevalence, impact, and interventions. *Nurse Educator, 40,* 194–198. doi:10.1097/NNE.0000000000000146

Buback, D. (2004). Home study program: Assertiveness training to prevent verbal abuse in the OR. *AORN Journal, 79*(1), 148–164.

Bureau of Justice Statistics. (2011, March). Special report. Workplace violence, 1993–2009. Retrieved January 18, 2018, from https://www.bjs.gov/content/pub/pdf/wv09.pdf.

Bureau of Labor Statistics. (2015). Injuries, illnesses, and fatalities. Fact sheet. Workplace homicides from shootings. Retrieved October 21, 2017, from https://www.bls.gov/iif/oshwc/cfoi/osar0016.htm.

Bureau of Labor Statistics. (2016a). News release. Nonfatal occupational injuries and illnesses requiring days away from work, 2015. Retrieved October 22, 2017, from https://www.bls.gov/news.release/archives/osh2_11102016.pdf.

Bureau of Labor Statistics. (2016b). Occupational employment statistics, May 2016. 29-0000 Healthcare Practitioners and Technical Occupations (Major Group). Retrieved January 18, 2018, from https://www.bls.gov/oes/current/oes290000.htm.

Bureau of Labor Statistics. (2016c). Occupational employment statistics, May 2016. 31-0000 Healthcare Support Occupations (Major Group). Retrieved January 18, 2018, from https://www.bls.gov/oes/current/oes310000.htm.

Bureau of Labor Statistics. (2016d). Occupational employment statistics, May 2016. 21-0000 Community and Social Service Occupations (Major Group). Retrieved January 18, 2018, from https://www.bls.gov/oes/current/oes210000.htm.

Bureau of Labor Statistics. (2017a). Industries at a glance. Health care and social assistance: NAICS 62. About the health care and social assistance sector. Retrieved October 21, 2017, from https://www.bls.gov/iag/tgs/iag62.htm.

Bureau of Labor Statistics. (2017b). Industries at a glance. Health care and social assistance: NAICS 62. Work-related fatalities, injuries, and illnesses. Retrieved October 21, 2017, from https://www.bls.gov/iag/tgs/iag62.htm.

California Division of Occupational Safety and Health. (2017). Workplace violent incident reporting system for hospitals. Retrieved October 26, 2017, from https://www.dir.ca.gov/dosh/workplace-violence-reporting-for-hospitals.html.

Capozzoli, T. K., & McVey, R. S. (1996). *Managing violence in the workplace.* Delray Beach, FL: St. Lucie Press.

Casella, S. M. (2015). Therapeutic rapport: The forgotten intervention. *Journal of Emergency Nursing, 41,* 252–254. doi:10.1016/j.jen.2014.12.017

Chipps, E., Stelmaschuk, S., Albert, N. M., Bernhard, L., & Holloman, C. (2013). Workplace bullying in the OR: Results of a descriptive study. *AORN Journal, 98,* 479–493. doi:http://dx.doi.org.ezproxy2.library.drexel.edu/10.1016/j.aorn.2013.08.015

Clements, P. T., DeRanieri, J. T., Clark, K., Manno, M. S., & Kuhn, D. W. (2005). WPV and corporate policy for health care settings. *Nursing Economics, 23*(3), 119–124.

Cowan, R. I. (2011). "Yes, we have an anti-bullying policy, but": HR professionals' understandings and experiences with workplace bullying policy. *Communication Studies, 62,* 307–327. doi:10.1080/10510974.2011.553763

Denenberg, R. V., & Braverman, M. (1999). *The violence-prone workplace.* Ithaca, NY: Cornell University Press.

Department of Homeland Security. (2017). Active shooter preparedness. Retrieved November 6, 2017, from https://www.dhs.gov/active-shooter-preparedness.

Duxbury, J., & Whittington, R. (2005). Causes and management of patient aggression and violence: Staff and patient perspectives. *Journal of Advanced Nursing, 50*(5), 469–478.

ECRI. (2017a). About ECRI. Retrieved October 21, 2017, from https://www.ecri.org/Pages/default.aspx.

ECRI. (2017b). Violence in healthcare facilities. Retrieved October 21, 2017, from https://www.ecri.org/components/HRC/Pages/SafSec3.aspx?tab=2.

Edward, K., Ousey, K., Warelow, P., & Lui, S. (2014). Nursing and aggression in the workplace: A systematic review. *British Journal of Nursing, 23,* 653–659.

Falcone, P. (2017). Progressive discipline: Answers to more of your common questions. *HRNews,* Retrieved May 3, 2018, from http://ezproxy2.library.drexel.edu/login?url=https://search-proquest-com.ezproxy2.library.drexel.edu/docview/2022274366?accountid=10559

Federal Bureau of Investigation. (n.d.[a]). 2016 crime in the United States. January-June preliminary semi-annual uniform crime report. Retrieved January 18, 2018, from https://ucr.fbi.gov/crime-in-the-u.s/2016/preliminary-semiannual-uniform-crime-report-januaryjune-2016/tables/table-3.

Federal Bureau of Investigation. (n.d.[b]). 2015 crime in the United States. Table 1. Crime in the United States by volume and rate per 100,000 inhabitants, 1996–2015. Retrieved January 18, 2018, from https://ucr.fbi.gov/crime-in-the-u.s/2015/crime-in-the-u.s.-2015/tables/table-1

Ferns, T., & Chojnacka, I. (2005). Reporting incidents of violence and aggression towards NHS staff. *Nursing Standard, 19*(38), 51–56.

Gallup News. (2017). Nurses keep health lead as most honest, ethical profession. Retrieved January 22, 2018, from http://news.gallup.com/poll/224639/nurses-keep-healthy-lead-honest-ethical-profession.aspx.

Gillespie, G. L., Gates, D. M., Kowalenko, T., Bresler, S., & Succop, P. (2014). Implementation of a comprehensive intervention to reduce physical assaults and threats in the emergency department. *Journal of Emergency Nursing, 40*, 586–591.

Goldberg, E. (2006). Fight social bullying. *Men in Nursing, 1*(3), 45–49.

Griffin, M. (2004). Teaching cognitive rehearsal as a shield for lateral violence: An intervention for newly licensed nurses. *Journal of Continuing Education in Nursing, 35*(6), 257–263.

Griffin, M., & Clark, C. M. (2014). Revisiting cognitive rehearsal as an intervention against incivility and lateral violence in nursing: 10 years later. *The Journal of Continuing Education in Nursing, 45*, 535–542. doi:10.3928/00220124-20141122-02

Haddon, W. (1968). The changing approach to the epidemiology, prevention, and amelioration of trauma: the transition to approaches etiologically rather than descriptively based. *American Journal of Public Health and the Nation's Health, 58*, 1431–1438. Retrieved October 28, 2017, from https://www.ncbi.nlm.nih.gov/pmc/articles/PMC1228774/.

Harrell, E. (2011, March). Special report. Workplace violence, 1993–2009. National Crime Victimization Survey and the Census of Fatal Occupational Injuries. Retrieved October 22, 2017, from https://bjs.gov/content/pub/pdf/wv09.pdf.

Hayes, L. J., O'Brien-Pallas, L., Duffield, C., Shamian, J., Buchan, J., Hughes, F., . . . North, N. (2006). Nurse turnover: A literature review. *International Journal of Nursing Studies, 43*, 237–263.

Health and Safety Executive. (n.d.). Violence in health and social care. Retrieved January 18, 2018, from http://www.hse.gov.uk/healthservices/violence/index.htm.

Hedin, B. (1986). A case study of oppressed group behaviour in nurses. *Image: Journal of Nursing Scholarship, 18*, 53–57.

Hollinworth, H., Clark, C., Harland, R., Johnson, L., & Partington, G. (2005). Understanding the arousal of anger: A patient-centered approach. *Nursing Standard, 19*(37), 41–47.

Hope Farm Medical Centre. (2016). Zero tolerance. Retrieved October 28, 2017, from http://hopefarmmedicalcentre.nhs.uk/practice/zero-tolerance.

Hospital Consumer Assessment of Healthcare Providers and Systems. (2017). HCAHPS fact sheet. Retrieved January 18, 2018, from http://www.hcahpsonline.org/globalassets/hcahps/facts/hcahps_fact_sheet_november_2017a.pdf.

Hospital Consumer Assessment of Healthcare Providers and Systems. (2018). *CAHPS® hospital survey.* Retrieved January 18, 2018, from http://www.hcahpsonline.org/en/.

Hutchinson, M., Vickers, M., Jackson, D., & Wilkes, L. (2005). "I'm gonna do what I wanna do." Organizational change as a legitimized vehicle for bullies. *Health Care Management Review, 30*(4), 331–336.

Hutchinson, M., Vickers, M., Jackson, D., & Wilkes, L. (2006). Workplace bullying in nursing: Towards a more critical organizational perspective. *Nursing Inquiry, 13*(2), 118–126.

Hutchinson, M., Wilkes, L., Vickers, M., & Jackson, D. (2008). The development and validation of a bullying inventory for the nursing workplace. *Nurse Researcher, 15*(2), 19–29.

Institute for Safe Medication Practices. (2004a, March 11). Intimidation: Practitioners speak up about this unresolved problem (Part I). ISMP Safety Alert. Retrieved January 18, 2018, from http://www.ismp.org/Newsletters/acutecare/articles/20040311_2.asp.

Institute for Safe Medication Practices. (2004b, March 25). Intimidation: Mapping a plan for cultural change in healthcare (Part II). ISMP Safety Alert. Retrieved January 18, 2018, from http://www.ismp.org/Newsletters/acutecare/articles/20040325.asp?ptr=y.

International Council of Nurses. (2007). Workplace bullying in the healthcare sector. Retrieved January 18, 2018, from http://www.icn.ch/images/stories/documents/publications/fact_sheets/19l_FS-Bullying_Health_Sector.pdf.

International Council of Nurses. (2017). Workplace violence. ICN statement. Retrieved January 18, 2018, from http://www.icn.ch/what-we-do/workplace-violence/workplace-violence.html.

Johnson, S., Boutain, D., Tsai, J., & de Castro, A. (2015). An investigation of organizational and regulatory discourses in workplace bullying. *Workplace Health & Safety, 63*, 452–461. https://doi.org/10.1177/2165079915593030.

Kelling, G. L. (2015). Don't blame my 'broken windows theory' for poor policing. *Politico Magazine.* Retrieved October 28, 2017, from https://www.politico.com/magazine/story/2015/08/broken-windows-theory-poor-policing-ferguson-kelling-121268.

Kelling, G. L., & Wilson, J. Q. (1982, March). Broken windows: The police and neighborhood safety. *Atlantic Monthly, 249*(3), 29–38.

Kling, R., Corbière, M., Milord, R., Morrison, J., Craib, K., Yassi, A., . . . Saunders, S. (2006). Use of a violence risk assessment tool in an acute care hospital. Effectiveness in identifying violent patients. *AAOHN Journal, 54*(11), 481–487.

Lanza, M. L., Zeiss, R. A., & Rierdan, J. (2006). Non-physical violence: A risk factor for physical violence in health care settings. *AAOHN Journal, 54*(9), 397–402.

Leong, Y. M., & Crossman, J. (2016). Tough love or bullying? New nurse transitional experiences. *Journal of Clinical Nursing, 25*, 1356–1366. doi:10.1111/jocn.13225

Longo, J., & Sherman, R. (2007). Leveling horizontal violence. *Nursing Management, 38*(3), 34–37, 50–51.

Love, C. C., Morrison, E., for the AAN Expert Panel on Violence. (2003). American Academy of Nursing Expert Panel on Violence Policy Recommendations on WPV (adopted 2002). *Issues in Mental Health Nursing, 24*, 599–604.

Malone, R. (2005). Assessing the policy environment. *Policy, Politics, and Nursing Practice, 6*(2), 135–143.

McGill, A. (2006). Evidence-based strategies to decrease psychiatric patient assaults. *Nursing Management, 37*(11), 41–44.

McPhaul, K., & Lipscomb, J. (2004). WPV in healthcare: Recognized but not regulated. *Online Journal of Issues in Nursing, 9*(3). Retrieved December 28, 2005, from http://www.nursingworld.org /ojin/topic25/tpc25_6.htm.

Nachreiner, N., Hansen, H., Akiko, O., Gerberich, S., Ryan, A., McGovern, P., . . . Watt, G. D. (2007). Difference in work-related violence by nurse license type. *Journal of Professional Nursing, 23*(5), 290–300.

National Health Service (1999). Health service circular. Campaign to stop violence against staff working in the NHS: NHS zero tolerance zone. Retrieved October 28, 2017, from http://webarchive .nationalarchives.gov.uk/20040218205543/http://www.dh.gov.uk:80/assetRoot/04/01/22/32/04012232.pdf.

National Health Service Wales. (2013). Health in Wales. Zero tolerance: The fresh clampdown on violence against ambulance staff. Retrieved January 18, 2018, fromhttp://www.wales.nhs.uk /news/29287.

National Institute for Occupational Safety and Health. (1996). Violence in the workplace. Purpose and scope. Retrieved July 11, 2006, from http://www.cec.gov/nisoh/violpurp.html.

National Institute for Occupational Safety and Health. (2002a). The changing organization of work and the safety and health of working people. Retrieved April 10, 2009, from http://www.cdc .gov/niosh/docs/2002-116.

National Institute for Occupational Safety and Health. (2002b). Violence: Occupational hazards in hospitals. Retrieved April 10, 2009, from http://www.cdc.gov/niosh/docs/2002-101.

National Institute for Occupational Safety and Health. (2006). WPV prevention strategies and research needs. Retrieved October 24, 2017, from https://www.cdc.gov/niosh/docs/2006-144 /pdfs/2006-144.pdf.

National Institute for Occupational Safety and Health. (2018). About NIOSH. Retrieved May 3, 2018, fromhttps://www.cdc.gov/niosh/about/default.html .

National Institute for Occupational Safety and Health. (2017a). Occupational violence. Fast facts. Retrieved October 21, 2017, from https://www.cdc.gov/niosh/topics/violence/fastfacts.html.

National Institute for Occupational Safety and Health. (2017b). Workplace violence prevention course for nurses. By Hartley, D., & Webb, S. Morgantown, WV: U.S. Department of Health and Human Services, Centers for Disease Control and Prevention, National Institute for Occupational Safety and Health. Retrieved October 22, 2017, from https://www.cdc.gov/niosh/docs/2017-114/.

National Institute for Occupational Safety and Health. (2017c). Occupational violence. Retrieved January 22, 2018, from https://www.cdc.gov/niosh/topics/violence/.

Needham, I., Abderhalden, C., Halfens, R., Fischer, J. E., & Dassen, T. (2005). Nonsomatic effects of patient aggression on nurses: A systematic review. *Journal of Advanced Nursing, 49*(3), 283–296.

Occupational Safety and Health Administration. (n.d.[a]). Worker safety in hospitals. Caring for our caregivers. Retrieved January 22, 2018, from https://www.osha.gov/dsg/hospitals/workplace _violence.html.

Occupational Safety and Health Administration. (n.d.[b]). OSH Act of 1970. Sec. 5. Duties. Retrieved October 24, 2017, from https://www.osha.gov/pls/oshaweb/owadisp.show _document?p_table=OSHACT&p_id=3359.

Occupational Safety and Health Administration. (n.d.[c]). Workplace violence prevention and related goals. Accreditation. Retrieved January 22, 2018, from https://www.osha.gov/Publications /OSHA3828.pdf.

Occupational Safety and Health Administration. (n.d.[d]). Workplace violence in healthcare. Understanding the challenge. Retrieved January 22, 2018, from https://www.osha.gov/Publications /OSHA3826.pdf.

Occupational Safety and Health Administration. (2017). The whistleblower protection programs. Retrieved October 24, 2017, from https://www.whistleblowers.gov/.

Patterson, K., Grenny, J., McMillan, R., & Switzler, C. (2005). *Crucial accountability. Tools for resolving violated expectations, broken commitments, and bad behavior* (2nd ed.). New York, NY: McGraw-Hill.

Patterson, K., Grenny, J., McMillan, R., & Switzler, C. (2012). *Crucial conversations. Tools for talking when stakes are high* (2nd ed.). New York, NY: McGraw-Hill.

Peter, E. H., Macfarlane, A. V., & O'Brien-Pallas, L. L. (2004). Analysis of the moral habitability of the nursing work environment. *Journal of Advanced Nursing, 47*(4), 356–367.

Pich, J., Hazelton, M., Sundin, D., & Kable, A. (2011). Patient-related violence at triage: A qualitative descriptive study. *International Emergency Nursing, 19*, 12–19. doi:10.1016/j.ienj.2009.11.007

Pryor, J. (2005). What cues do nurses use to predict aggression in people with acquired brain injury? *Journal of Neuroscience Nursing, 37*(2), 117–121.

Relias (Formerly AHC Media). (2016, January 1). OSHA lists new violence prevention strategies for healthcare. Retrieved January 22, 2018, from https://www.ahcmedia.com/articles/136812 -osha-issues-new-violence-prevention-strategies-for-healthcare.

Rew, M., & Ferns, T. (2005). A balanced approach to dealing with violence and aggression at work. *British Journal of Nursing, 14*(4), 227–232.

Rippon, T. J. (2000). Aggression exposure and mental health among nurses. *Australian E-Journal for the Advancement of Mental Health, 1*(2). Retrieved April 10, 2009, from www.auseinet.com /journal/vol1iss2/Lam.pdf

Roberts, S. (1983). Oppressed group behavior: Implications for nursing. *Advances in Nursing Science, 5*(4), 21–30.

Roberts, S. (2000). Development of a positive professional identity. Liberating oneself from the oppressor within. *Advances in Nursing Science, 22*(4), 71–82.

Roberts, S. (2015). Lateral violence in nursing: A review of the past three decades. *Nursing Science Quarterly, 28*, 36–41. doi:10.1177/0894318414558614.

Roman, L. (2007). Aftermath of a shooting. Tightened security in our ED. *RN, 70*(12), 39–42.

Rowe, M. M., & Sherlock, H. (2005). Stress and verbal abuse in nursing: Do burned out nurses eat their young? *Journal of Nursing Management, 13*, 242–248.

Rugala, E. A., Isaacs, A. R. (Eds.), for the National Center for the Analysis of Violent Crime. (2003). WPV issues in response. Quantico, VA: Critical Incident Response Group, NCAVC, FBI Academy. Retrieved October 24, 2017, from https://www.fbi.gov/file-repository/stats -services-publications-workplace-violence-workplace-violence.

Runyan, C. W. (1998). Using the Haddon matrix: Introducing the third dimension. *Injury Prevention*. Retrieved July 11, 2006, from http://ip.bmjjournals.com/cgi/content/full/4/4/302#otherarticles

Safety + Health. (2016, July 13). Labor unions petition OSHA for standard to prevent workplace violence in health care. Retrieved October 21, 2017, from http://www.safetyandhealthmagazine .com/articles/14383-labor-unions-petition-osha-for-standard-to-prevent-workplace-violence-in -health-care.

Safety Lit. (n.d.). The Haddon matrix. Retrieved October 28, 2017, from https://www.safetylit.org /haddon.htm.

Shea, T., Sheehan, C., Donohue, R., Cooper, B., & De Cieri, H. (2017). Occupational violence and aggression experienced by nursing and caring professionals. *Journal of Nursing Scholarship, 49*, 236–243.

Spector, P. E., Zhou, Z. E., & Che, X. X. (2014). Nurse exposure to physical and nonphysical violence, bullying, and sexual harassment: A quantitative review. *International Journal of Nursing Studies, 51*, 72–84. doi:10.1016/j.ijnurstu.2013.01.010

The Joint Commission. (2016). OSHA and worker safety. Assault halt. OSHA and The Joint Commission offer guidance and resources to curb workplace violence. Retrieved January 22, 2018, from https://www.jcrinc.com/assets/1/7/ECN-OSHA-Apr-16.pdf.

The Joint Commission, Division of Health Care Improvement. (2014, August). Preventing violent and criminal events. *Quick safety. An advisory on safety & quality issues, 5*. Retrieved October 24, 2017, from https://www.jointcommission.org/assets/1/23/Quick_Safety_Issue_Five_Aug_2014 _FINAL.pdf.

Trossman, S. (2006). Nurses want to put an end to workplace violence. *The American Nurse, 38*(2), 1, 6–7.

Trotto, S. (2014). Workplace violence in health care. *Safety + Health*. Retrieved October 21, 2017, from http://www.safetyandhealthmagazine.com/articles/11172-workplace-violence-in-health-care -nurses.

Turner, M. G., & Gelles, M. G. (2003). *Threat assessment. A risk management approach.* Binghamton, NY: Haworth Press.

Van De Griend, K. M., & Messias, D., K. (2014). Expanding the conceptualization of workplace violence: Implications for research, policy, and practice. *Sex Roles, 71*, 33–42. doi:10.1007/s11199-014 -0353-0.

Way, M., & MacNeil, M. (2006). Organizational characteristics and their effect on health. *Nursing Economics, 24*(2), 67–76. Retrieved July 5, 2006, from CINAHL—Database of Nursing and Allied Health Literature.

Winstanley, S., & Whittington, R. (2002). Anxiety, burnout and coping styles in general hospital staff exposed to workplace aggression: A cyclical model of burnout and vulnerability to aggression. *Work & Stress, 16*(4), 302–315.

Wolf, L. A., Delao, A. M., & Perhats, C. (2014). Nothing changes, nobody cares: Understanding the experience of emergency nurses physically or verbally assaulted while providing care. *Journal of Emergency Nursing, 40*, 305–310. doi:http://dx.doi.org/10.1016/j.jen.2013.11.006

World Health Organization. (2015). Almost 500 health worker deaths in Ebola outbreak. Retrieved January 22, 2018, from http://www.who.int/life-course/news/occupational-health-in-ebola -outbreak/en/.

World Health Organization, International Confederation of Midwives, & White Ribbon Alliance. (2016). WHO and partners call for better working conditions for midwives. Retrieved January 18, 2018, from http://www.who.int/mediacentre/news/releases/2016/midwives-better-conditions/en/.

Zhou, C., Mou, H., Xu., W., Li, Z., Liu, X., Shi, L., . . . Fan, L. (2017). Study on factors inducing workplace violence in Chinese hospitals based on the broken window theory: A cross-sectional study. *BMJ Open, 7*, e016290. doi:10.1136/bmjopen-2017-016290. Retrieved October 28, 2017, from http://bmjopen.bmj.com/content/bmjopen/7/7/e016290.full.pdf.

Zuzelo, P., Curran, S., & Zeserman, M. (2012). Registered nurses' and behavior health associates' responses to violent inpatient interactions on behavioral health units. *Journal of the American Psychiatric Nurses Association, 18*, 112–126.

Supplemental Resource Publication

U. S. Department of Labor Occupational Safety and Health Administration. (n.d.). WPV: Hazard Awareness. Retrieved January 22, 2018, from http://www.osha.gov/SLTC/workplaceviolence /recognition.html

CHAPTER 6

Environmentally Conscientious Healthcare: Opportunities to Improve Sustainability and Reduce Resource Consumption

Patti Rager Zuzelo, EdD, RN, ACNS-BC, ANP-BC, CRNP, FAAN

A dvanced nurses are well positioned to lead initiatives designed to improve and protect the environment by reducing or altering consumption practices, encouraging clean energy use, and incorporating ecofriendly considerations into the forefront of planning decisions. Advanced practice registered nurses (APRNs) may influence environmental health by counseling patients to reduce meat intake, not only for personal health benefits but also for environmental reasons. They may educate patients, families, and the public about strategies to reduce indoor and outdoor air pollutants. Nurses in other advanced roles also have opportunities to contribute to conservation efforts by wise product-purchasing decisions that include packaging and disposal considerations. They may consider opportunities to influence menu choices available in the care setting and encourage policies that advance green efforts. Administrators may demonstrate environmental conscientiousness by ensuring that there are opportunities for recycling and by insisting that wastage is minimized when possible. New building plans might be influenced by sustainability concerns, including carbon dioxide emissions. Influential advanced nurses have many opportunities to wield formal and informal power in ways that could potentially improve environmental practices and outcomes.

Environmentalism is a high-priority concern that is not often addressed in nursing education, whether at undergraduate, graduate, or doctoral levels of study. Riedel (2016) asserts that sustainability of interventions and the associated use of materials need to be ensured a place in ethical reflection and decision making in professional nursing practice. Sustainability is a complex concept that has not been well defined and is inconsistently applied to ethical considerations about resource distribution (Riedel, 2016). It is inadequately considered in practice and poorly addressed or ignored in nursing academics. This *green-gap* in knowledge and practice supports a system of waste and consumption that could likely be improved by a more ecologically proactive and measured approach to health care delivery. Certainly advanced nurses have a stake in protecting the environment, as Earth inhabitants, resource stewards, and role models for good health practices.

Nurses use a holistic approach during encounters with care recipients. Holism must also include an interest in environmental stewardship, careful and limited resource consumption, and protection of nature so that the fresh air, sunlight, pure water, and rich earth that are essential to basic life-supporting health practices continue to be freely available (Zuzelo, 2016). This chapter provides ideas for consideration and resources for review so that advanced nurses can work with others to improve the ecosensitivity of care practices and to influence systems in more ecofriendly directions. Environmental initiatives provide ideal opportunities for advanced nurses to work with interprofessional colleagues on projects that are uniquely different from the more typical activities that address administrative or practice concerns. The potential for team building across a health care network, including participation of patients and families, offers many powerful partnership possibilities devoted to environmental stewardship.

▶ The Case for Prioritizing Ecologically Sound Care Practices

The natural world is under tremendous pressure as a result of many influences, largely man-made, particularly greenhouse gases but also poor urban planning, plastics, chemical usage, and consumption practices. Leading scientific organizations agree that global warming trends over the past century are very likely the result of human activity (National Aeronautics and Space Administration [NASA], n.d.). Although some individuals and groups deny the science supporting climate change, 97% or greater of actively publishing climate scientists concur that weather-warming trends are related to human activities (Cook et al., 2013).

Global warming and climate change are contemporary issues profoundly important to health. Green conversations are occurring across a wide swath of systems ranging from individual homes and workplaces to international communities. The *2015 United Nations Climate Change Conference* worked to establish a binding and universal agreement on climate change with the intent of reducing greenhouse gas emissions and avoiding catastrophic changes in nature (Climate Action, n.d.). Hundreds of thousands of people across the world marched during this conference period clamoring for environment protections. The World Health Organization (WHO, n.d.) recognizes climate change as "the greatest threat to global health in the 21st century."

Moral and religious world leaders are adding to the discussion and these conversations influence secular efforts. The papal encyclical letter *Laudata Si'* on *Care for Our Common Home* was released in 2015. Pope Francis comments, "When we speak of the 'environment', what we really mean is a relationship existing between nature and the society which lives in it. Nature cannot be regarded as something separate from ourselves or as a mere setting in which we live. We are part of nature, included in it and thus in constant interaction with it" (2015, p. 104). The Dalai Lama is also concerned about climate change and has framed the battle against climate change as a "matter of survival of humanity" (Manadhana, 2015). The confluence of these perspectives from religious leaders contributes to an appreciation for the complex interconnections between a healthy planet and human health and, in partnership with scientific findings, supports the premise that advanced nurses have a role to play in environmentally friendly initiatives that cumulatively have the potential to make a real difference in carbon outlays and waste volume.

Advanced nurses should keep in mind that Florence Nightingale (1946) recognized the interplay between environment and health. She asserted that sunlight, fresh air, pure water, and effective sewage management were important to health and healing. Nightingale (1946) recognized the influence of the environment on patient outcomes and called for nurses to use the environment to hasten recovery and promote wellness.

It makes sense that an extension of the premise that environmental factors influence health is the parallel responsibility of nurses to protect the environment so as to ensure that sunlight, clean air, pure water, and other natural gifts remain available for future generations. Furukawa, Cunha, Pedreira, and Marck (2016) observe that health services exist to promote health and to preserve life. These charges are compromised when hospitals and other agencies contribute to resource depletion by inefficiently utilizing energy or poorly managing waste streams because these unsustainable practices threaten human health. Furukawa et al. point out that nurses comprise the largest group of hospital employees and, as such, are major resource consumers and waste generators. The upside to these large nursing numbers is that there is great potential to make a difference by committing to improving sustainability efforts, including those directly related to medication processes (Furukawa et al., 2016).

Zuzelo (2016) comments on nurses' use of the Earth's rich biodiversity and natural beauty to restore and promote health through meditation, herbal remedies, homeopathy, and allopathic medications. Advanced nurses often employ a variety of holistic practices, including guided imagery with its frequent focus on the natural world and "relaxation techniques based on deeply breathing oxygen-rich air, envisioning green spaces and tranquil water and beach scenes" (p. 187). Nurses are often drawn to nature as a source of healing, and their reliance on the natural world requires intentional engagement in sustainability efforts and green practice initiatives.

In sharp contrast to the *desired* state of the environment is the stark reality of health care systems' adverse impact on environmental health. The U.S. health care system annually generates more than 4 billion pounds of waste (Wormer et al., 2013). This is a particularly staggering total given that about 70% of this waste ends as biohazardous waste (Wormer et al., 2013), a fiscally and environmentally horrific outcome. Much of this waste is from the disposable supplies used in operating rooms (ORs) (Southorn, Norrish, Gardner, & Baxandall, 2013; Wormer et al., 2013).

Medical waste is an international problem and the 4 billion pounds of American waste needs to be considered in addition to total worldwide waste. The United

Kingdom annually contributes more than 400,000 tons at great ecological and fiscal cost (Southorn et al., 2013). WHO (2015) reports that of all health care generated waste, approximately 85% is nonhazardous. The hazardous remainder is toxic, infectious, or radioactive and is composed of many types of waste products that have potentially far-reaching environmental consequences (**TABLE 6-1**). Incinerated health care waste emits dioxins, furans, and other toxins into the air while landfill waste can pollute ground water. There are other environmental concerns, including infection.

WHO (2015) estimates that 16 billion injections are provided on an annual basis around the world and not all of the needles and syringes are disposed in safe fashion. As a result, in 2010, unsafe injections accounted for approximately 33,800 new human immunodeficiency virus (HIV) infections, 1.7 million hepatitis B infections, and 315,000 hepatitis C infections (WHO, 2015). The volume of waste and the risks associated with its improper disposal and expense is staggering, particularly considering that these figures are estimates that likely do not include the full volume of waste generated by all types of health-related agencies, including dental, animal research, blood banks, nursing homes, and others.

There are diverse opportunities for advanced nurses to initiate, lead, and contribute to ecology efforts within health care agencies and institutions. Projects and programs may be implemented at individual, department, and system levels of care. There are many creative ecosensitive and ecosustaining initiatives currently underway in health care and other venues that are likely transferrable to health care systems. Exploring

TABLE 6-1 Waste Typology

Type	Selected Components
Infectious	Contaminated with blood, body fluids, waste from patients in isolation, discarded diagnostic samples
Pathological	Human tissues, organs, fluids, body parts, contaminated animal carcasses
Sharps	Syringes, needles, disposable scalpels, blades
Chemicals	Laboratory solvents, disinfectants, heavy metals from devices, including mercury and batteries
Pharmaceuticals	Expired, unused, and contaminated drugs and vaccines
Genotoxic	Mutagenic, teratogenic I or carcinogenic drugs, including those used in cancer therapies and their metabolites
Radioactive	Radioactive diagnostic materials or testing materials
Nonhazardous or general	Poses no direct harm

conservation and green possibilities may provide advanced nurses with new ideas or opportunities for replication within their health care enterprises. Keep in mind that students may also be interested in participating in environmentally conscientious programs and these sorts of efforts may encourage cross-disciplinary team building while improving environmental outcomes (**EXEMPLAR 6-1**).

EXEMPLAR 6-1 Building a Team Around Environmental Action

Alana Cuellar, DNP, RN, ACNS-BC, was frustrated with her unit's work environment. Numerous complaints to environmental services and to nursing staff had not fully addressed the cleanliness of the nurses' station, storage areas, staff lounge and bathroom, or patient rooms. She noticed that there appeared to be a lot of waste—lights were always on, computers were rarely turned off, trash contained many plastic bottles, plastic cutlery, and coffee pods. Dr. Cuellar reflected on the contrast between the wastefulness demonstrated in routine fashion throughout the hospital and her careful approach to recycling in her home. She was increasingly disturbed by this environmental chaos and wastefulness and decided to reframe the issues into a possible opportunity for exploring a team-based approach to improving the unit's environment by implementing ecologically focused initiatives.

Alana decided that exploring published literature and science-based websites was likely the best way to devise a tentative plan. She categorized the search yield into carbon offset, consumption, and waste; and then clustered specific opportunities into "green buckets" that were small, manageable, and relevant to her unit. Once she had a preliminary familiarity of low-resource project endeavors that were described in the literature, she considered those that offered good opportunities for immediate success. She then reached out to her unit team.

Alana realized that the *team* could be broadly and inclusively defined. Ecology-focused opportunities offered a chance for housekeeping, environmental services, nursing staff, house staff, clerical and other support personnel to join together to begin efforts designed to clean up the unit and improve the environmental context of their work lives while also potentially triggering a ripple effect throughout the hospital. Dr. Cuellar pulled together a steering committee of five employees who represented a variety of interested nursing staff and other employees. She also personally asked nursing faculty who instructed undergraduate and graduate students on the unit if they might be interested. This request yielded two students and a nursing professor. Alana then began planning for the inaugural environmental task force meeting.

The group reviewed the evidence and resources that had been compiled by Dr. Cuellar. Team members conducted a preliminary survey of the physical area and spent some time observing work processes as time permitted. Each team member spoke with department colleagues to solicit ideas and recommendations. The task force developed a plan that included:

- Organizational structure based on ad hoc subcommittees. Each subcommittee would have its own unique charge and a timeline for assignment completion. Subcommittee plans would be shared with the leadership task force. The two groups would collaboratively develop strategies, secure resources as needed, and determine outcomes that could be measured to demonstrate progress and/or success in the specific endeavor.

(continues)

EXEMPLAR 6-1 Building a Team Around Environmental Action *(continued)*

- Ad hoc subcommittee membership would be based on interest. Subcommittees would be diverse, interprofessional, and collegial. Ad hoc subcommittees would select their own leaders or coleaders. Ad hoc committees would be structured to address projects of no longer than 6 months' duration with most anticipated to require 3–4 months.
- Publications, abstracts, and posters would be shared ventures with authorship and credit sorted out prior to any meaningful work effort. The general rule would be that if an individual could not describe meaningful project contributions, the person could not receive authorship credit. Otherwise, ad hoc committee members were each eligible for institutional recognition and professional opportunities, if so desired. While Dr. Cuellar did not anticipate an immediate need for these guidelines, she recognized that there were certainly possible venues available to subcommittees to share their project ideas.

The task force held a unit kickoff ceremony to rally support from external administrators, other unit staff, and anyone else with an interest in ecological and environmental improvements. The task force placed two suggestion boxes on the unit, created a unit environment blog, and constructed an image presentation, entitled "State of the Unit Address." The festivities ended with a 15-minute brainstorming session to identify "green activities" that could be rapidly implemented and readily sustained. Participants identified the following first steps:

1. Ink cartridge recycling
2. Plastic recycling
3. Eliminating disposable foam cups from the nurses' lounge
4. Turning off office computers as permitted by information technology
5. Office paper recycling

Three ad hoc committees were formed: One group was charged with establishing paper recycling opportunities within the unit; a second group was assigned responsibility for plastics recycling; the final committee was delegated with responsibility for reducing electricity consumption, including energy used for computer powering.

Alana was pleased with the initial enthusiasm and anticipated that the groups would have a positive impact on the resource consumption and recycling efforts of the unit. As a direct result of the kickoff event, several nurses suggested that the annual small gifts given to nurses on Nurses' Day could connect to environmental health and specific ideas included reusable lunch bags or refillable water bottles. One staff member brought in sustainable locally sourced food items for snacking during a staff meeting and soon others expressed interest in sharing other healthy food options. Of course, Dr. Cuellar recognized that there was still much work to be done and she hoped that the team's enthusiasm would influence the larger hospital system.

Reflection

- Consider opportunities for environmental improvements in your care setting.
- Reflect on small, relatively easy changes with comparably large benefits (*low-hanging fruit*).
- Identify possible approaches to ecologically sensitive projects that might do well with an interprofessional approach.

> 👤 **EXEMPLAR 6-1** Building a Team Around Environmental Action *(continued)*
>
> ■ Explore options for ideas and support within your agency but also external to your care delivery system.
> ■ Engage others in conversations and activities around environmental improvements, including food sourcing, resource consumption reduction opportunities, enhanced recycling options, and decreased use of toxic chemicals and environmentally unfriendly products.
> ■ Contemplate possible team-building activities constructed around improving the health of the workplace environment.

▶ Ecological Project Possibilities: Partnering Health and Planet Sustainability

Health care systems contribute to environmental polluting and resource depletion predominately through resource consumption and waste disposal practices (**FIGURE 6-1**). Advanced nurses may find it useful to consider ecology initiatives within these broad categories. There are many ways to reduce or revise resource consumption patterns. Waste disposal practices can also be modified in ways that can have an incrementally powerful effect on an institution's carbon footprint. Some current initiatives have advantaged the environment through green activities that beautify the local environment and offset carbon production while also promoting efforts that support positive health practices. Each possibility offers multiple benefits, no matter how seemingly small. Nurses in advanced roles need to consider the indirect ripple effect that their ecofriendly efforts may have on the people, places, and things that are integral to health care as it is very likely that small labors will contribute to larger efforts that cumulatively affect the workplace culture specific to sustainability.

Influencing Consumption Patterns

Advanced nurses may influence consumption patterns by working to reduce consumption or by revising consumption choices from those that adversely affect the ecosystem in particularly negative ways to those that have less of a net negative effect. A few examples of opportunities to alter consumption include changing cooked and processed meat menu options available to patients, visitors, and employees in the hospital cafeteria or through food services; and eliminating or limiting plastic-bottled water purchase choices and encouraging refillable container options with easily located water container fill-up stations. The water stations will encourage employees to reuse containers and reduce waste while encouraging healthy water intake rather than sodas, thus eliminating the need for countless plastic containers.

Advanced nurses are creative and intelligent people with a keen eye for improvement opportunities. The Environmental Protection Agency (EPA, 2018) advocates "Reduce, Reuse, and Recycle" as a mantra for modifying consumption and waste management behaviors. Advanced nurses are well advised to look at the

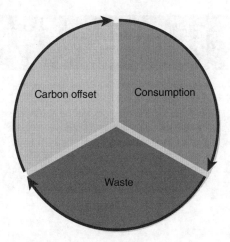

FIGURE 6-1 Typology of Eco-Friendly Sustainability Efforts

many facets of health care delivery systems and consider how the process can be modified in response to the EPA challenge. Excellent exemplars of successful ecofriendly programs are available for consideration and replication on the Web and in the published literature.

Opportunities to Reduce the Consumption of Resources

The Healthier Hospitals Initiative (HHI) was founded in 2012 by 12 of the largest and most influential U.S. health care systems in partnership with key agencies, including Practice Greenhealth, Health care Without Harm (HCWH), and the Center for Health Design (Healthier Hospitals [HH], 2013). Its purpose was to provide guidance for hospitals to learn data-driven practices for energy and waste reduction, to make safer and less toxic product selection decisions, and to purchase and serve healthier foods (HH, 2013). The HHI was designed in similar fashion to the Institute for Healthcare Improvement's successful 100,000 Lives Campaign. It was built on the triple aim of the Centers for Medicare and Medicaid Services (CMS): better health, better care, and lower costs. The program has been so successful, now boasting 1,200 enrolled members (HH, 2013), that it has been established as a permanent partner of Practice Greenhealth as Healthier Hospitals (HH, n.d.). The HH program continues to use data-driven, evidence-based environmentally conscientious strategies around six key challenges updated in 2015: engaged leadership, healthier food, leaner energy, less waste, safer chemicals, and smarter purchasing (HH, n.d.); and is easily accessible via the Practice Greenhealth website (https://practicegreenhealth.org/) under the "Tools & Resources" tab (Practice Greenhealth, 2018a).

The *2014 Milestone Report* (HH, 2014) provides evidence as to the significant progress that hospitals can make on indicators reflecting improved sustainability practices. The report builds on 3 years of data collected from the 1,200-member organizations, including 970 hospitals (HH, 2014). Outcomes offer inspiring possibilities for advanced nurses to consider (e.g., in a single year, 38 hospitals collectively reduced their meat utilization by 1,359.61 pounds equating to a reduction of 21,093 metric tons of carbon dioxide). Other outcomes reflect progress on decreasing medical waste, increasing the percentage of compound-free furniture purchases rather than compound-containing products, and redesigning surgical kits to improve ecofriendliness and to reduce costs (HH, 2014). These outcomes measures support the value of sustainability in nursing and health care practice.

One important component of a sustainability plan is a communication structure that supports data collection, reporting mechanisms, goal-setting, and tracking and provides for the comprehensive baseline assessment that informs progress measurement (HH, 2014). The report notes that engaged leadership is a necessity and this leadership needs to create "a culture of possibility" (HH, 2014, p. 7) that can positively affect the integration of sustainability into everyday care decisions as a routine aspect of health care decision making. Although sustainability and consumption are currently popular ideas, advanced nurses and their colleagues need to give careful thought as to how to begin and sustain environmentally conscientious programs and decision-making processes; organized communication systems need to be considered as integral to these efforts.

Healthy and Sustainable Food and Drink Programs

The *2014 Milestone Report* (HH, 2014) offers multiple examples of projects that reduce or alter hospitals' consumption patterns. Healthier food is one of the six challenge categories prioritized by the HH program (2014). This particular category focuses on revising consumption patterns by increasing healthy food opportunities and encouraging people to move from highly processed or high-sugar content foods to choices that are local, sustainable, and healthier. Consumption reduction efforts are exemplified by a *less meat, better meat* program that is designed to decrease the volume of purchased meat products while also increasing the quality of meats to include those that are free of antibiotics and more sustainably produced.

Several participating hospitals worked to improve transparency of food purchasing decisions and mounted efforts to reduce the use of antibiotics in meat production and to improve living conditions of animals raised in meat production facilities. Hospitals increased options for grass-fed beef, antibiotic-free chicken, and locally secured produce that was farmed using sustainable practices. These successful efforts often galvanized other hospitals to begin similar initiatives (HH, 2014).

The *Healthy Beverages* goal of the healthier food challenge category is focused on reducing sugary drink consumption and encouraging a switch to tap water (HH, 2014). Participating agencies are addressing vending machine options, tap water access, and swaps between sugary beverages to full fruit juice options. Another HH goal relates to local sourcing of food products as a mean to support the local economy and encourage sustainable food practices (HH, 2014). Many of the participating hospitals improved their baseline local sourcing percentages by responding to this challenge.

Healthy Food Options: Insect-Based Products as a High-Protein Food Source

Switzerland has recently allowed specific insect-based food products, mealworms, locusts, and crickets to be sold commercially providing that national food safety requirements are followed (The Local, 2017). Switzerland's decision reflects a growing trend, entomophagy or insect consumption. Insects are rich in protein and have been a common food source in some countries, particularly those regions that are non-Western. Some other insect foods include spider legs, crickets, grasshoppers, and larvae. These food options are often locally popular and culturally unique. As likely anticipated, a major barrier to entomophagy is food palatability when insects are plated and prepared for consumption. "Bugs" are often perceived as pests and this negative viewpoint influences reactions to palatability (Zuzelo, 2017).

Advanced nurses working in Western countries are not going to see insect-laden food choices appearing on hospital and health care system menus any time in the near future; however, as concerns increase about food costs, meat production expenses, environmental and financial costs, chronic illness risks associated with meat (including cancers), and animal production conditions that are often cruel and abusive, there will likely be momentum toward some forms of entomophagy (Zuzelo, 2017).

Insect consumption offers positive ecological opportunities to advanced nurses who are interested in exploring this dietary option and, perhaps, considering some small steps in this area even if as an initially novel dining experience to acquaint colleagues and others with this possibility. Insect proteins do not need to be provided in whole form although this is certainly an option. In some countries, insects are boiled, fried, and roasted and may be served as snacks (van Huis et al., 2013). A more appealing strategy for incorporating insect powder into foodstuffs may be to grind them into a powder that may be used in baking.

Although entomophagy may be perceived by some advanced nurses as atypical or an extreme food option, the fact is that these food products are widely available and judged by many as tasty and appealing. A quick search on Amazon.com reveals cricket bites with buffalo wing sauce flavoring; mixed insect samples including grasshoppers, crickets, sago worms, and silk worms; and a roasted scorpion mix. There are many insect-based food snacks and flours that can be used for smoothies or baked goods. Consider the health implications of a rich protein supplement that is reasonably priced without environmental costs and sustainably produced without worries about potential animal abuse and harvesting conditions!

In Vitro Meat: Producing Meat in the Lab

Laboratory produced meat is another possible way to provide animal meat without harming animals or the environment. This meat is cultured from the muscle cells of animals and the in vitro process allows for the opportunity to alter the meat's fat content while controlling the pathogens that contribute to foodborne illness (Laestadius & Caldwell, 2015). Cultured meat is not yet currently available for purchase and, like insect consumption, may be met with some general public resistance. However, as concerns about animal treatment and carbon dioxide emissions increase, particularly given the concurrent increase in world population thereby requiring even more food production, the opportunities provided by insects and in vitro meat need to be considered. Informed advanced nurses will best serve their colleagues and patients by keeping abreast of food trends and their various advantages and disadvantages.

Advanced nurses may consider devising program options that include all or part of these efforts as first steps in a sustainability advocacy program within hospitals and other agencies. There is much public awareness on the risks of obesity, cardiovascular disease, and diet-related cancers. These programs may provide an initial vehicle for propelling forward a commitment to improved sustainability practices given public interest.

Targeting Energy Consumption

The HH (2014) program has prioritized lean energy use as a major category of change. Energy consumption is recognized as malleable through the use of more efficient technologies that are better maintained as well as via decreased use, particularly unnecessary use. HH (2012) recognizes that energy consumption measurements require robust data and detailed analysis that allow for comparisons and evidence-based decision making. Advanced nurses may consider how energy use can be reduced by conservation policies and also how ecofriendly energy sources and products can be substituted for dirtier or inefficient energy types.

Reducing Consumption of Toxic Chemicals

Reducing the number of products containing polyvinyl chloride (PVC) or bis(2-ethylhexyl) phthalate (DEHP) is one goal of the HH (2015) Safer Chemicals Challenge. The particular product targets include "breast pumps, enteral nutrition products, parenteral infusion devices and sets, general urological (irrigation/urology sets and solutions, urinary catheters), exam gloves, umbilical vessel catheters, and vascular catheters" (HH, 2014, p. 18). Another chemical initiative addresses ecofriendly cleaning solutions for bathroom, general purpose, carpet, and window cleaners rather than using traditional, less environmentally friendly products. HH (2014) recommends Green Seal or EcoLogo Certified products.

Hospital furniture purchases often contain toxic chemicals that are used as flame retardants. HH (2016) recommends avoiding furniture that has been treated with halogenated flame retardants, formaldehyde, perfluorinated compounds, and PVC. These chemicals were initially used when cigarette smoking was common in public spaces. HH (2014) notes that these chemicals have been demonstrated to poorly perform as flame retardants and they emit toxic chemicals into the environment that are linked to cancer, birth defects, and asthma. HH (2016) is working with hospitals to pressure manufacturers for increased chemical transparency and is using purchasing power pressure to encourage companies to change chemical usage.

These efforts target the interior hospital environment, including patient care areas and nursing work settings. Advanced nurses may want to consider the recommendations of the HH program and include chemical scrutiny in furniture, equipment, and product purchasing decisions. Specific vendors that have met the HH interior environment chemical challenge are available on its furniture list (www.HealthierHospitals.org/hhichallenges/furniturelist) (HH, 2016). This is good information to use in conversation with colleagues who work in administration and purchasing departments. Given that nursing staff spend the most time in direct patient care settings, working toward a healthy interior environment is a reasonable employee health expectation.

Partners Healthcare (n.d.) provides an excellent example of environmental sustainability in action. This newly constructed 850,000 square feet of office space houses 4,200 employees that provide the administrative supports of a large health care system. Its energy usage is efficient and it is a Leadership in Energy and Environmental Design (LEED) Gold Version 4 candidate. Demonstrating its commitment to ecofriendly purchasing and to reducing harmful chemical usage, 70% of the $22 million spent on facility furnishings is free of flame retardants, formaldehyde, perfluorinated chemicals, and PVC, consistent with the Interior Goals of the Healthier Hospitals organization (Partners Healthcare, n.d.).

This new construction example demonstrates a pledge to sustainability. Natural lighting, energy efficiency, avoidance of toxic chemicals, environmentally friendly design and construction, and LEED candidacy are opportunities in whole or in part that may be considered by advanced nurses and raised during discussions with team members and leadership during building construction or unit remodeling. Addressing these opportunities is important and advocating for environmentally sustainable and ecofriendly choices when purchasing new furniture, selecting mattresses, linens, cleaning products, lighting, and many other products influences the market when product lines are less or more successful depending on their environmental impact.

Waste Management Practices: Reducing and Recycling

Published literature on waste management practices and reduction efforts in health care reports that there is serious need for altering resource consumption and waste disposal practices. The problem is international and knowing where to begin can be challenging. Advanced nurses are wise to explore the "low-hanging fruit" opportunities and pursue them so that change takes on momentum and projects scaffold into larger, systemwide initiatives.

One service line that may be a good place to start is surgical services, particularly the OR. ORs use many disposable equipment sets and have significant quantities of disposable packing materials. Southorn et al. (2013) report that nearly 20% of all hospital waste in the United Kingdom is produced by OR suites and most of this waste is incinerated. Recycling efforts in hospitals on a worldwide basis are inconsistent. The United States recycles approximately 50% but the United Kingdom lags at less than 10% (Southorn et al., 2013).

A major waste management challenge relates to waste classification practices. When waste is deemed "clinical waste," incineration is required. Southorn et al. (2013) comment that clinical waste is an overused designation that is often applied even to OR-generated waste that is clean and safe. The majority of OR waste is actually generated in preparation for the surgical procedure; hence, as long as sharps are excluded, the waste is clean and incineration is not necessary (Southorn et al., 2013).

Southorn et al. (2013) investigated the feasibility and effectiveness of a change in waste management practices for select surgical cases—specifically, total hip replacement, total knee replacement, and facet joint injections. These high-frequency procedures generate a large amount of waste. Data were collected prior to and after revisions in waste collecting and sorting activities. Waste analysis over a 2-week period revealed that 47% was recyclable dry paper and cardboard; an additional 47% was potentially recyclable plastic; 6% was not recyclable. The waste was monitored and carefully scrutinized and there was not one occasion of contaminated waste being improperly discarded. The researchers extrapolated from these results that if waste from these specific procedures were separated and recycled, the carbon footprint associated with incineration would be decreased by 75% (Southorn et al., 2013).

Wormer et al. (2013) also explored waste reduction strategies in the OR in an effort to reduce its environmental impact. Consistent with the UK experiences described by Southorn et al. (2013), Wormer et al. note that the majority of regulated medical waste comes from the OR and most of this volume consists of disposable surgical materials. This volume substantively contributes to the 4 billion pounds of waste annually produced by the American health care system (Wormer et al., 2013). This project explored the impact of the Green Operating Room Committee on waste reduction and recycling yield. The committee was initiated by a surgeon and nurse and its membership was interprofessional.

The Green Operating Room Committee implemented a variety of ecological initiatives; and, over an approximate 5-year period, diverted 6.5 tons of medical waste (Wormer et al., 2013). Recycling efforts focused on all single-use devices with a solid waste decrease of approximately 12,860 pounds per annum. Disposable foam padding was substituted with reusable gel padding that saved over $50,000 per year and batteries that would previously have been thrown out were salvaged and donated to other departments or to local organizations thereby yielding a $9,000 per year savings. The committee initiated a "Power Down" program designed to reduce energy consumption; and it reduced carbon emissions by 234.3 metric tons annually while also saving $33,000 per year. Water usage reductions by converting from soap to an alcohol-based water-free scrub further contributed to the tremendous reduction in resource utilization by saving 2.7 million liters of water per year (Wormer et al., 2013). The efforts of this single OR-based committee produced impressive savings that reflect reduced consumption, reduced waste, and a reduced carbon footprint. Advanced nurses should consider how this initiative might be used as an exemplar for similar efforts in high-resource utilization care areas across health care systems. The implications for practice changes are staggering!

The OR is one practice area that offers opportunities for successfully yielding dramatic improvements following fairly simple practice changes. Peregrin (2015) notes that *green* sustainability initiatives are also *green* dollars savings and that fiscal and ecological concerns are not mutually exclusive. One suggestion is for providers to look around the clinical practice setting and determine how the department or practice setting is contributing to the carbon footprint of the institution (Peregrin, 2015). Single-use devices are costly both in dollars and in waste disposal expenses. Advanced nurses may find it useful to conduct unit-based or service line audits to determine the volume of single-use devices that are purchased and discarded on an annual basis. Certainly this is an example of low-hanging fruit that may provide a big yield with comparatively little difficulty. Challenges may present in setting up a process for recycling, but recycling is safe provided that requirements are followed and markedly less expensive in dollars, resource consumption, and discard expense than purchasing a device to use one time and subsequently throwing it out.

Peregrin (2015) offers other examples and suggestions specific to the surgical environment; however, these recommendations could be easily applied to other health care settings. Prepackaged surgical packs offer opportunities for review and reduction and these efforts pay off in terms of packaging and trash reductions as well as decreased resource consumption associated with unnecessarily sterilizing equipment that was not needed during a procedure but was opened at the start of the operative case (Peregrin, 2015).

Ecology efforts should be interdisciplinary and are best served with input from all members of the team; the more diverse and inclusive, likely the better the ideas and outcomes! Peregrin (2015) reports that one physician recommendation is to utilize a peer-to-peer communication model so that there is a green committee member representing each practice role and these committee members disseminate information to their respective role group members. This model avoids the contest of wills and resentment that may occur when professionals feel that they are being imposed upon by another professional group. Rather, the work efforts are communicated via the particular professional group by a representative of that group. It would make sense to consider extending this model to include not only various direct care providers but also indirect care providers and ancillary staff who are responsible for providing the physical and organizational context of care.

One example provided in the Peregrin (2015) discussion highlighted the positive impact of a recommendation put forth by a custodian. Red trash bags are used for contaminated waste and this type of waste requires incineration, a contributor to dioxin in the atmosphere and to considerable fiscal expense. The custodial staff observed that the red bag–lined trashcans were the largest cans in the OR and were the closest to the surgical team. They recommended using the smaller trash cans for contaminated waste and positioning these cans in the corners of the room so that there was some effort involved in the discard process. Larger cans were no longer red bag lined and were used for general trash; specifically, no incineration process required for disposal. The interviewee shared that this simple change yielded a cost savings of $50,000 per annum with a reduction of 75% in red bag trash volume (Peregrin, 2015)!

As previously noted, HH is partnered with Practice Greenhealth (2018a), a nonprofit membership organization created to support and promote positive environmental stewardship and best ecological practices in the health care sector. Its mission, to "transform health care worldwide so that it reduces its environmental footprint, becomes a community anchor for sustainability and a leader in the global movement for environmental health and justice", relates to the critical need for improved ecological practices in health care (Practice Greenhealth, 2018b).

Practice Greenhealth's (2018a) organizational goals include to prevent and reduce waste; to achieve carbon neutrality; to reduce energy and water consumption; to build, renovate, and purchase responsibly; to increase recycling, incrementally eliminate hazardous substances, and toxic chemicals; and to address other aspects related to leadership and mission engagement. The organization offers individual facility or health system membership. Fees vary depending upon need and institutional characteristics and organizational members receive full agency support. Advanced nurses will find many ideas and opportunities through this organization and its richly detailed website. The scope of membership benefits may be reviewed on its website under the "Membership" tab.

Advanced nurses are encouraged to consider ecological improvement opportunities in their practice settings that are parallel to Practice Greenhealth's objectives. Simple changes in waste disposal practices can yield significant reductions in carbon emissions. Recycling packaging from disposable equipment and exploring opportunities for plastic recycling may yield significant improvements in resource consumption and waste generation with little effort.

The Practice Greenhealth (2018a) website provides information, best practices, and solutions to a number of topics that directly relate to its goals. There are also tools that will appeal to advanced nurses (e.g., the *Less Waste* section offers a member-only toolkit containing case studies, presentations with scripts, evidence-based practice resources, and other resources that are designed to assist with implementing *Less Waste* strategies within an organization) (Practice Greenhealth, 2018c).

The Greenhealth Academy (Practice Greenhealth, 2018d) offers e-learning, phone call supports, webinars, and other supports in the interest of supporting green teams in the health care sector that are working to improve sustainability and reduce

BOX 6-1 Greenhealth Academy Selected Webinar Topics

Starting or growing a sustainability internship program
Sustainability and the role of human resources
Hello there. Get ready to share! What's new to do for Earth Day 2018
Environmental Excellence Awards question and answer session #1 and #2
When leaders say "yes" to energy
Connecting climate and health co-benefits to community benefit strategies
Inspiration hour: Hospital farm to hospital plate
Health care plastic recycling—It's not all rainbows and unicorns

Data from Greenhealth Academy. Retrieved from https://practicegreenhealth.org/sites/default/files/upload-files/greenhealth -academy-calendar.pdf

adverse environmental effects of the health care system. Webinar topics are interesting and cutting edge, and they offer opportunities to support and nurture green teams that have varying expertise and diverse project goals (**BOX 6-1**). Practice Greenhealth (2017) may be an ecological opportunity for advanced nurses to consider, particularly when searching for tangible, structured supports. Pricing information is not publicly available but there is contact information, and fees are described as influenced by the needs of the institution or system.

Another example of an interesting project addressed opportunities to improve environmentally sustainable medication processes at a hospital in Brazil (Furukawa et al., 2016). This project applied Six Sigma methodology to the medication processes performed by nurses in an intensive care unit setting. Nurses often administer pharmaceuticals that negatively influence the environment and the vehicles of medication administration delivery consume materials and contribute to medical waste and trash. Preintervention data were collected and compiled based on observations of the nursing team during medication use system processes across four shifts.

Following baseline observation and data collection, several ecologically favorable improvements were implemented specific to various aspects of the medication delivery system. These interventions, treated as independent variables, included installing water flow–regulating devices on room faucets, placing medication labels directly on the medication blister pack rather than on the outer plastic bags to ensure that the bags could be recycled, delivering single-dose medications and materials from the pharmacy without plastic bags, standardizing smaller doses of hormone-based anti-inflammatory medications to avoid disposal of excess drugs, utilizing containers in the rooms for nonrecyclable waste, and training and alerting the team as to the sustainability efforts (Furukawa et al., 2016). Data were collected before and after the interventions.

Of particular note to advanced nurses was a reduction in material usage including plastic bags and leftover hormonal anti-inflammatory drugs. There were also improvements in appropriate waste disposal and the rate of label removal to allow for recycling of plastic bags. There was sharp decrease in total waste generation. Overall, the study provided a glimpse at the contributions of medication use systems to waste creation and resource utilization. The study also suggests that there are institutional barriers to ecological practices that require consideration by professionals other than or in addition to staff (Furukawa et al., 2016).

Advanced nurses working in all types of roles can positively influence the carbon footprint of the health care sector by building on the work of predecessors and taking full advantage of the rich resources freely available online. Published successes provide examples of projects, large and small, that could be implemented as first steps toward enhancing or creating interprofessional team experiences. The Green Operating Room Committee structure (Wormer et al., 2013) may offer a strategy for advanced nurses to create and lead a unit-based or department-based committee arrangement so that employees have an arrangement within which to work with colleagues to strategize novel and simple ways to reduce resource utilization or increase recycling productivity. Advanced nurses may also find support and ideas via coalitions and nonprofit organizations focused on sustainability and ecology efforts in the health care sector.

International Health Care Coalitions to Improve Environmental Stewardship

The Centre for Sustainable Healthcare (n.d.[a]) is a UK-registered charity that is working to support the National Health Service's efforts to reduce its carbon footprint by 80% by the year 2020. It offers programs designed to support sustainable health care models. The center is highly recognized for its sustainable specialties program and operates with four principles of sustainable clinical practice: specifically, prevention, patient empowerment and self-care, lean systems, and low carbon alternatives (Centre for Sustainable Healthcare, n.d.[b]). The center also runs a greenspace program designed to assist health care agencies with improving their natural environments and connecting their stakeholders, including the local community, with the health benefits derived from natural settings. One of the greenspace programs is NHS Forest, a popular initiative that works to open public access to health care organizations' green spaces while also planting trees, dementia gardens, orchards, and other sorts of naturally therapeutic environments in an effort to increase community health benefits gained from engaging with nature (Centre for Sustainable Healthcare, n.d.[c]).

Advanced nurses will find a variety of thought-provoking and useful resources freely available to them through the Centre for Sustainable Healthcare's website "Resource" tab (n.d.[d]). The resources include peer-reviewed publications that address a variety of topics that relate to sustainability efforts encompassing a wide range of topics, including but not limited to education, health care redesign effort, quality improvement, and climate change. There are interesting opportunities to explore sustainability efforts related to particular clinical care activities (e.g., green strategies used in kidney [dialysis] units). Some posted resources are PowerPoint presentations, case studies, videos, and other teaching aides that may be incorporated into health profession educational programs. These resources would likely serve as interesting additions to continuing education (CE) programs or self-study modules. Resources are freely shared; and because the Centre for Sustainable Healthcare is based in the United Kingdom, the international perspectives are interesting and thought provoking.

HCWH (2018a) is an international organization that seeks to transform the worldwide health care sector into an ecologically sustainable enterprise that provides uncompromisingly safe and effective patient care while protecting environmental health and justice. Its mission is to "[t]ransform health care worldwide so that it reduces its environmental footprint, becomes a community anchor for sustainability and a leader in the global movement for environmental health and justice" (HCWH, 2018a). The organization works to protect the public from climate change, to transform the supply chain across the globe to one that is ethical and sustainable in its practices, and to build leadership focused on environmental health. These goals are addressed through programs that include similar priorities of other health care groups interested in ecofriendly practices and sustainability, including efforts related to building design, chemicals, energy efficiency and cleanliness, food, pharmaceuticals, transportation, waste, and water (HCWH, 2018a).

HCWH (2017a) makes available its position paper on antimicrobial resistance via its website. The paper, "Antimicrobial Resistance: A HCWH Europe Position Paper," specifically addresses issues of antimicrobial resistance across Europe and around the world and asserts that this issue is one of the most concerning global public health threats. A key concern is the lack of alternative antimicrobial research and development over the past three decades leaving the global public at risk as increasing numbers of microbes develop resistance to the antimicrobial therapies that are currently available. This antimicrobial resistance is a priority HCWH concern and the position paper clearly describes the factors that contribute to the problem beginning with the drug manufacturing processes.

Advanced nurses are well advised to read this paper addressing antimicrobial resistance (HCWH, 2017a) and consider how each provider and health care system could participate in reducing the threat of antimicrobial resistance by targeting contributing factors that could be improved upon within the particular agency. While individual hospitals do not largely contribute to active pharmaceutical ingredient discharge into the environment via wastewater, they do have a responsibility to educate patients about the need to avoid improper disposal of antimicrobials in an effort to reduce the risk of resistance. There is also a need to increase public awareness of the dangers of unnecessarily prescribing antibiotic therapy for viral illnesses. Providers often need support from colleagues and agencies so that when they decline (sometimes insistent) requests for antibiotics to treat a viral illness, they have the very public support of the health care system and its leaders. The Centers for Disease Control and Prevention (CDC) offers materials for public display on viruses versus bacteria that are attractive, clearly written, and available at no cost other than printing expense (**FIGURE 6-2**).

Antibiotics are frequently used in the food chain to prevent infections that are largely the result of poor animal living conditions and to promote animal growth (HCWH, 2017b). A majority of the antibiotics used for livestock are important to human health. Some antibiotics are infrequently used in humans but are critically important as "last-ditch" efforts to combat infection that is not responding to first-line therapies. As livestock antibiotics are absorbed into the food chain, microbes develop resistance. Animal sources of human antimicrobial exposures are not the only trigger for resistance as nonanimal food sources may also be exposed to antimicrobials, including probiotics and raw food products (HCWH, 2017b).

Advanced nurses may be interested in opportunities to address antimicrobial resistance by reviewing the HCWH Europe recommendations and applying relevant recommendations to practice environments. The CDC (2017a) has created public information materials addressing antibiotic resistance and food safety (**FIGURE 6-3**). Its website provides useful information about how the public can protect itself from

Viruses or Bacteria
What's got you sick?

Antibiotics are only needed for treating certain infections caused by bacteria. Viral illnesses cannot be treated with antibiotics. When an antibiotic is not prescribed, ask your healthcare professional for tips on how to relieve symptoms and feel better.

Common Condition	Common Cause			Are Antibiotics Needed?
	Bacteria	Bacteria or Virus	Virus	
Strep throat	✔			Yes
Whooping cough	✔			Yes
Urinary tract infection	✔			Yes
Sinus infection		✔		Maybe
Middle ear infection		✔		Maybe
Bronchitis/chest cold (in otherwise healthy children and adults)*		✔		No*
Common cold/runny nose			✔	No
Sore throat (except strep)			✔	No
Flu			✔	No

* Studies show that in otherwise healthy children and adults, antibiotics for bronchitis won't help you feel better.

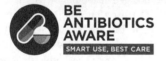

BE ANTIBIOTICS AWARE
SMART USE, BEST CARE

To learn more about antibiotic prescribing and use, visit www.cdc.gov/antibiotic-use.

FIGURE 6-2 Viruses or Bacteria: What's Got You Sick

foodborne illness and also makes available interesting educational materials, including audiovisual clips, instructing viewers on antibiotic resistance and food (CDC, 2017a).

One HCWH Europe (2017a) recommendation that is a potentially good first step as a hospital-based initiative is to establish awareness campaigns to (1) educate the public on correct administration and disposal of antimicrobials; (2) educate health professionals, prescribing and nonprescribing personnel, about responsible prescribing practices; and (3) educate farmers on the responsible use of antimicrobial drugs in agriculture and animal husbandry. Advanced nurses may have other ideas that relate to these awareness campaign content recommendations. Certainly spinoff projects could be tailored at unit and department levels in addition to hospital and health care system potential initiatives. The HCWH (2017a) recommendations are consistent with

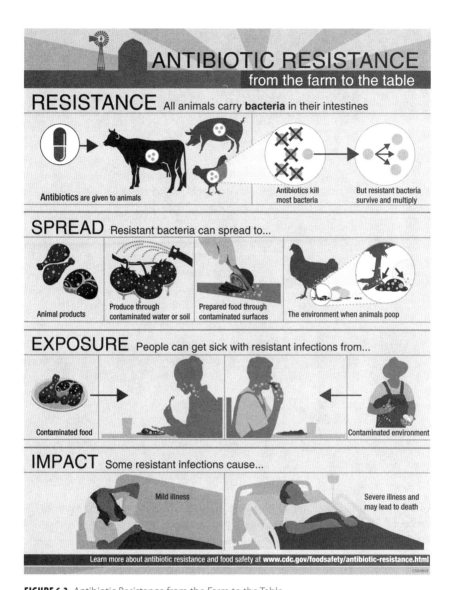

FIGURE 6-3 Antibiotic Resistance from the Farm to the Table

Reproduced from CDC. Antibiotic Resistance From The Farm To The Table. Retrieved January 23, 2018, from https://www.cdc.gov/foodsafety/pdfs/ar-infographic-508c.pdf

the CDC (2018) "Be Antibiotics Aware" national effort to curb antibiotic resistance and improve antibiotic prescribing and usage patterns (**TABLE 6-2**).

HCWH (2017b) offers a blog on its website that addresses many far-ranging topics that offer interesting and realistic ideas for advanced nurses to consider. One blog entry describes the major positive developments in animal welfare specific to boiler chicken production and the associated implications for health care systems (HCWH, 2017c). Sourcing animals from farmers via food service management companies that require antibiotic-free farming and humane animal husbandry practices is good for public health in general and certainly is a program that hospitals could tout as a component

TABLE 6-2 HCWH and CDC Public and Professional Antibiotic Resistance Information Campaigns

HCWH (2017a)	CDC (2018)
■ Educate the public on correct administration and disposal of antimicrobial therapies	■ U.S. Antibiotic Awareness Week (https://www.cdc.gov/antibiotic-use/week/index.html) ■ Federal Drug Administration (FDA): Disposal of Unused Medicines. What You Should Know (https://www.fda.gov/Drugs/Resources ForYou/Consumers/BuyingUsingMedicine Safely/EnsuringSafeUseofMedicine/Safe DisposalofMedicines/ucm186187.htm) ■ CDC refers public to FDA for drug wastage information
■ Educate prescribing and nonprescribing health professionals about responsible prescribing practices	■ Antibiotic Prescribing and Use in Doctors' Offices (https://www.cdc.gov/antibiotic-use/community/index.html) ■ Antibiotic Prescribing and Use in Hospitals and Long-term Care (https://www.cdc.gov/antibiotic-use/healthcare/index.html)
■ Educate farmers on the responsible use of antimicrobial drugs in agriculture and animal husbandry	■ Antibiotic Use and Food Safety (https://www.cdc.gov/foodsafety/challenges/antibiotic-resistance.html)

of its green initiatives. Another blog post touts the efforts to remove meat from the center of the hospital plate in an effort to promote good health while also addressing environmental concerns associated with meat production.

Nurses often educate patients and the public about the benefits of avoiding red meat, in particular, and usually construct this message within the context of cardio-vascular health. Embellishing this instruction with information about the cancer risks that are associated with some processed and highly salted meats and the adverse environmental effects of the meat production industry that is supported by meat consumption is an important responsibility of nurses, including those in advanced roles (Zuzelo, 2017). Deforestation, significant water consumption, and increased greenhouse gas emissions are also associated with the meat production industry; greenhouse emissions are estimated at 18% to 50%, as a direct outcome of animal production, not including the industrial wastage (Beverland, 2014; Cicatiello, De Rosa, Franco, & Lacetera, 2016). The ideas shared by bloggers on HHWH and other sites may lay the groundwork for hospital system or department discussions about strategies for enlarging the typical food service and dietary department choices to increase the variety of sustainably produced, local food products, including a greater variety of vegetable-based products.

Clean Energy Efforts in Health Care

The Hospital Energy Alliance (HEA) was launched by the Department of Energy (DOE) in 2009 and charged with increasing energy efficiency in the health care sector (Federal Information & News Dispatch, Inc., 2009). This federal partnership is designed to encourage the amalgamation of advanced energy efficiency and renewable technologies in the design, building, retrofit, operations, and maintenance of hospitals (Federal Information & News Dispatch, Inc., 2009). The press announcement notes that hospitals have more than 2.5 times the energy intensity and carbon dioxide emissions of commercial office buildings. Advanced nurses likely recognize the accuracy of this point given the technologies and supplies used on a routine basis to deliver around-the-clock care to patients often admitted with conditions that require significant resource utilization.

The HEA 2012 Annual Report notes 57 members and the creation of 15 technology fact sheets offering case studies and information about energy-efficient technologies as well as practices that hospitals and health care facilities might adopt. The report information is technical although readily understood. It does not address topics that are typically related to the work of advanced nurses; however, having an informed sense of the sorts of efforts that are moving ahead to encourage sustainability and energy efficiency in the health care sector is important to best appreciate the multifaceted approach, currently in relatively early stages, that stakeholders, including policy makers, regulatory agencies, and government departments, are using to address the significant energy consumption patterns of hospitals (HEA, 2012).

Advanced nurses may consider these initiatives and raise questions during hospital construction and refurbishing efforts. For example, the HEA 2012 report offers photos and brief descriptions of light-emitting diode (LED) technology for parking lots or LED refrigerated display cases. These two examples, parking lots and refrigerator cases in hospital food courts and cafeterias, are certainly relevant to the physical setting in which advanced nurses work. An appreciation for these efforts may facilitate informed conversations with colleagues and other professionals and provide a jump-off point for future chats about energy-saving possibilities.

▶ Tools Advanced Nurses Can Use to Support an Ecofriendly Agenda

There are many Web-based tools available to advanced nurses, most with no associated costs. Many websites offer opportunities to connect with like-minded health professionals and maximize benefits often obtained through networking.

The Nurses Climate Change Toolkit

There are toolkits, a package or bundle of resources, available to those nurses interested in working to improve the ecological circumstances of their practice and public environments. HCWH (2018b) offers *The Nurses Climate Change Toolkit* and makes the point that nurses are inevitably going to be at the front end of care delivery during health disasters that are the result of climate change (HCWH, 2018b). Given the complexities of climate changes, the toolkit addresses a broad array of topics and provides linkages to relevant organizations that can lead a nurse to resources and supports that are of particular interest to whatever initiative the nurse is considering.

HCWH's (2018b) toolkit resources offer links to scientific reports, webinars, *The Inconvenient Truth* video, and many peer-reviewed and science-driven publications. A primer (Maibach, Nisbet, & Weathers, 2011) is freely available to inform conversations, policy, and education efforts that health practitioners, including advanced nurses, need to have with the public and with officials about the impact of climate change on societal health outcomes. The primer is clearly written and offers guidance to health care professionals regarding effective messaging. For example, Maibach et al. (2011) make the point that these sorts of discussions are often more effective when the key premise relates to climate change as a health concern rather than as an environmental issue. The authors assert that it is important for nurses to make the case that climate change is a local issue, not only a global or planet concern. The primer suggests that nurses and other health professionals need to engage in policy-level work, including writing letters to the editor, speaking to policy makers, contributing to social media, and searching for opportunities to share expertise on climate change and its impact on human health (Maibach et al., 2011). There are many opportunities for advanced nurses to contribute to the public dialogue of climate change and health. These opportunities also provide platforms for advanced nurses to partner with other health professionals in creating collaboratively developed messaging within a health care system and in the public and policy domains.

The Alliance of Nurses for Healthy Environments (ANHE) provides resources and networking opportunities via its website (http://envirn.org/) (ANHE, 2017a) and its social media connections, including Facebook page (ANHE, 2017b). ANHE emphasizes the powerful responsibility that nurses have to the public specific to environment health in light of nurses' status as the public's most trusted information source (ANHE, 2017a). Its mission is "[p]romoting healthy people and healthy environments by educating and leading the nursing profession, advancing research, incorporating evidence-based practice, and influencing policy" (AHNE, 2017a). ANHE (2017a) began in 2008 and was organized using working group structure, including four main groups: Education, Practice, Research, Policy/Advocacy. It is a global organization and is rich with resources for nurses striving to positively influence environmental health.

Advanced nurses practicing in roles with an educational focus will find helpful the electronic textbook, *Environmental Health in Nursing* (Leffers, Smith, Huffling, McDermott-Levy, & Sattler, 2016). This e-textbook was selected as the 2017 AJN Book of the Year in the environmental nursing category (ANHE, 2017c). It is freely available for download in portable document format (pdf) and is appropriate for worldwide use. The hyperlinks are robust and connect the reader to leading environmental organizations and cutting-edge science and reports. The e-book was developed to address the 1995 Institute of Medicine (IOM) recommendations offered in its report, *Nursing, Health, and The Environment*. Leffers et al. (2016) point out that the IOM report notes the lack of mandatory education on the environment and health in nursing education. The book delivers this content in a style and format that advanced nurses will find useful across various types and levels of nursing education and, likely, in CE program departments as well.

The ANHE Practice Workgroup's efforts focus on assisting nurses to practice in an environmentally safe and healthy fashion (ANHE, 2017d). The group has a listserv available to those who sign up for the Practice Workgroup. The group seeks to develop networks and provides webinars. Advanced nurses may be interested in joining this group and sharing project possibilities, successes, and challenges.

Nurses are increasingly called upon to maximize their voices by participating in policy and advocacy efforts. These efforts may be in the board room or may be manifested through expert testimony, leadership efforts in practice settings, or engaged participation in professional organizations. The Policy-Advocacy Workgroup of ANHE (2017e) aspires to advocate for public and environmental health. As with the Practice Workgroup, there is a listserv available to those who join the workgroup. Keep in mind that this organization was initiated less than 10 years ago. The work is important and certainly offers an opportunity for advanced nurses to begin in small ways while incrementally building their networks, supporting coalitions, and crafting expert messages based on developing expertise. Relatively new organizations often provide many opportunities and getting to know colleagues and work with like-minded people can be a terrific way for advanced nurses to move in new or interesting professional directions!

ANHE also provides CE opportunities that advanced nurses may want to consider as individual learning experiences or, perhaps, as a CE possibility for staff or colleagues. One topic, "Advancing Clean Air, Climate, & Health: Opportunities for Nurses," includes media modules and a workbook. Another 1-hour CE program addresses "Defending the EPA—How Nurses Can Take Action and Make a Difference." CE posttests are provided to ensure knowledge acquisition and to satisfy CE credit requirements (ANHE, 2017f).

Other ANHE (2017a) engagement opportunities include an active blog, periodic newsletter, and opportunity to donate to forward the organizational cause. The blog posts often provide good information that would be useful to advanced nurses looking for a place to begin environmental efforts within their departments or systems. One posting offers recommendations for reducing energy consumption and discusses the impact of purchasing decisions on sustainability (Schenk, 2017). Another blog shares the writer's experience with advocacy and makes the case that many people often find themselves in situations that are unknown to them but there are people and resources available if you reach out (Campbell, 2017). The blog post was a clear reminder that many environmental issues would benefit from nurses' keen problem-solving abilities. These blogs provide opportunities for advanced nurses who are feeling some uncertainty and trepidation but a determination to positively influence environmentally friendly health care practices.

Collaborative on Health and the Environment

The Collaborative on Health and the Environment (CHE) is a network of health-related groups and others with a common interest in environmental influences on health conditions. The CHE mission is to "cultivate a learning community based on the latest, evidence-based science to share knowledge and resources, and improve individual and collective health" (2018a). CHE is focused on how environmental risks can impact human health. By informing and connecting affected and interested groups, CHE hopes to build a groundswell of demand for prevention-focused behaviors and policies, as well as economic and legal structures that protect public health (CHE, 2018a). The organization prioritizes science efforts related to chemical exposures and its relationship to certain health outcomes. It provides open-access, science-driven information. CHE values the contributions of diverse organizations with an interest in environmental health. It is a rigorous, science-based network that offers unbiased, critically analyzed science-based findings to facilitate environmentally focused initiatives that promote human and ecological health (CHE, 2018a). It is interesting to note that some CHE founders are active leaders in previously mentioned environmental groups, including HCWH.

The CHE webinar resources are rich and available for viewing in multimedia format with links to slides, publications, and other resources. Recent webinars include the presentations "Chemicals in Consumer Products: Exposure Science at the Forefront of Regulation," "Successive Generations of Estrogenic Exposure and Male Reproductive Health," and "How Trump's Proposed EPA Budget Cuts Threaten Clean Air, Clean Water, and Public Health" (CHE, 2017b). CHE (2017b) also provides numerous podcasts of *Partnership Calls* that cover an array of topics to provide opportunities for sharing and exploring emerging science on environmental contributors to disease and disability. There are many opportunities for learning posted in the "News and Announcements" section of the website (CHE, 2017c) and the publications and reports have linkages to Medscape or other access sources (e.g., a summary of what is currently known about Alzheimer's prevention, the relationship of autism and the environment, or findings from a study linking the nicotine in e-cigs to an increased risk of heart disease are readily available via the CHE-provided hyperlinks).

CHE (2018d) provides a searchable *Toxicant and Disease Database* that describes the linkage between chemicals and close to 200 human diseases or conditions. The database represents the current understanding about toxicants and disease. Information is categorized by the strength of evidence and is labeled as strong, good, or limited/conflicting. The database was last updated in 2011 and while some information may be outdated, it is a dynamic database and work is underway to ascertain how maintenance should be best handled. Nonetheless, the database is a useful start and there are plenty of materials and links to other databases and resources.

Advanced nurses with a particular interest in evidence-based practice, science, and particular chemicals or diseases/chronic illness may find CHE's (2018e) SciencScience eServs useful. CHE has crafted the ScienceServs listservs as collaborative networking opportunities for nurses, advocates, researchers, public health professionals, and other providers (CHE, 2018e). There are many listserv topics, including asthma, autism, cancer, children's environmental health, climate and planetary issues, diabetes and obesity, electromagnetic fields, environmental health science, healthy aging, integrative healthy, learning and developmental disabilities, and reproductive health (CHE, 2018e). Instructions to join are provided for each individual list topic. There is also a signup opportunity for quarterly newsletters and monthly webinar announcements. Interested advanced nurses may wish to subscribe to the CHE newsfeed as well.

The American Nurses Association: Practice Safe Practice Healthfully

The American Nurses Association (ANA, 2018) provides some resources addressing environmental health, although these Web-based reserves are few in number. Online resources include a link to the CDC National Center for Environmental Health (NCEH) and its robust big data resources (CDC, 2017b). This repository for environmental public health data provides access for data that can be downloaded directly from the

Internet. There are data sets that relate to health, biomonitoring, and environment with links to available query engines. The engines can search and locate information about watersheds, toxins, cancer incidence and survival rates, and other data that may be of interest to advanced nurses. The National Environmental Public Health Tracking Network (2017b) is also linked to the ANA website, and it may be used to examine health and environmental data by utilizing the query tool or to view information that is sorted by county. Links are also provided to state and local tracking websites.

The ANA also provides other links to the EPA's website, *Children's Environmental Health: Online Resources for Healthcare Providers* (EPA, 2017). This EPA resource provides robust, current information that pertains to many environmental issues that affect children's health including mercury, lead, asthma, and other topics. A pediatric environmental health toolkit, training package for health care providers, and multimedia products are also available via this EPA site.

Several ANA resolutions addressing environmental policies and positions are available via the Environmental Health webpage (**TABLE 6-3**). There is also a printable document describing the Principles of a Healthy, Sustainable Food system that was developed by the ANA in a collaborative partnership with the Academy of Nutrition

TABLE 6-3 ANA Resolutions Related to Environmental Health		
Resolution Name	**Year**	**Web Address**
Global Climate Change and Human Health	2008	http://www.nursingworld.org/MainMenu Categories/WorkplaceSafety/Healthy-Work -Environment/Environmental-Health /GlobalClimateChangeandHuman Health.pdf
Healthy Food in Health Care	2008	http://www.nursingworld.org/MainMenu Categories/WorkplaceSafety/Healthy-Work -Environment/Environmental-Health /HealthyFoodinHealthCare.pdf
Nurses' Role in Recognizing Educating and Advocating for Health Energy Choices	2012	http://www.nursingworld.org/MainMenu Categories/WorkplaceSafety/Healthy-Work -Environment/Environmental-Health/ nurses-role-in-recognizing-educating -advocating-healthy-energy-choices.pdf
Inappropriate Use of Antimicrobials in Agriculture	2004	http://www.nursingworld.org/MainMenu Categories/WorkplaceSafety/Healthy -Work-Environment/Environmental-Health /ANAResolution.pdf
Safety and Effectiveness of Reprocessed Single Use Devices in Health Care	2010	http://www.nursingworld.org/MainMenu Categories/WorkplaceSafety/Healthy-Work -Environment/Environmental-Health/Single -Use-Devices.pdf

and Dietetics, American Planning Association (APA), and American Public Health Association. The end product of this collaboration provides a comprehensive overview of critical components necessary to a healthy, sustainable food system (APA, 2010).

The ANA provides a link to ANHE and describes it as a global network of nurses who are acting on the idea that environment and health are inextricably bound. Other links and policy updates or newsfeed information related to environmental health is available via the website but locating them is easiest using the search feature to guide the effort. There is not much else available to an advanced nurse on the ANA website specific to environmental health but one key reminder is that practicing in an environmentally safe and healthy manner is a standard of nursing care and it needs to be followed as such (ANA, 2015).

The Medical Society Consortium on Climate and Health

The Medical Society Consortium on Climate and Health (the Consortium) is an interesting and health-relevant site with a name that belies its relevance to nursing practice. Its website speaks to "doctors and nurses" as well as the broader "medical community." The consortium represents a variety of professional organizations that represent approximately 400,000 clinical practitioners with the goal of relaying three key messages to the public: (1) Climate change is harming Americans and these adverse effects will continue to increase if not addressed; (2) decreasing fossil fuel usage, increasing energy use efficiency, and using clean energy sources are the ways to reduce the harms of climate change; and (3) making these changes in energy choices will improve air and water quality and facilitate immediate health benefits (the Consortium, 2017a).

The Consortium offers many multimedia resources that are visually powerful and interesting. Resources are presented in a variety of formats including presentation slides, posters, and fact sheets. Content is consistent with the Consortium's three-point messaging priorities. Educational materials are designed for community residents, patients, and colleagues (the Consortium, 2017b). One presentation for colleagues, entitled *Communicating Effectively as a Health Professional*, provides well-crafted instruction on effectively conveying important ideas and emphasizes, "Simple clear messages, repeated often, by a variety of trusted voices" as a guiding principle (Maibach, 2017, slide 2). The presentation provides the viewer with excellent advice on *how* to deliver climate change messages in ways that attract and entice listeners rather than turning them off from the message.

Most advanced nurses have not been exposed to this sort of instruction about effective message delivery and would likely benefit from this presentation. Science informs the presentation, and Maibach (2017) takes into account key beliefs about climate change and recognizes the wide range of beliefs, worries, and motivation in the public related to the climate change message. Overall, this presentation is one example of many powerful opportunities for nurses in advanced roles to enhance their messaging effectiveness on environmental influences on health outcomes.

The patient education resources (the Consortium, 2017c) are available in downloadable pdf format. Topics include heat, asthma, asthma and climate change in both English and Spanish forms, and a health fact paper on the effects of global warming on ragweed allergies, air pollution, and asthma. The patient education resources are from outside agencies including the American Thoracic Society, Natural Resources Defense Fund, Kendrick Fincher Hydration Foundation, and others (the Consortium, 2017c).

The Consortium's resources are robust, likely advantaged by the partnering across an array of health-related organizations including, but not limited to, physician-driven member organizations (specifically the National Medical Association, American Academy of Pediatrics, American Academy of Family Physicians and affiliate groups that include the ANHE, Asthma and Allergy Foundation of America, Health Professionals for a Healthy Climate, and HCWH). The Consortium encourages physicians, nurses, and other professionals to become activists and promoters for climate and health in their communities. Advanced nurses may wish to sign up to become an advocate. The Consortium's overarching goal is to connect with health professionals who are willing to step up and explain to their community stakeholders—including government officials, journalists, local business leaders, and others—about the harmful effects of climate change and the positive health effects associated with rapid transitioning to clean renewable energy sources (the Consortium, 2017d).

The Consortium offers tangible supports for advanced nurses who may be interested in this advocacy role. Resources are provided for contacting policy makers and for writing editorials. Questions on climate change and health are offered by the Consortium as a resource to guide conversations with policy makers. These queries are based on the climate change and health position paper of the American College of Physicians (Crowley, 2016). The Consortium provides a sample letter addressing state-level clean power plan possibilities and also linkages to congressional representatives. The "Write Letters to the Editor" section (the Consortium, 2017e) of the website provides excellent examples of opinion editorials that have been authored by physicians. Frankly, advanced nurses and professional nursing staff need to be encouraged to contribute to editorial submissions. Nurses are trusted, persuasive, and pragmatic; people hold nurses in high esteem and believe that nurses have the public's best interests at heart. This sentiment is evidenced by the numerous Gallup polls, including the December 2016 survey that found nurses rated as having higher honesty and ethical standards than most other professionals (Gallup, Inc., 2017). Advocating for the climate and better health is a reasonable extension of the health promotion and disease prevention expertise of advanced nurses and it is likely that community members will respond to the message in part because of the messenger!

The Consortium published a report on the adverse effects of climate change on health (Sarfaty, Gould, & Maibach, 2017). The report is endorsed by many medical societies and it flows between reader-friendly data summarization, well-written narratives by preeminent physicians, and personal accounts of harmful climate change experiences on health. Overall, it is a report that makes an impression. Photos provide visual context and help the reader identify with the message. The report does not mention nurses and, given that the member organizations of the Consortium are physician associations, the lack of inclusivity is not surprising. However, the report has an influential and relevant message that could be used as one part of an advanced nurse's efforts to educate colleagues, patients, administrators, and communities. It is a downloadable report that is freely available.

▶ Conclusion

Advanced nurses are confronted with many opportunities to encourage ecological health care practices. Small, incremental changes in sustainability practices and reduced consumption patterns contribute to dramatic systemwide environmental benefits. Advanced nurses are in an ideal position to persuade and encourage colleagues, patients, and administrators to step up and contribute to environmental improvements that benefit the greater good, locally and internationally. Nursing students and other health care profession students need to be more fully educated about environmental stewardship and advanced nurses can certainly contribute to this effort via the formal roles as educators, instructors, managers, and providers but also through informal role modeling. Environmental workplace projects provide ideal circumstances for interprofessional collaboration efforts that could include students and even involve practice–academic partnerships. With much at stake, advanced nurses are encouraged to consider available possibilities for correcting green-gaps by leading or collaborating on environmental issues. Professional organizations, Web-based materials, and networking offer supports needed for beginning the sustainability, deconsumption journey.

References

Alliance of Nurses for Healthy Environments. (2017a). About. Retrieved January 23, 2018, from http://envirn.org/about/.

Alliance of Nurses for Healthy Environments. (2017b). Facebook homepage. Retrieved January 23, 2018, from https://www.facebook.com/allianceofnursesforhealthyenvironments/?ref=nf&hc_ref=ARRk2zi4PYMtLDtMk_dvnRPs41fAE0Ig8Xv_ghyFQ5hkn1mM8sbiGLgJ8w6Qi2YZhGI

Alliance of Nurses for Healthy Environments. (2017c). E-textbook. Environmental health in nursing. Retrieved January 23, 2018, from https://envirn.org/e-textbook/.

Alliance of Nurses for Healthy Environments (2017d). Practice workgroup. Retrieved January 23, 2018, from http://envirn.org/practice/.

Alliance of Nurses for Healthy Environments. (2017e). Policy-advocacy. Retrieved January 23, 2018, from https://envirn.org/policy-advocacy/.

Alliance of Nurses for Healthy Environments. (2017f). Continuing education. Retrieved January 23, 2018, from http://envirn.org/category/continuing-education/.

American Nurses Association. (2015). Scope and standards of practice (3rd ed.). Silver Spring, MD: ANA NursesBooks, Publishers.

American Nurses Association. (2018). Environmental health. Retrieved January 23, 2018, from http://www.nursingworld.org/rnnoharm.

American Planning Association. (2010). Principles of a healthy, sustainable food system. Retrieved January 23, 2018, from https://planning-org-uploaded-media.s3.amazonaws.com/legacy_resources/nationalcenters/health/pdf/HealthySustainableFoodSystemsPrinciples_2012May.pdf.

Beverland, M. B. (2014). Sustainable eating: Mainstreaming plant-based diets in developed economies. *Journal of Macromarketing, 34,* 369–382. doi:10.1177/0276146714526410 Campbell, L. (2017. May 19). Blog. A call to advocacy! Oh my goodness now what do I do? Retrieved January 23, 2018, from http://envirn.org/a-call-to-advocacy-oh-my-goodness-now-what-do-i-do/.

Centers for Disease Control and Prevention. (2017a). Antibiotic resistance and food safety. Retrieved January 23, 2018, from https://www.cdc.gov/foodsafety/challenges/antibiotic-resistance.html.

Centers for Disease Control and Prevention. (2017b). National Environmental Public Health Tracking Network. Retrieved January 23, 2018, from https://ephtracking.cdc.gov/showHome.action.

Centers for Disease Control and Prevention. (2018). Antibiotics prescribing and use. Be antibiotics aware. Retrieved January 23, 2018, from https://www.cdc.gov/antibiotic-use/.

Centre for Sustainable Healthcare. (n.d.[a]). Who we are. Retrieved January 23, 2018, from http://sustainablehealthcare.org.uk/who-we-are.

Centre for Sustainable Healthcare. (n.d.[b]). What we do. Retrieved January 23, 2018, from http://sustainablehealthcare.org.uk/what-we-do.

Centre for Sustainable Healthcare. (n.d.[c]). NHS forest. Retrieved January 23, 2018, from http://sustainablehealthcare.org.uk/what-we-do/green-space/nhs-forest.

Centre for Sustainable Healthcare. (n.d.[d]). Resources. Retrieved January 23, 2018, from https://sustainablehealthcare.org.uk/resources.

Cicatiello, C., De Rosa, B., Franco, S., & Lacetera, N. (2016). Consumer approach to insects as food: Barriers and potential for consumption in Italy. *British Food Journal, 118*, 2271–2286. doi:10.1108/BFJ-01-2016-0015

Climate Action. (n.d.). Find out more about COP21. Retrieved January 22, 2018, from http://www.cop21paris.org/about/cop21.

Collaborative on Health and the Environment. (2018a). Mission, vision, & values. Retrieved May 3, 2018, from https://www.healthandenvironment.org/about/mission-vision-and-values/

Collaborative on Health and the Environment. (2018b). Webinars. Retrieved January 23, 2018, from https://www.healthandenvironment.org/our-work/webinars/.

Collaborative on Health and the Environment. (2018c). In the news. Retrieved January 23, 2018, from https://www.healthandenvironment.org/environmental-health/in-the-news.

Collaborative on Health and the Environment. (2018d). Toxicant and disease database. Retrieved January 23, 2018, from https://www.healthandenvironment.org/our-work/toxicant-and-disease-database/.

Collaborative on Health and the Environment. (2018e). ScienceServs overview. Retrieved January 23, 2018, from https://www.healthandenvironment.org/our-work/scienceservs.

Cook, J., Nuccitelli, D., Green, S. A., Richardson, M., Winkler, B., Painting, R., . . . Skuce, A. (2013). Quantifying the consensus on anthropogenic global warming in the scientific literature. *Environmental Research Letters, 8*(2), 1–7. doi:10.1088/1748-9326/8/2/024024

Crowley, R. A., for the Health and Public Policy Committee of the American College of Physicians. (2016). Climate change and health: A position paper of the American College of Physicians. *Annals of Internal Medicine, 164*, 608–610. doi:10.7326/M15-2766

Environmental Protection Agency. (2018). Reduce, reuse, recycle. Retrieved January 22, 2018, from https://www.epa.gov/recycle.

Federal Information & News Dispatch, Inc. (2009). Department of energy announces the launch of the hospital energy alliance to increase energy efficiency in the healthcare sector. Retrieved January 23, 2018, from https://www.energy.gov/articles/department-energy-announces-launch-hospital-energy-alliance-increase-energy-efficiency.

Furukawa, P., Cunha, I., Pedreira, M., & Marck, P. (2016). Environmental sustainability in medication processes performed in hospital nursing care. *Acta Paul Enferm, 29*, 316–324. doi:10.1590/1982-0194201600043

Gallup, Inc. (2017). *Honesty/ethics in professions*. Retrieved October 3, 2017, from http://news.gallup.com/poll/1654/honesty-ethics-professions.aspx.

Healthcare Without Harm. (2017a). Antimicrobial resistance. A HCWH Europe position paper. Retrieved January 23, 2018, from https://noharm-europe.org/sites/default/files/documents-files/5037/2017-10-09_HCWH_Europe_PositionPaper_AMR.pdf.

Healthcare Without Harm. (2017b). Latest blog content. Retrieved January 23, 2018, from https://noharm-uscanada.org/feeds/article/blog.

Healthcare Without Harm. (2017c). Major food service management companies help to fill the GAP for hospital chicken needs. Retrieved January 23, 2018, from https://noharm-uscanada.org/articles/blog/us-canada/major-food-service-management-companies-help-fill-gap-hospital-chicken-needs.

Healthcare Without Harm. (2018a). About us. Retrieved May 3, 2018, from https://noharm-uscanada.org/content/us-canada/mission-and-goals.

Healthcare Without Harm. (2018b). Nurses climate change toolkit. Retrieved January 23, 2018, from https://noharm-uscanada.org/content/us-canada/nurses-climate-change-toolkit.

Healthier Hospitals. (2012, January 25). Leaner energy. Retrieved May 3, 2018, from http://healthierhospitals.org/hhi-challenges/leaner-energy.

Healthier Hospitals. (2013, April 4). About. Retrieved January 22, 2018, from http://healthierhospitals.org/about-hh.

Healthier Hospitals. (2014). 2014 milestones report. Retrieved January 22, 2018, from https://practicegreenhealth.org/sites/default/files/upload-files/fnl_hhi_milestone_report_061015_lores.pdf.

Healthier Hospitals. (2015, December 3). Safer chemicals. Retrieved May 3, 2018, from http://healthierhospitals.org/hhi-challenges/safer-chemicals.

Healthier Hospitals. (2016). *List of furniture and materials that meet the HH healthy interiors goal, version 1.0*. Retrieved from http://www.healthierhospitals.org/hhi-challenges/safer-chemicals/list-furniture-and-materials-meet-hh-healthy-interiors-goal/version.

Healthier Hospitals. (n.d.). HH challenges. Retrieved January 22, 2018, from http://healthierhospitals.org/hhi-challenges.

Hospital Energy Alliance. (2012). *2012 annual report.* Retrieved January 23, 2018, from https://www1
.eere.energy.gov/buildings/publications/pdfs/alliances/hea_annual_report_2012.pdf.

Laestadius, L. I., & Caldwell, M. A. (2015). Is the future of meat palatable? Perceptions of in vitro
meat as evidenced by online news comments. *Public Health Nurse, 18,* 2457–2467. doi:10.1017
/S1368980015000622

Leffers, J., Smith, C. M., Huffling, K., McDermott-Levy, R., & Sattler, B. (Eds.). (2016). *Environmental
health in nursing.* Mount Rainier, MD: Alliance of Nurses for Healthy Environments.

Maibach, E. (2017, May). Communicating effectively as a health professional about climate change,
clean energy & health. PowerPoint presentation. Retrieved January 23, 2018, from http://
medsocietiesforclimatehealth.org/wp-content/uploads/2017/06/CommunicatingClimateHealth
-20171.pdf.

Maibach E., Nisbet, M., & Weathers, M. (2011). Conveying the human implications of climate change: A
climate change communication primer for public health professionals. Fairfax, VA: George Mason
University Center for Climate Change Communication.

Manadhana N. (2015, October 20). Dalai Lama: Combating climate change a matter of 'survival of
humanity.' *Wall Street Journal.* Retrieved January 22, 2018, from http://www.wsj.com/articles/dalai
-lama-combating-climate-change-a-matter-of-survival-of-humanity-1445358872.

National Aeronautics and Space Administration. (n.d.). Global climate change. Vital signs of the
planet. 2016. Retrieved January 22, 2018, from http://climate.nasa.gov/scientific-consensus.

Nightingale, F. (1946). *Notes on nursing: What it is, and what it is not.* New York: Appleton-Century.

Partners Healthcare. (n.d.). Sustainable campus at Assembly Row. Retrieved January 23, 2018, from
http://www.partners.org/Innovation-And-Leadership/Sustainability/Sustainable-Campus-AR.aspx.

Peregrin, T. (2015, May 1). Strategies for sustainability: Going green in the OR. *Bulletin of the
American College of Surgeons.* Retrieved October 5, 2017, from http://bulletin.facs.org/2015/05
/strategies-for-sustainability-going-green-in-the-or/.

Practice Greenhealth. (2018a). About. Retrieved January 22, 2018, from https://practicegreenhealth.org/

Practice Greenhealth. (2018b). Mission and vision. Retrieved January 22, 2018, from https://
practicegreenhealth.org/about/mission.

Practice Greenhealth. (2018c). Less waste. Retrieved January 23, 2018, from https://practicegreenhealth
.org/topics/less-waste.

Practice Greenhealth. (2018d). Greenhealth academy. Retrieved January 23, 2018, from https://
academy.practicegreenhealth.org/index.php.

Riedel, A. (2016). Sustainability as an ethical principle: Ensuring its systematic place in professional
nursing practice. *Healthcare, 4*(1), 2. doi:10.3390/healthcare4010002

Sarfaty, M., Gould, R., & Maibach, E. (2017). Medical alert! Climate change is harming our health.
The Medical Society Consortium on Climate and Health. Fairfax, VA: George Mason University
Center for Climate Change Communication. Retrieved January 23, 2018, from https://medsocieties
forclimatehealth.org/wpcontent/uploads/2017/03/gmu_medical_alert_updated_082417.pdf.

Schenk, B. (2017, March 7). Blog. Reducing the environmental impacts of healthcare and nursing
practice. Retrieved January 23, 2018, from http://envirn.org/reducing-the-environmental
-impacts-of-healthcare-and-nursing-practice/.

Southorn, R., Norrish, A. R., Gardner, K., & Baxandall, R. (2013). Reducing the carbon footprint of
the operating theatre: A multicenter quality improvement report. *The Journal of Perioperative
Practice, 23,* 6, 144–146.

The Holy Father Francis. (2015). Encyclical letter. *Laudato si' of the Holy Father Francis on care for our
common home* (official English-language text of encyclical). Rome, Italy: Vatican Press. Retrieved
January 22, 2018, from http://w2.vatican.va/content/dam/francesco/pdf/encyclicals/documents
/papa-francesco_20150524_enciclica-laudato-si_en.pdf.

The Local. (2017, May 1). Locusts for dinner? Switzerland allows sale of insect-based foods. Retrieved January 22,
2018, from https://www.thelocal.ch/20170501/locusts-for-dinner-switzerland-allows-sale-of-insect-based-foods.

The Medical Society Consortium on Climate and Health. (2017a). About. Retrieved January 23, 2018,
from https://medsocietiesforclimatehealth.org/about/.

The Medical Society Consortium on Climate and Health. (2017b). For your colleagues. Resources for
educating your colleagues. Retrieved January 23, 2018, from http://medsocietiesforclimatehealth.
org/educate/colleagues/.

The Medical Society Consortium on Climate and Health. (2017c). For your patients. Retrieved January 23, 2018, from http://medsocietiesforclimatehealth.org/educate/patients/.

The Medical Society Consortium on Climate and Health. (2017d). Become an advocate for climate and health. Retrieved January 23, 2018, from https://medsocietiesforclimatehealth.org/become -champion-climate-health/.

The Medical Society Consortium on Climate and Health. (2017e). Write letters to the editor. Retrieved October 3, 2017, from http://medsocietiesforclimatehealth.org/take-action/write-op-eds-letters-editor/.

World Health Organization. (n.d.). Climate change and human health. Retrieved January 22, 2018, from http://www.who.int/globalchange/global-campaign/cop21/en/.

World Health Organization. (2015). Media-centre. Health-care waste. Fact sheet number 253. Retrieved January 22, 2018, from www.who.int/mediacentre/factsheets/fs253/en/.

Wormer, B., Augenstein, V., Carpenter, C., Burton, P., Yokeley, W., Prabhu, A., . . . Heniford, B. (2013). The green operating room: Simple changes to reduce cost and our carbon footprint. *The American Surgeon, 79*, 666–671.

van Huis, A., Itterbeeck, J. V., Klunder, H., Mertens, E., Halloran, A., Muir, G., & Vantomme, P. (2013). Edible insects: Future prospects for food and feed security. Food and Agriculture Organization of the United Nations: Rome. Retrieved January 23, 2018, from http://www.fao.org/docrep/018 /i3253e/i3253e.pdf.

Zuzelo, P. R. (2016). Sustaining nature's healing powers. *Holistic Nursing Practice, 3*, 187–189.

Zuzelo, P. R. (2017). Animal proteins: Challenges and opportunities beyond "avoiding red meat." *Holistic Nursing Practice, 31*, 201–212.

CHAPTER 7

Effectively Educating to Transform Health and the Healthcare System

Patti Rager Zuzelo, EdD, RN, ACNS-BC, ANP-BC, CRNP, FAAN

Education is a critically important enterprise to the health care system and is presumed to directly affect the quality of patient care, systems functions, and institutional efficiencies. It can be expensive to develop effective, meaningful education programs, but it is also expensive to educate poorly. High costs associated with a failure to educate include the select liabilities associated with failures in practitioner competency, deteriorating health of patients unable to adequately manage self-care activities due to knowledge deficiencies, and poor publicity or civil suits associated with discriminatory practices or privacy violations in part based on underlying knowledge gaps.

Traditional modes of formal staff education and in-service programming include classroom lecture, continuing education articles with posttests, and unit-based workshops. For the most part, these learning opportunities are packaged in a one-size-fits-all format with little attention paid to experience, age, preferred learning style, culture, or gender. Learning disabilities are rarely, if ever, considered.

Staff is assigned or compelled to attend programs deemed as mandatory. Programs are often offered while nurses have colleagues cover their patient assignments, and attendance at many workshops is often poor. Educators, including advanced nurses responsible for staff development, quality improvement, and educational programming of other sorts, charged with providing these programs typically lament the poor participation and the low rate of return on the expensive investment of time. Oftentimes administrators and other nurse leaders insist on repeated program offerings to increase attendance figures and demonstrate competence so as to satisfy accrediting and regulatory agencies and to reduce liability exposure.

Advanced nurses often have responsibilities for teaching patients and families, either directly or indirectly. Patient education concerns differ from those associated with staff education, and yet there are commonalities. Classroom-based instructional programs for patients, families, and community residents are not uncommon. Teaching experiences often follow established routines, including the use of pamphlets, videotapes, and lecture with pretest and posttest evaluation designs. Attendance at post discharge or preadmission programs is not a guarantee, and health care professionals decry the perceived disinterest or other barriers to learning. Discharge teaching is offered quickly and supplemented by printed instructions, possibly designed with grade-level readability in mind but perhaps without consideration of overall health literacy concerns.

Nursing students, particularly undergraduates, are taught in clinical settings and are influenced by advanced nurses, including clinical nurse specialists, unit educators, charge nurses, staff development specialists, managers, and other leaders. These advanced professionals facilitate a context of learning within the institution or teach as adjunct faculty, instructors, or professors of nursing. Those who educate may teach as they have been taught using traditional methods of instruction in tried-and-true formats. These teaching strategies may include preconferences, postconferences, or instructor-directed labs and lectures. Advanced practice registered nurses (APRNs) are in an ideal position to teach graduate nursing students during clinical practicum experiences because their role requires a current knowledge base and the wherewithal to recognize and promote safe clinical decision making. Other advanced nurses may teach didactic content to graduate students or both clinical and classroom materials to undergraduate students. However, many APRNs and other nurses with advanced educational preparation are unfamiliar with the role of the adjunct faculty member and its associated responsibilities, including processes of student evaluation. They may also be unfamiliar with active teaching strategies, including problem-based learning or simulation. It may be quite difficult for advanced nurses to keep up with nursing education literature in addition to the role and specialty content that is critical to their practice. As a result, nurses with some stake in direct education may be unaware of cutting-edge topics in education.

Relatively new computer technologies are affecting several of these scenarios in positive ways. Web-enhanced learning, distance education learning platforms, intranet opportunities, patient model simulations, and smart classrooms are enhancing the attractiveness of education programs by engaging learners in a variety of instructional modalities that appeal to multiple senses. The need for real-time or synchronous education is often minimized with Web-based or distance teaching/learning and nurses can take advantage of completing academic work efforts at a time that suits individual schedules. The Web has dramatically increased the amount of information available to patients, families, and staff. While patients and providers are satisfied with the easy information access, professionals worry about potential misinformation and overwhelming volumes of data. Many hospitals offer patients, families, and community residents various opportunities to access health materials via learning laboratories and public computer stations.

This chapter addresses issues relevant to the education component of advanced nursing practice. Many nurses with graduate degrees are practicing in staff development roles within nursing education departments. Advanced nurses working within a product line or care program practice arrangement may find themselves participating in or orchestrating programs for nursing staff, patients and family, community, interdisciplinary team members, and other individuals operating within the health care system. Many nurses with master's or doctoral degrees teach undergraduate or graduate students of nursing. Advanced nurses with doctoral preparation are often employed as professors of nursing, with some having opportunities to practice in joint arrangements with clinical affiliates.

▶ Patient and Community Education

A Description of the Challenge: Literacy in the United States

Nurses are generally aware of the complexities of the English language and recognize that it is a difficult language to master, particularly once people have reached adulthood (**BOX 7-1**). Becoming literate is a more challenging endeavor than the acquisition of conversation skills (**FIGURE 7-1**). Health literacy is related to language literacy but is different, both in its components and in its usages. Health literacy is an important concern with significant practice implications for nurses in advanced roles and for those at the sharp point of direct care.

Many advanced nurses are directly involved in patient education programs, either inpatient, outpatient, or through public health initiatives. This involvement requires them to have a clear understanding of health literacy and its influence on patient education. Nurses in education roles are often familiar with literacy concerns specific to readability and grade level of written materials but may not have a clear

---

BOX 7-1   Reasons Why the English Language Is Hard to Learn

1. The bandage was wound around the wound.
2. The farm was used to produce produce.
3. The dump was so full that it has to refuse more refuse.
4. We must polish the Polish furniture.
5. He could lead if he would get the lead out.
6. The soldier decided to desert his dessert in the desert.
7. Since there is no time like the present, he thought it was time to present the present.
8. A bass was painted on the head of the bass drum.
9. When shot at, the dove dove into the bushes.
10. I did not object to the object.
11. The insurance was invalid for the invalid.
12. There was a row among the oarsmen about how to row.
13. They were too close to the door to close it.
14. The buck does funny things when the does are present.
15. A seamstress and a sewer fell down into a sewer line.
16. To help with planting, the farmer taught his sow to sow.
17. The wind was too strong to wind the sail.
18. After a number of injections, my jaw got number.
19. Upon seeing the tear in the painting I shed a tear.
20. I had to subject the subject to a series of tests.
21. How can I intimate this to my most intimate friend?

Data from Plain Language Action and Information Network

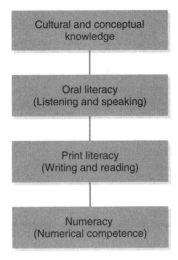

FIGURE 7-1 Literacy Components.

Data from Health Literacy: A Prescription to End Confusion by the National Academy of Sciences, courtesy of the National Academies Press, Washington, DC. 2004.

grasp of the enormity of the literacy problem in the United States. Advanced nurses need understanding of the most recent comprehensive examination of adult literacy in the United States, although last conducted approximately 15 years ago, and its relationship to health literacy.

The National Assessment of Adult Literacy (NAAL) was conducted in 2003 to assess English literacy among a nationally representative probability sample of American adults age 16 and older (National Center for Education Statistics [NCES], n.d.[a]). Data were collected from over 19,000 adults. Subjects were solicited from homes and prisons, both federal and state. NAAL results were compared to the 1992 results of the National Adult Literacy Survey (NALS).

NALS was conducted in three parts and included a national survey of 13,600 people, a 12-state survey of 1,000 people per state, and a prison survey of 1,100 inmates incarcerated in 80 federal and state prisons. Respondents were scored in three areas: prose, document, and quantitative literacy. The results were ranked into five levels ranging from least to most proficient as designated by levels 1 through 5 (NCES, n.d.[b]).

A comparison of NAAL to NALS results provides a decade point progress indicator for national adult literacy. Advanced nurses should be aware of these results, as they provide a meaningful description of challenges specific to health literacy and they support the need for professionals in the health care system to carefully consider the average skillset of the nation that is dependent on it for services. The NAAL has several components that examine the breadth of adult literacy (NCES, n.d.[a]) (**TABLE 7-1**).

The NAAL results are concerning, as they demonstrate no significant changes in prose and document literacy when compared with the NALS. There was some improvement in quantitative literacy. Literacy is currently ranked using levels ranging from below basic to basic, intermediate, and proficient (**TABLE 7-2**) (NCES, n.d.[b]).

Findings reveal that 93 million Americans, or approximately 43%, are functioning at below basic or basic levels of literacy (NCES, n.d.[c]) (**FIGURE 7-2**). These levels denote an ability to perform tasks at the most basic, uncomplicated level. Tasks include locating information in a short news article or totaling the entry on a bank deposit

TABLE 7-1 NAAL Components

Component	Description
1. Background Questionnaire	Describes relationships between adult literacy and select respondent characteristics
2. Prison Component	Identifies literacy skills of incarcerated adults
3. State Assessment of Adult Literacy (SAAL)	Statewide literacy estimates for participating states
4. Health Literacy	Ability to use literacy skills in understanding health-related materials and forms
5. Fluency Addition	Measures basic reading skills by examining decoding ability, word recognition, and reading fluency
6. Adult Literacy Supplemental Assessment	Describes the ability of the least-literate adults to identify letters and numbers and to comprehend simple prose and documents

Data from National Center for Education Statistics. (n.d.). National Assessment of Adult Literacy. What is NAAL? Retrieved January 23, 2018, from https://nces.ed.gov/naal/.

TABLE 7-2 Literacy Levels

Literacy Level	Skillset
Below Basic	No more than the most simple and concrete literacy skills
Basic	Able to perform simple and everyday literacy activities
Intermediate	Can perform moderately challenging literacy activities
Proficient	Able to perform complex and challenging literacy activities

Reproduced from National Center for Education Statistics. (n.d.). Performance levels. Overview of the literacy levels. Retrieved January 23, 2018, from http://nces.ed.gov/naal/perf_levels.asp

slip. People with a basic level of literacy have considerable difficulty carrying out tasks requiring them to read and comprehend long texts, and two-step calculations may be beyond their capabilities (NCES, n.d.[d]). A worrisome finding related to the below basic in prose group is that its members are also at greatest risk for compromised health status or societal disenfranchisement (**TABLE 7-3**).

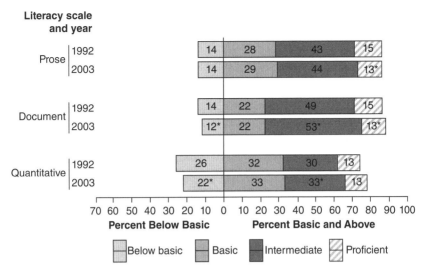

Literacy scale and year

Prose	1992	14	28	43	15
	2003	14	29	44	13*
Document	1992	14	22	49	15
	2003	12*	22	53*	13*
Quantitative	1992	26	32	30	13
	2003	22*	33	33*	13

Percent Below Basic   **Percent Basic and Above**

Below basic   Basic   Intermediate   Proficient

FIGURE 7-2 Number of Adults in Each Prose Literacy Level (NCES, n.d.[d]).

* Significantly different from 1992.
Note: Detail may not sum to totals because of rounding. Adults are defined as people 16 years of age and older living in households or prisons. Adults who could not be interviewed due to language spoken or cognitive or mental disabilities (3% in 2003 and 4% in 1992) are excluded from this figure.
U.S. Department of Education, Institute of Education Sciences, National Center for Education Statistics, 1992 National Adult Literacy Survey and 2003 National Assessment of Adult Literacy.

TABLE 7-3 Characteristics of Adults with Below Basic Prose Literacy

	Percent in Prose Below Basic Population	Percent in Total NAAL Population
Did not graduate from high school	56	15
No English spoken before starting school	44	13
Hispanic adults	39	12
Black adults	20	12
Age 65+	26	15
Multiple disabilities	21	9

Data from National Center for Education Statistics. (n.d.). National assessment of adult literacy—demographics. Overall. Retrieved November 30, 2017, from https://nces.ed.gov/naal/kf_demographics.asp.

Health Literacy: A Challenge within the Context of Literacy

Health literacy is a shared function of social and individual factors (Institute of Medicine [IOM], 2004) that influence the extent to which individuals are able to obtain, process, and understand basic health information and the services needed to make appropriate health decisions (Office of Disease Prevention and Health Promotion [ODPHP], 2010). Health literacy is not independent of general literacy skills (Rudd, 2007). Health literacy includes the ability to decode instructions, charts, and diagrams; analyze risks to benefits; and make decisions that lead to actions (National Institutes of Health, n.d.). Numeracy, or quantitative literacy, is important to the management of daily medications, extracting nutrition information from food product labels, calculating insurance copayments, or monitoring quantitative data specific to chronic conditions (Wolf, Davis, & Parker, 2007).

The IOM of the National Academies convened the *Committee on Health Literacy* to examine the problem of health literacy. The committee's report, *Health Literacy: A Prescription to End Confusion* (IOM, 2004), offers a comprehensive, detailed description of health literacy with potential interventions. The report is an excellent resource for nurses who are interested in examining this problem and developing a better sense of the enormity of the challenge to design effective, targeted patient and family education programs.

The Committee on Health Literacy developed a framework that characterizes health literacy as a synergistic relationship between culture and society, health system, education system, and health outcomes and costs (IOM, 2004). During its work, the committee examined the customary measures of literacy and health literacy and found them lacking. Responding to these deficiencies, the committee identified three potential points for intervening in the health literacy framework and potentially improving health literacy (**FIGURE 7-3**). The committee identified that the health system cannot bear full responsibility for health literacy and that efforts must include both culture and society. The health system and education system were also viewed as important partners in health literacy. This finding needs to influence the ways that advanced nurses assess and address patient teaching.

Health literacy incorporates a variety of factors, not the least of which includes listening, speaking, writing, reading, cultural influences, conceptualizations, and arithmetic. When advanced nurses critically examine patient education materials, they typically use traditional readability measures, such as the simple measure of gobbledygook (SMOG) or Gunning–Fog indices. These measures are imprecise estimates that do not take into account the broad context of literacy. As a result, materials may seem suitable in terms of word usage and grade-level readability and yet may not represent patients' understanding of the essential truths necessary for health management. Advanced nurses should keep in mind that there are many times when newly developed or traditionally utilized teaching materials are not evaluated for readability at any point in time. These sorts of aides may be ineffective resources for patients not only because of unsuitable clarity for people struggling with health

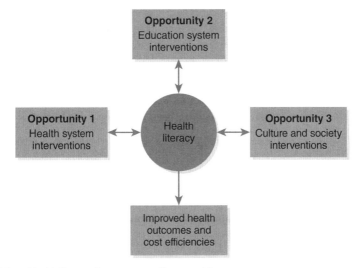

FIGURE 7-3 Health Literacy Improvement Opportunities.

Data from Health Literacy: *A Prescription to End Confusion* by the National Academy of Sciences, courtesy of the National Academies Press, Washington, DC. 2004.

literacy but also because they are written at a grade level that is inappropriate for the intended audience.

Patients with English as a second language have additional challenges that may be worsened by limited education. The committee interpreted available data as suggesting that there is a relationship between health literacy, health care use, and health care costs. In other words, limited health literacy is expensive fiscally and personally. The Committee on Health Literacy (IOM, 2004) recognized that shame and stigma related to limited literacy skills cause people to refrain from seeking resources to improve health literacy. As a result, adults with limited health literacy have less knowledge of health promotion, disease prevention, and disease management and use preventive services at a comparably lower rate (IOM, 2004).

The committee asserted that hundreds of studies have demonstrated that health information cannot be understood by most of the people for whom it was intended (IOM, 2004). The education system does not prepare people for a basic appreciation of anatomy and physiology. Therefore, when a patient experiences pathologies requiring self-management, he or she may not understand even the simple mechanics of functioning that are vital to making decisions about drug dosing, contacting a health care professional for follow-up, or returning to the hospital.

For example, a patient with congestive heart failure and coronary artery disease needs to understand the basic premise of coronary artery blood flow, ischemia, anticoagulation, heart rate, and pumping ability. This foundation informs self-management and facilitates recognition of the signs and symptoms that require medical or nursing review. Much of this information is couched in scientific terminologies that are not taught in basic education programs. The knowledge deficit worsens the challenges facing health professionals as they attempt to provide the education needed for self-care efficacy in a time frame that is constrained by inadequate personnel and fiscal resources.

Literacy Resources for Nurses in Advanced Roles

Health literacy is gaining a lot of attention from both private and public agencies and corporations. As a result, many Web-based resources are available at a low cost. These resources may be used to positively affect patient outcomes by influencing the expertise of health professionals within the health care system. Resources may also be used to empower patients by helping them to better understand and act on provided health information. Advanced nurses should explore the many available resources and keep in mind that most government sites allow for the free use of materials, providing that they are properly acknowledged (**TABLE 7-4**).

One important idea upon which advanced nurses need to reflect is that health literacy is more than the development of materials and resources that are

TABLE 7-4 Recommended Health Literacy Web Resources		
Name	**Web Address**	**Comments**
Pfizer principles for clear health communication (2nd ed.)	https://www.pfizer.com/files/health/PfizerPrinciples.pdf	Downloadable for no charge. Packed with concise information, including readability formulas, and recommendations
National Institutes of Health. Clear communication. Health literacy	https://www.nih.gov/institutes-nih/nih-office-director/office-communications-public-liaison/clear-communication/health-literacy	Links to trainings, toolkits, and workshops
Agency for Healthcare Research and Quality. Health literacy universal precautions toolkit (2nd ed.)	https://www.ahrq.gov/professionals/quality-patient-safety/quality-resources/tools/literacy-toolkit/index.html	Tools (N = 21), presentations, guidelines, toolkit companion addressing clinical implementation

Name	Web Address	Comments
NC Program on Health Literacy	http://www.nchealthliteracy.org/toolkit/	Provides disease-specific health literacy toolkits and other resources in addition to the fully downloadable AHRQ health literacy universal precautions toolkit (2nd ed.)
EthnoMed	http://ethnomed.org/patient-education	Addresses health literacy by providing patient education materials in many languages as well as culture-specific information needed to inform health literacy efforts
Centers for Disease Control and Prevention. Health literacy resources	https://www.cdc.gov/healthliteracy/learn/resources.html	Provides array of materials and links related to scientific reports, research, special population groups, and standards
American Health Information Management Association. Health literacy resources. Resources for becoming an empowered patient	http://www.myphr.com/HealthLiteracy/resources.aspx	Provides many different resources targeting the health care consumer with the goal of increasing empowerment and ownership of personal health

readily understandable to people. It is also more than working with individuals and the public to increase familiarity with key components of literacy as related to health. Rather, advanced nurses need to recognize that the communication abilities of the health professional who is responsible for delivering the message, regardless of the form, has a major influence on message effectiveness. Rudd (2015) describes health literacy as in a state of evolution. Health literacy has been considered an important determinant of health and there has been a good bit of attention over the past few decades on the health literacy capabilities of the public. At some point a bit later but parallel to efforts describing and addressing individual and public literacy, researchers initiated study on health information and the fit between health materials' readability and understandability and the public's reading skills (Rudd, 2015).

Rudd (2015) makes the case that these past few decades have largely been composed of literacy investigation and ascertaining readability/understandability of materials and resources; however, there has been little attention paid to the communication skills of health professionals or the context within which teaching and coaching were occurring. This is an important point because factors that influence health literacy include the communication skills of the agent and the environment context. Advanced nurses need to consider health literacy program opportunities that pay attention to the intended message recipient, the message itself, and the messenger.

One opportunity that uniquely addresses the message recipient is the *Ask Me 3*® program. This program was developed by the Partnership for Clear Health Communication, a committee established in 2002 and composed of 19 organizations and individuals working in close collaboration with health literacy experts to improve communication between providers and patients and to address the relationship between low health literacy and its negative impact on health status (ODPHP. Healthfinder.gov, 2013). *Ask Me 3*® is currently run by the Institute for Healthcare Improvement (IHI) since its merger with the National Patient Safety Foundation (NPSF), the original administrative agency for *Ask Me 3*® (IHI, 2018).

Ask Me 3® promotes three simple questions for patients to ask their health care provider during every encounter:

1. What is my main problem?
2. What do I need to do?
3. Why is it important for me to do this?

The program's website (http://www.npsf.org/page/askme3) offers a variety of resources for providers, patients, large-scale implementers, and media. Numerous materials are available to freely download and distribute to assist in supporting health literacy efforts. There is a registration process to which advanced nurses need to respond and following this step, a zip folder is available for download that contains a variety of posters (**FIGURE 7-4**), flyers in both English and Spanish, teaching materials, health literacy educational module slides and transcript, and terms and conditions for downloading (IHI, 2018).

Another helpful Web-based resource is PlainLanguage.gov, a federal government employee initiative designed to facilitate the use of plain language to improve communication. In 1995, a group of federal employees joined together with an agenda to spread the use of plain language. The Plain Language Action and Information Network (PLAIN) (n.d.[a]) created the website (www.plainlanguage.gov/index.cfm) to help people learn about and use plain language. The site is accessible in modern browsers. The Plain Writing Act of 2010 requires federal agencies to use clear government communication that the public can understand and use (PLAIN, n.d.[a]). Advanced nurses likely recognize the similar need for plain language in health care and may find the various templates and exemplars to be quite useful when developing educational resources for patients and their families but also for students, staff, and interprofessional colleagues.

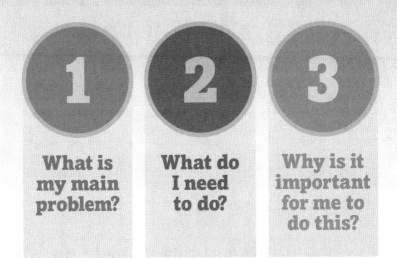

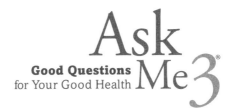

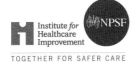

FIGURE 7-4 Sample "Ask Me 3" Poster.

PLAIN provides an excellent exemplar of a revised document in plain language as compared to its original state (**BOXES 7-2** and **7-3**) and the example selected by Doak and Doak (2004) from the U.S. Department of Health and Human Services provides a clear illustration of the powers of plain language efforts on breast examination teaching materials. Wonderful tools are available via the plainlanguage.gov website; and health

---

BOX 7-2 Comparison of Breast Cancer Patient Information After Revision Using Principles for Clear Health Communication

Original Information Based on the Medical Model

An extra step: Mammography
Women in the three high-risk categories—age 50 or more, age 40 or more with a family history of breast cancer, and age 35 or more with a personal history of breast cancer—may consider an additional routine screening method. This is x-ray mammography. Mammography uses radiation (x-rays) to create an image of the breast on film or paper called a mammogram. It can reveal tumors too small to be felt by palpation. It shows other changes in the structure of the breast, which doctors believe point to very early cancer. A mammographic examination usually consists of two x-rays of each breast, one taken from the top and one from the side. Exposure to x-rays should be carried out to ensure that the lowest possible dose will be absorbed by the body. Radiologists are not yet certain if there is any risk from one mammogram, although most studies indicate that the risk, if it does exist, is small relative to the benefit. Recent equipment modifications and improved techniques are reducing radiation absorption and thus the possible risk.

Revised Information Based on the Health Belief Model

What is a mammogram and why should I have one?
A mammogram is an x-ray picture of the breast. It can find breast cancer that is too small for you, your doctor, or nurse to feel. Studies show that if you are in your 40s or older having a mammogram every 1–2 years could save your life.

How do I know if I need a mammogram?
Talk with your doctor about your chances of getting breast cancer. Your doctor can help you decide when you should start having mammograms and how often you should have them.

Why do I need one every 1–2 years?
As you get older, your chances of getting breast cancer get higher. Cancer can show up at any time—so one mammogram is not enough. Decide on a plan with your doctor and follow it for the rest of your life.

Where can I get a mammogram?
To find out where to get a mammogram:

- Ask your doctor or nurse
- Ask your local health department or clinic
- Call the National Cancer Institute's Concern Information Service at 1-800-4-CANCER

Reproduced from U.S. Department of Health and Human Services, National Cancer Institute/National Institutes of Health. Breast Exams: What you should know. 1997. Readability: 5th grade. Doak, L. G. & Doak, C. C. (Eds.). (2004). *Pfizer Principles for Clear Health Communication*. (2nd ed.). Retrieved January 24, 2018, from https://www.pfizer.com/files/health/PfizerPrinciples.pdf

literacy is a popular topic. PLAIN offers a checklist for plain language on documents (**BOX 7-4**) (PLAIN, n.d.[b]) and for Web pages (PLAIN, n.d.[c]). Each item may be selected using the hyperlink to acquire additional details. There are opportunities for online training that could be incorporated into staff education modules; alternatively, advanced nurses might want to consider developing familiarity with or expertise in plain language. Several health agencies and government departments have made their plain language resources available for public use (**TABLE 7-5**).

BOX 7-3   Before and After Comparisons: Losing Weight Brochure

Before

The Dietary Guideline for Americans recommends 30 minutes or more of moderate physical activity on most days, preferably every day. The activity can include brisk walking, calisthenics, home care, gardening, moderate sports exercise, and dancing.

After

Do at least 30 minutes of exercise, like brisk walking, most days of the week.

Data from Plain Language Action and Information Network

BOX 7-4   Document Checklist for Plain Language Documents

1. Written for the average reader
    Know the expertise and interest of your average reader, then write to that person. Do not write to the experts, the lawyers, or your management, unless they are your intended audience.
2. Organized to serve the reader's needs
    Organize your content in the order the reader needs—the two most useful organization principles, which are not mutually exclusive, are to put the most important material first, exceptions last; or to organize material chronologically.
3. Has useful headings
    Headings help the reader find the way through your material. Headings should capture the essence of all the material under the heading—if they do not, you need more headings! You should have one or more headings on each page.
4. Uses "you" and other pronouns to speak to the reader
    Using pronouns pulls the reader into the document and makes it more meaningful to him or her. Use "you" for the reader ("I" when writing question headings from the reader's viewpoint) and "we" for your agency.
5. Uses active voice
    Using active voice clarifies who is doing what; passive obscures it. Active voice is generally shorter, as well as clearer. Changing our writing to prefer active voice is the single most powerful change we can make in government writing. Active sentences are structured with the actor first (as the subject), then the verb, then the object of the action.

(continues)

BOX 7-4 Document Checklist for Plain Language Documents   *(continued)*

6.   Uses short sections and sentences
     Using short sentences, paragraphs, and sections helps your reader get through
     your material. Readers get lost in long dense text with few headings. Chunking
     your material also inserts white space, opening your document visually and
     making it more appealing.
7.   Uses the simplest tense possible—simple present is best
     The simplest verb tense is the clearest and strongest. Use simple present when
     possible—say, "We issue a report every quarter," not "We will be issuing a report
     every quarter."
8.   Uses base verbs, not nominalizations (hidden verbs)
     Use base verbs, not nominalizations—also called "hidden verbs." Government writing
     is full of hidden verbs. They make our writing weak and longer than necessary.
     Say, "We manage the program" and "We analyze data" not "We are responsible for
     management of the program" or "We conduct an analysis of the data."
9.   Omits excess words
     Eliminate excess words. Challenge every word—do you need it? Pronouns,
     active voice, and base verbs help eliminate excess words. So does eliminating
     unnecessary modifiers—in "HUD and FAA issued a joint report" you do not need
     "joint." In "This information is really critical" you do not need "really."
10. Uses concrete, familiar words
     You do not impress people by using big words, you just confuse them. Define
     (and limit!) your abbreviations. Avoid jargon, foreign terms, Latin terms, and legal
     terms. Avoid noun strings. See our alphabetized list of complex words and simple
     subjects in the "word suggestions" page on this website.
11. Uses "must" to express requirements; avoids the ambiguous word "shall"
     Use "must" not "shall" to impose requirements. "Shall" is ambiguous and
     rarely occurs in everyday conversation. The legal community is moving to a
     strong preference for "must" as the clearest way to express a requirement or
     obligation.
12. Place words carefully (avoids large gaps between the subject, the verb, and the
     object; puts exceptions last; places modifiers correctly)
     Placing words carefully within a sentence is as important as organizing your
     document effectively. Keep subject, verb, and object close together. Put
     exceptions at the end. Place modifiers correctly—"We want only the best" not
     "We only want the best."
13. Uses lists and tables to simplify complex material
     You can shorten and clarify complex material by using lists and tables. And
     these features give your document more white space, making it more appealing
     to the reader.
14. Uses no more than two or three subordinate levels
     Readers get lost when you use more than two or three levels in a document.
     If you find you need more levels, consider subdividing your top level into
     more parts.

Data from Plain Language Action and Information Network

TABLE 7-5 Government Plain Language Instructional Resources (plainlanguage.gov, 2017)

Agency/ Department/ Service	Web Address	Description
Federal Aviation Administration	https://www.faa.gov /about/initiatives /plain_language/media /toolkit.pdf	Provides links to plain language resources and helpful tips, including formatting tools; word usage tools; and evaluation queries to assist with keeping the writer on track.
National Institutes of Health (NIH) plain language training	https://plainlanguage .nih.gov/CBTs /PlainLanguage/login.asp	Offers online training with or without a certificate of completion following successful conclusion of the course. Registration is free. The modules include: how people read, concise writing, clarity, format, organizing your ideas, choosing words, tone, and optional exercises. The modules may be completed in any order and the program may be stopped and started as the learner prefers.
Centers for Disease Control and Prevention's Health Literacy for Public Health Professionals	https://www.cdc.gov /healthliteracy/training/	This user-friendly online course provides 1.0 contact hour upon successful completion. The course consists of an introduction followed by three lessons. Each lesson is composed of videos, case studies, and knowledge check questions.
Centers for Medicare and Medicaid Services' Toolkit for Making Written Material Clear and Effective	https://www.cms .gov/Outreach-and -Education/Outreach /WrittenMaterialsToolkit /index.html	This toolkit consists of 11 components, including discussion about readability formulas, things to know if writing for older adults, before and after exemplars, and guidelines for culturally appropriate translation.

Data from Plain Language Action and Information Network, Online Training. Retrieved from https://www.plainlanguage.gov /training/online-training/.

Pfizer, Inc. (2018a) supports health literacy efforts through its Web-based resources targeting consumer education. The website (https://www.pfizer.com /health-wellness) is organized by audience type and provides relevant, accessible health literacy materials for patients and families, health care professionals, and public policy/researchers (Pfizer, Inc., 2018b). Topics within the patients and families category include (1) education about the nature of health literacy; (2) a plan for responding to this concern; (3) a description of clear health communication; (4) information about low health literacy as a high-frequency problem; and (5) important connections between low health literacy and health outcomes. The various topics are described and YouTube video hyperlinks are provided. Connections to *Ask Me 3®* program opportunities are provided so that consumers can better understand how they can learn to secure the information needed to make good health care decisions (Pfizer, Inc., 2018b).

Pfizer, Inc. (2018c) provides health care professionals with excellent descriptive data about health literacy as well as with tools and recommendations for practice. Topics are interesting and presented using a clearly written style. Universal precautions for health communication address the importance of simple, straightforward communication and acknowledge the challenges that health professionals may face when attempting to use plain language. Public communication recommendations are shared and this informational section links to the Centers for Disease Control and Prevention's (CDC) health literacy training program for health professionals (https://www.cdc .gov/healthliteracy/gettraining.html). The health professionals' section guides readers to resources that are suitable when advising patients and families toward online content. Hyperlinks are provided to Medline Plus and the *EZ to Read* materials as well as other sites (**TABLE 7-6**).

The content designed for public policy researchers is interesting and provides advanced nurses with opportunities to access current research in health literacy via a streamlined approach. This section includes an overview of health literacy and clear health communication, particularly as informed by NAAL data. There is a selected research bibliography, although the cited materials stop at 2011. Some important reports relevant to researchers and policy stakeholders are described and linked within this section (e.g., the IOM's Innovations in Health Literacy 2011 roundtable discussion).

One other particularly useful tool is a downloadable handbook for creating patient education materials, entitled *Pfizer Principles for Clear Health Communication* (2nd ed.). Doak and Doak (2004) edited this handbook to explore health literacy and offer suggestions, strategies, and examples. The downloadable pdf is written in an easy-to-read format that exemplifies the simple yet meaningful recommendations it puts forth. This is an excellent resource for advanced nurses with responsibility for developing, leading, using, or evaluating patient education materials and it may also be a useful tool for interprofessional educational endeavors.

The Agency for Healthcare Research and Quality (AHRQ, 2017a) offers a variety of health literacy resources for health professionals. The tools are designed to make information easier to understand. There are 10 categories of content (**BOX 7-5**) and each provides helpful resources for advanced nurses who are seeking to understand and respond to health literacy concerns. One tool that falls within the first category, *Tools for Health Care Professionals, Delivery Organizations, and Systems*, is the second edition of the *AHRQ Health Literacy Universal Precautions Toolkit* (DeWalt et al., 2010).

Experts recommend using a universal precautions approach to health literacy. Similar to the assumption of infection risk associated with bodily fluid exposures

TABLE 7-6 Consumer-Oriented Websites Recommended by Pfizer, Inc.

Site Name (Copyright Date)	Web Address	Brief Content Description
Healthfinder.gov (2017)	https://healthfinder.gov/	Health information
Medline Plus (2017)	https://medlineplus.gov/	Health information, including easy-to-read materials, organizations, directors, and materials in multiple languages
Health.gov (2017)	https://health.gov/	Health information about food and nutrition, physical activity, health literacy, health care quality, healthy people, and a link to healthfinder (a prevention and wellness resource developed in English and Spanish)
National Institute on Aging's (NIA) Health Information (n.d.)	https://www.nia.nih.gov/health	Health information and ordering information for print publications; clinical trials, contact information to NIA
KidsHealth® from Nemours (2017)	http://kidshealth.org/	Health information for parents, kids, and teens, in both Spanish and English versions
National Council on Patient Information and Education (NCPIE) (2017)	http://www.bemedwise.org/	Smart medication use, medication adherence, medicine risk reduction, and better communication with providers regarding safe medication use

BOX 7-5 AHRQ'S Health Literacy Resources

Health Literacy Content Categories

Tools for Health Care Professionals, Delivery Organizations, and Systems
Professional Education and Training
Patient Education Resources
Assessing the Patient Experience
Health Information Technology
Tools for Researchers
Articles, Papers, and Reports
Podcasts and Videos
Impact Case Studies
Related Department of Health and Human Services Resources

Reproduced from Agency for Healthcare Research and Quality. (2018). Health Literacy. Retrieved from https://www.ahrq.gov/topics/health-literacy.html.

and universal precautions as the required response, the health literacy toolkit builds on the premise that practices should assume that all patients and caregivers will have difficult comprehending health information. In response, providers should communicate in ways that are universally understandable by using simple communication within easily navigated systems so that patients' efforts to seek health improvements are supported (AHRQ, 2015a).

The toolkit is designed for use by all types of primary care practice staff who work with pediatric and adult patients, including caregivers and parents (DeWalt et al., 2010). The kit is divided into four domains that include 21 tools to make for manageable implementation. A companion guide is provided and at least one person with some expertise in quality improvement or health literacy is encouraged to read this guide before the toolkit is applied to the practice setting. AHRQ (2015a) recommends starting the health literacy practice improvement project by forming a team, creating a health literacy improvement plan, and raising awareness. However, recognizing that some practices may prefer to start right away by trying a tool, a *Quick Start Guide* is provided to assist (**FIGURE 7-5**).

The *Quick Start Guide* includes a 6-minute health literacy video that sets the stage for the viewer. Advanced nurses might consider sharing the provided video with staff and colleagues as a first step in selecting health literacy improvement areas charged to work groups or interprofessional teams. This toolkit is a particularly

---

Quick Start Guide

(1) **Watch a short video.**
This 6-minute **health literacy video** is sponsored by the American College of Physicians (ACP) Foundation and has some vivid examples of why addressing health literacy is so important.

(2) **Pick a tool and try it.**
Link to one of these tools and review it. Pick a day and try it out on a few patients.

- I want to be confident my patients are taking their medications correctly.   **Brown Bag Medication Review**

- I want to be confident that I am speaking clearly to my patients.   **Tips for Communicating Clearly**

- I want to be confident that my patients understand what they need to do regarding their health when they get home.   **The Teach-Back Method**

(3) **Assess your results.**
How did it go? Do you need to make some adjustments? Do you want to address another statement from the list above and try another tool?
    Or, you may want to take this to the next step by going to the **Overview** and learning about health literacy universal precautions and this toolkit.

FIGURE 7-5 Quick Start Guide.

Reproduced from Health Literacy Universal Precautions Toolkit. AHRQ Pub. No. 10-0046-EF, page 7.

rich resource that could easily be used to assist individuals and teams to reach a shared baseline of health literacy expertise before focusing on particular areas of identified needs.

The Healthy Literacy Studies program of the Department of Social and Behavioral Sciences at the Harvard T. H. Chan School of Public Health, Health Literacy Studies (2015) offers a variety of health literacy resources (https://www.hsph.harvard.edu /healthliteracy/). The website provides information specific to health literacy, health literacy literature, research and policy, innovative materials, overview presentation slides (Rudd, 2015), health literacy curricula, links, contact information, and up-dated notifications of talks, presentations, and health literacy studies in the news. The website also offers a variety of teaching materials available for downloading, printing, and distributing. A few of the Harvard T. H. Chan School of Public Health's (2018) Web-based materials available for download include disease-specific plain language glossaries specific to arthritis, lupus, and asthma. Assessment tools for readability and understandability are available and general usage guidelines are provided as well.

EthnoMed offers patient education materials tailored to a variety of cultures including Amharic, Cambodian, Chinese, Eritrean, Hispanic, Somali, and others (University of Washington, Harborview Medical Center, 2018). Signified cultures represent immigrant and refugee groups living in Seattle and other parts of the United States. Cross-cultural links are available. The EthnoMed project began in 1994 with the goal of bridging cultural and language barriers during medical encounters. The project's objective is to make information about culture, language, health, illness, and local resources readily available to health care providers working with diverse ethnic groups.

EthnoMed (2018) offers advanced nurses a menu of various cultures. The nurse selects the culture of interest and is presented with options for a cultural profile, clinical topics, or patient education materials. As an example, if a nurse is working with a Vietnamese patient with a cancer diagnosis but has no experience with this cultural group, the EthnoMed site provides a detailed overview of Vietnamese culture. A list of common Vietnamese symptoms is offered as well as health and illness topics. If the nurse is looking for education materials for this patient, the "Patient Education" link reveals many resources written in Vietnamese, including a *What Is Cancer?* document available in both Vietnamese and English. The site is an ongoing activity and encourages providers to share information about treatments, resources, and cultural perspectives with the Eth-noMed group. This Web-based tool is a terrific resource for advanced nurses to use directly in their practice or for those advanced nurses practicing in indirect roles to incorporate into patient education repositories, nursing education experiences, or other patient care vehicles.

An additional resource is fee-based patient education materials. Some vendors create patient education materials for purchase. Many hospitals and other health organizations choose to purchase patient education materials in the form of text pamphlets with visual aids, website development, and specialty program development. These types of products may be useful for streamlining education material resources and protecting the accuracy and consistency of the information provided during health care encounters. Vendors also provide databases that may be used to develop individualized discharge instructions for a variety of settings, including emergency departments. If this option is interesting, advanced nurses should request a vendor list from the purchasing expert at the health care institution. Vendor information is also available at professional nursing conferences, particularly the larger regional, national, and international conference venues.

A Word About Teach-Back

Teach-back is an easy method that may be used to evaluate patients' understanding of taught information. The method consists of asking patients how they would explain the pertinent procedure, treatment, or other self-care activity to their spouse or family member (AHRQ, 2015b). Patients should explain by using their own words. If the patient is incorrect, the nurse should provide clarification using different phrases rather than repeating the previously provided information. To avoid patient feelings of foolishness or defensiveness, nurses should phrase the request for the patient to "teach back" by requesting feedback on the nurse's performance. For example, the advanced nurse teaching the patient how to administer a daily insulin dose might consider saying, "I want to make certain that I did a good job of explaining this insulin dosing to you. Would you please show me how you're going to do this when you get home?"

Frankly, advanced nurses may want to emphasize this respectful approach when soliciting honest evaluation from patients given that Rudd (2015) has made a strong case for the role of skillful communication in health literacy outcomes. "Studies linking literacy and health outcomes should include variables from both sides of the coin—the literacy skills of individuals as well as the communication skills of the professionals; the communication skills of professionals as well as the policy related constraints/ facilitators set by the institutions within which they practice" (Rudd, 2015, p. 8).

The patient teach-back moment is critical to the process. Studies demonstrate that 40% to 80% of medical information shared with patients during office visits is immediately forgotten and the information that is retained is incorrect nearly half the time (AHRQ, 2015b). Unless patients, caregivers, and family members are gently encouraged to feel comfortable and share their understanding of the instruction, the method will prove to be ineffective—in other words, the teach-*back* is an imperative step!

AHRQ (2015b) provides Web-based opportunities to learn the teach-back method and to track user confidence progression and skill acquisition. The Always Use Teach-Back! Toolkit provides detailed information about the principles of plain language, teach-back, and other contextual concerns needed to encourage the consistent use of teach-back. Key points about the teach-back method are provided (**BOX 7-6**). There are video exemplars of correct teach-back technique and other informational videos as well. Although this technique is particularly touted as useful for primary care settings, it has been used in hospital settings as well and has been demonstrated to encourage marked improvement in teaching and learning outcomes (Centrella-Nigro & Alexander, 2017).

A systematic review of the effectiveness of the teach-back method as a strategy to prevent 30-day readmissions in patients with heart failure revealed some specific benefits of this tool at low cost but also revealed a need for more research support (Almkuist, 2017). Given that there are likely benefits to the teach-back method, certainly the technique is low risk, it is a recommended strategy to support patient

BOX 7-6 Teach-Back Method: Key Points

- Keep in mind this is not a test of the patient's knowledge. It is a test of how well you explained the concept.
- Plan your approach. Think about how you will ask your patients to teach back the information. For example: "We covered a lot today and I want to make sure that I explained things clearly. So let's review what we discussed. Can you please describe the three things you agreed to do to help you control your diabetes?"
- "Chunk and Check." Do not wait until the end of the visit to initiate teach-back. Chunk out information into small segments and have your patient teach it back. Repeat several times during a visit.
- Clarify and check again. If teach-back uncovers a misunderstanding, explain things again using a different approach. Ask patients to teach-back again until they are able to correctly describe the information in their own words. If they parrot your words back to you, they may not have understood.
- Start slowly and use consistently. At first, you may want to try teach-back with the last patient of the day. Once you are comfortable with the technique, use teach-back with everyone, every time!
- Practice. It will take a little time, but once it is part of your routine, teach-back can be done without awkwardness and does not lengthen a visit.
- Use the show-me method. When prescribing new medicines or changing a dose, research shows that even when patients correctly say when and how much medicine they will take, many will make mistakes when asked to demonstrate the dose. You could say, for example: "I've noticed that many people have trouble remembering how to take their blood thinner. Can you show me how you are going to take it?"
- Use handouts along with teach-back. Write down key information to help patients remember instructions at home. Point out important information by reviewing written materials to reinforce your patients' understanding. You can allow patients to refer to handouts when using teach-back, but make sure they use their own words and are not reading the material back verbatim.

Reproduced from Health Literacy Universal Precautions Toolkit, 2nd Edition. Content last reviewed February 2015. Agency for Healthcare Research and Quality, Rockville, MD. http://www.ahrq.gov/professionals/quality-patient-safety/quality-resources/tools/literacy-toolkit/healthlittoolkit2.html

education (Almkuist, 2017). Although use of the teach-back technique is advocated by health literacy experts, a survey of health care professionals attending plenary sessions on health literacy/health communication at 12 different state and national conferences on patient safety and health care quality revealed that less than 40% of total respondents (N = 356) used the teach-back technique during patient education encounters (Schwartzberg, Cowett, VanGeest, & Wolf, 2007). Although these findings are from a decade ago, it seems reasonable to suspect that teach-back technique underutilization persists.

Advanced nurses should share this simple strategy with nurses and other health providers. As an aside, this may also be a useful method to use when teaching nursing students and professional nurses, as the technique is similar to an effective "bottom-line" teaching approach recommended by Zuzelo (1999) to assist students in learning essential information required for success with the National Council of State Boards of Nursing Examination-RN (NCLEX-RN).

▶ Levels of Literacy

Managed care requires people to be increasingly autonomous in self-care practices. Ownership of self-care responsibilities demands health literacy. Many areas of health management are connected to health literacy (**BOX 7-7**).

Levels of literacy are described by fairly common terms. Advanced nurses should think about these descriptive terms and consider the demographics of the practice setting within the context of these literacy levels. Low literacy is also referred to as marginally literate or marginally illiterate and designates individuals who are able to read, write, and comprehend information at the fifth- through eighth-grade level of difficulty (Bastable, 2013). Functional illiteracy describes adults with reading, writing, and comprehension skills that are below the fifth-grade level. Literacy categorizations should not be interpreted as akin to intelligence (Bastable, 2014).

Health literacy is one of the health communication objectives in Healthy People (HP) 2020 (ODPHP, 2010). Health literacy falls within the scope of Health Communication and Health Information Technology (HC/HIT). Objective HC/HIT-1 is "improve the health literacy of the population" and Objective HC/HIT-2 calls to "increase the proportion of persons who report that their health care providers have satisfactory communication skills" (ODPHP. HealthyPeople.gov, 2018). These objectives particularly relate to the previous discussion regarding the impact of the message recipient, message, and communicator on health literacy. The expanded objectives for the HC/HIT topic address the many aspects of health literacy in its broadest sense (**TABLE 7-7**).

Assessing Patient Education Materials

Advanced nurses should be aware of established and common screening instruments used to determine a patient's literacy and to ascertain the readability and appropriateness of available teaching materials. Nurses need to be comfortable selecting the best-fit instruments and using these tools. Readability is frequently discussed in nursing textbooks, and most nurses are familiar with issues specific to the level of difficulty of materials; however, they may be less familiar with the concept of health literacy.

BOX 7-7 Health Literacy Self-Care Impact Areas

1. Patient–health care provider communication: health histories, advanced directives, untoward drug reactions, discharge instructions
2. Medication labeling: prescription drug dosing and scheduling, empty stomach instructions, drug interaction precautions
3. Equipment labeling: using durable medical equipment safely and correctly
4. Health information publications and other resources: self-care pamphlets, public health precautions, hazardous materials warnings, household items warnings concerning mixing materials
5. Informed consent
6. Responding to medical and insurance forms
7. Nutrition: food labeling, avoiding allergens, proper food storage, expiration dates, handling instructions

TABLE 7-7 Health Communication and Health Information Technology (HC/HIT) Healthy People 2020 Detailed Objectives

Objective	Related Sub-Objectives
HC/HIT-1 Improve the health literacy of the population	HC/HIT-1.1 Increase the proportion of persons who report their health care provider always gave them easy-to-understand instructions about what to do to take care of their illness or health condition HC/HIT-1.2 Increase the proportion of persons who report their health care provider always asked them to describe how they will follow the instructions HC/HIT-1.3 Increase the proportion of persons who report their health care providers' office always offered help in filling out a form
HC/HIT-2 Increase the proportion of persons who report that their health care providers have satisfactory communication skills	HC/HIT-2.1 Increase the proportion of persons who report that their health care providers always listened carefully to them HC/HIT-2.2 Increase the proportion of persons who report that their health care providers always explained things so they could understand them HC/HIT-2.3 Increase the proportion of persons who report that their health care providers always showed respect for what they had to say HC/HIT-2.4 Increase the proportion of persons who report that their health care providers always spent enough time with them
HC/HIT-3 Increase the proportion of persons who report that their health care providers always involved them in decisions about their health care as much as they wanted	
HC/HIT-4 (Developmental) Increase the proportion of patients whose doctor recommends personalized health information resources to help them manage their health	

(continues)

TABLE 7-7 Health Communication and Health Information Technology (HC/HIT) Healthy People 2020 Detailed Objectives *(continued)*

Objective	Related Sub-Objectives
HC/HIT-5 Increase the proportion of persons who use electronic personal health management tools	HC/HIT-5.1 Increase the proportion of persons who use the Internet to keep track of personal health information, such as care received, test results, or upcoming medical appointments HC/HIT-5.2 Increase the proportion of persons who use the Internet to communicate with their health provider
HC/HIT-6 Increase individuals' access to the Internet	HC/HIT-6.1 Increase the proportion of persons with access to the Internet HC/HIT-6.2 Increase the proportion of persons with broadband access to the Internet HC/HIT-6.3 Increase the proportion of persons who use mobile devices
HC/HIT-7 Increase the proportion of adults who report having friends or family members with whom they talk about their health	
HC/HIT-8 Increase the proportion of quality, health-related websites	HC/HIT-8.1 Increase the proportion of health-related websites that meet three or more evaluation criteria for disclosing information that can be used to assess information reliability HC/HIT-8.2 Increase the proportion of health-related websites that follow established usability principles
HC/HIT-9 Increase the proportion of online health information seekers who report easily accessing health information	
HC/HIT-10 Increase the proportion of medical practices that use electronic health records	
HC/HIT-12 Increase the proportion of crisis and emergency risk messages intended to protect the public's health that demonstrate the use of best practices	HC/HIT-12.1 Increase the proportion of crisis and emergency risk messages embedded in print and broadcast news stories that explain what is known about the threat to human health

Objective	Related Sub-Objectives
	HC/HIT-12.2 Increase the proportion of crisis and emergency risk messages embedded in print and broadcast news stories that explain what is NOT known about the threat to human health
	HC/HIT-12.3 Increase the proportion of crisis and emergency risk messages embedded in print and broadcast news stories that explain how or why a crisis or emergency event happened
	HC/HIT-12.4 Increase the proportion of crisis and emergency risk messages embedded in print and broadcast news stories that promote steps the reader or viewer can take to reduce their personal health threat
	HC/HIT-12.5 Increase the proportion of crisis and emergency risk messages embedded in print and broadcast news stories that express empathy about the threat to human health
	HC/HIT-12.6 Increase the proportion of crisis and emergency risk messages embedded in print and broadcast news stories that express commitment from the responsible or responding entity
HC/HIT-13 Increase social marketing in health promotion and disease prevention	HC/HIT-13.1 Increase the number of state health departments that report using social marketing in health promotion and disease prevention programs

Reproduced from U.S. Department of Health and Human Services. 2018. Health Comunication and Health Information Technology: Objectives. Retrieved from https://www.healthypeople.gov/2020/topics-objectives/topic/health-communication-and-health-information-technology/objectives.

Understandability is another critical characteristic of quality teaching materials. Both measures plus the communication skills of the educator should be carefully examined when planning patient education.

AHRQ (2015c) cautions that readability formulas should be warily used to evaluate text because they are narrowly focused and address the mechanics of words and sentences, not the understandability or reading ease. There are also differences in calculated reading scores based on the selected evaluation tool. Tools typically generate grade-level scores based on average length of word and sentence. Judicious advanced nurses looking for a readability formula need to consider that the formulas do not measure comprehension, reading ease, and overall suitability as related to the particular audience (AHRQ, 2015c). However, there are options that are better than others, depending on the rationale for ascertaining the score.

One other caveat related to readability and ease of use is to consider the intended audience. Estimate the likely reading skill level based on years of education and, perhaps, the NALS results based on demographics, keeping in mind that the results are from 2003 (NCES, n.d.[a]). AHRQ (2015c) notes that experts usually recommend a general approach to grade-level scores and analyses that compare the anticipated average reading skills of the intended reader versus the earned grade-level score. If the comparison reveals concerning differences, long words and lengthy sentences should be shortened and syntax should be simplified. Generally, materials scored at grades 4–6 are considered easy to read; those at grades 7–9 are evaluated as average level of difficulty; and anything written at or above grade 10 is considered difficult (AHRQ, 2015c).

Readability

Advanced nurses may be familiar with readability tools including the Flesch–Kinkaid Grade Level score and the Flesch Reading Ease score, as these options are available in the readability scores feature of Microsoft Word. The Center for Health Care Strategies, Inc. (CHCS) offers health literacy fact sheets that provide clinicians with various useful resources, including a number of print communication readability scores (Mahadevan, CHCS, 2013). Two examples of popular readability measures are the SMOG and Fog formulas.

The SMOG index is based on average sentence length and the number of words with three or more syllables in a total of 30 sentences (Mahadevan, CHCS, 2013). SMOG is fast and easy to use and has well-established validity. SMOG is based on 100% comprehension of material read, so if the index calculates the readability level to be grade 6, it means that 100% of readers able to read at the sixth-grade level should fully comprehend the material. Other formulas rely on 50% to 75% of all persons reading at the sixth-grade level, which explains why SMOG results are often about two grade levels higher than those determined by other indices (Bastable, 2014; CHCS, 2013). The SMOG index follows simple calculation steps (**BOX 7-8**) that may be cumbersome when applied to lengthy documents. Resources are available for passages longer and shorter than 30 sentences that offer conversion tables for ease of use (Bastable, 2013; CHCS, 2013). The SMOG index is the most common readability formula used and is recommended by the National Cancer Institute (Hedman, 2008). It is applicable to the English language only.

The Fog index or the Gunning–Fog index (Bastable, 2013) measures readability of print materials ranging from fourth grade to college level. The formula calculates grade level based on average sentence length and the percentage of multisyllabic words in a 100-word passage. It is an easy formula to use, and the resulting number indicates the number of years of formal education that a person needs to easily understand the text on the first reading (Bastable, 2013).

The Flesch Reading Ease score rates the text on a 100-point scale, with a high score indicating greater understandability. Microsoft recommends a target score of

---

BOX 7-8 SMOG Index

To calculate the SMOG index:
1. Count the number of complex words (words containing three or more syllables).
2. Multiply the number of complex words by a factor of 30/number of sentences.
3. Take the square root of the resultant number.
4. Add 3 to the resultant number.

approximately 60–70 for standard documents (**BOX 7-9**). The Flesch–Kincaid Grade Level score rates text on a U.S. grade-school level. A score of 8 indicates that the text can be understood by an individual with the skillset of an eighth grader. For a standard document, the recommended grade level is between seven and eight (**BOX 7-10**). This recommended grade level should be determined by the average reading level of the typical patient with whom the advanced nurse practices.

Readability scores in Microsoft Word are not provided as a default function. To take advantage of this feature, it must be selected. Given its usefulness, advanced nurses, particularly those with education responsibilities of any type, should consider adding the feature to the spell-check function to verify the grade level of written work that directly affects patients, families, or staff. To turn on this function in Word, depending on the version, select "Review" from the tool bar. Select "Language" and then select "Language Preferences; Proofing." There is a box next to "Readability Statistics." Check this box and select "OK." Readability statistics will now be presented with completed spell-checks. The steps for accessing these statistics vary by software version but may be found in the Help feature of most programs.

Understanding how the reading ease and grade-level scores are calculated will assist in improving the appropriateness of Word documents by reducing the grade level or enhancing the understandability of the document. In general, a sixth-grade level (rather than an eighth-grade level) may be more appropriate for a large patient audience, depending on the typical demographic profile of the patient group. If needed, consider a fourth-grade level.

The readability tools in software programs may be inaccurate and underestimate the level of text difficulty (Doak & Doak, 2004). Pfizer recommends using the manual Fry formula because it is not copyrighted, uses a reasonably small sample size of 100 words, has respectability within the reading community, and takes only

---

BOX 7-9 Flesch Reading Ease Score Formula

The formula for the Flesch Reading Ease score is

$$206.835 - (1.015 \times ASL) - (84.6 \times ASW)$$

Where:
ASL = average sentence length (the number of words divided by the number of sentences)
ASW = average number of syllables per word (the number of syllables divided by the number of words)

BOX 7-10 Flesch–Kincaid Grade-Level Score Formula

The formula for the Flesch–Kincaid Grade Level score is

$$(0.39 \times ASL) + (11.8 \times ASW) - 15.59$$

Where:
ASL = average sentence length (the number of words divided by the number of sentences)
ASW = average number of syllables per word (the number of syllables divided by the number of words)

15–20 minutes to obtain results (Doak & Doak, 2004). The Pfizer Principles for Clear Health Communication manual (Doak & Doak, 2004) offers step-by-step instructions for using the Fry formula and provides the Fry chart for ease of use. Pfizer's, Inc. (2018c) health literacy resources for health care professionals provide excellent resources that offer good information to nurses who are interested in developing written communication expertise.

Online resources enable opportunities for advanced nurses to cut and paste text into text boxes and have the selection evaluated for readability. Wikipedia.com, a free online encyclopedia, provides external links to tools that evaluate the Fog index, Flesch–Kincaid scores, and other readability measures and offers suggestions for enhancing readability (Wikipedia, 2017).

AHRQ has available the *Patient Education Materials Assessment Tool* (PEMAT) (Shoemaker, Wolf, & Brach, 2014), an instrument designed to assess the understandability and actionability of print and audiovisual patient education materials. A user guide is also available as are the two tools, one for printable materials and one for audiovisual materials. The intent of the PEMAT is to use a systematic method for the evaluation and comparison of the understandability and actionability of patient education materials (AHRQ, 2017b). PEMAT has established content validity and construct validity (Shoemaker et al., 2014). The final PEMAT demonstrated strong internal consistency ($\alpha = 0.71$; average item-total correlation $= 0.62$). PEMAT was developed to provide a better measure of reading comprehension than the grade-level indicator calculated by most readability formulas. The PEMAT was demonstrated to have strong interrater reliability when used by untrained laypeople and by health professionals.

Shoemaker et al. (2014) defined understandability as "patient education materials are understandable when consumers of diverse backgrounds and varying levels of health literacy can process and explain key messages" (p. 3). Actionability builds on this understanding by evaluating how well "consumers of diverse backgrounds and varying levels of health literacy can identify what they can do based on the information presented" (p. 3). PEMAT is composed of items from two scales; understandability (n = 19) and actionability (n = 7). PEMAT scores educational materials on a 100-point scale. One major advantage of the tool is its ease of administration given that there is no required training for instrument application.

Formatting for Appeal and Impact

In addition to grade level and understandability, advanced nurses must consider the overall look of printed materials. Graphics can be important visual cues that enhance learning. Elderly patients provided with a leaflet that included graphics were five times more likely to receive a pneumococcal vaccine than were those elders in a control group who received a text-only brochure. They were also more likely to speak with their physicians about receiving the immunization (Jacobson et al., 1999).

Nurses should keep in mind that the average patient is probably a poor reader and this is why the universal precautions for health communication notion is so important to patient education endeavors (Pfizer, Inc., 2018d). Clear headings, bullets rather than full paragraphs, and ample white space are important. Short sentences, active voice, and familiar language with pictures and examples also facilitate engagement and learning. Pfizer, Inc. (2018d) recommends written materials with a 14-point font and contrasting colors. When developing critical materials, it may be useful to consider bringing together a group of intended audience members and field testing materials to solicit feedback about the effectiveness and appeal of the written product. Pfizer, Inc. cautions that while culturally appropriate visual images can intrigue readers and help to clarify important concepts, excessive details can be distracting so avoid visual clutter.

Assessing the Learner

There are several health literacy measurement tools that may be useful to advanced nurses, including those who are designing or participating in research projects around the subject of health literacy. One database of health literacy measures, the *Health Literacy Tool Shed*, is made available through a collaboration involving Boston University, CommunicateHealth, Inc., and RTI International. The database provides details about various measures, including their psychometric properties, and bases this information on peer-reviewed literature. The tools are not necessarily free so advanced nurses need to pay attention to permission or fee requirements (Health Literacy Tool Shed, 2018).

The Tool Shed offers search tools that include filter measures based on lead author; health literacy domain; specific context; modern approach for tool development; number of items; approximate administration time, sample size, sample population age, mode of administration, and language in validation study; assessment; and measure style. A glossary is provided to facilitate understanding of relevant vocabulary and terminology. There is also a recommended references list with hyperlinks that directly connects to health literacy resources (CommunicateHealth, Boston University, & RTI International, 2018).

Validated measures for ascertaining health literacy include the Rapid Estimate of Adult Literacy in Medicine (REALM), REALM-Short Form (SF), and the Test of Functional Health Literacy in Adults (TOFHLA). REALM measures a person's ability to recognize and pronounce common health and medical terms. REALM does not measure understanding but can be used to assist health professionals in selecting appropriate educational materials and instructions. This scale is one of the most frequently used instruments to measure healthy literacy, particularly because it requires only a few minutes to administer and score. Dumenci, Matsuyama, Kuhn, Perera, and Siminoff (2013) investigated the validity of the Shortened REALM to make inferences about health literacy and found that although it is a highly consistent tool, it is most accurately a measure of reading and pronunciation ability rather than providing an accurate measure of health literacy. Dumenci et al. point out that the test does not address major health literacy content areas, including comprehension of printed materials, numeracy, and information seeking and navigation. The authors recommend that the Shortened REALM not be used for health literacy measurement.

REALM comprises 66 items and takes 2–3 minutes to administer and score. Subjects read from a list of 66 medical words arranged in order of complexity as determined by the number of syllables and pronunciation difficulty. Patients read aloud as many words as they can from the first word and continue until they reach words that they cannot pronounce correctly. REALM yields a score that estimates a grade level for reading. A sample kit and pricing information can be obtained by writing to the developer. REALM has established validity and reliability (Davis et al., 1991, 1993) and is available only in English. REALM-SF is a revised, shortened version of REALM that consists of a seven-item word recognition test (AHRQ, 2016; Arozullah et al., 2007).

The TOFHLA is available in both English and Spanish (Parker, Baker, Williams, & Nurss, 1995; Weiss, 2007). It measures the functional literacy of patients using real-to-life health care materials. Examples of these materials include prescription bottle labels, diagnostic test instructions, and patient education information. The TOFHLA is a valid and reliable method for establishing the patient's ability to read health-related materials.

The TOFHLA has 67 items and measures numeracy and reading comprehension. Scores categorize patients into low, marginal, or adequate health literacy skill groups. It takes 22 minutes to complete both constructs. A short form is available in a variety of languages (CommunicateHealth, Inc., Boston University, & RTI International, 2018).

Culturally and Linguistically Appropriate Health Care

The Joint Commission (TJC) views culturally and linguistically appropriate health services as critical to quality and safety (Jordan, 2016). Many TJC standards support this requirement, including interpreter and translation services, food preferences, equal standard of care, informed consent, among others. TJC recognizes that health literacy is a broader concern than reading ability but, rather, refers to a complex set of skills and abilities necessary when navigating health situations. Health literacy is viewed as dynamic, influenced by illness, age, stress level, and other fluctuating variables (Jordan, 2016). TJC requires that determination of patients' health literacy needs must build on their identified learning needs, including learning barriers and preferred learning methods. The education plan for patients must be consistent with patients' health literacy needs (Jordan, 2016). TJC requires that an interactive process or methodology be used to ascertain patients' health literacy levels. Tools may be used as well but not in lieu of interaction.

▶ Educating Nurses to Support Practice Excellence

Advanced nurses are frequently engaged in nursing staff education. Teaching activities are often informal and spontaneous—that is, spur-of-the-moment opportunities to provide new information about any number of topics, including practice concerns, new technologies, policies, or patient care–related concerns. Continuing education is critically important to ensure competent care delivery and few providers would dispute this caveat. However, effectively educating within a demanding context of perpetual change, stressful work requirements, and limited resources challenges nurses in advanced roles and the nurses and colleagues that they need to instructionally support.

Education Programs: Not a Cure-All

Advanced nurse educators, advanced practice nurses, staff development experts, and other nursing authorities are frequently charged with creating educational programs to correct an identified patient care or indirect care problem. These program requests are often triggered by the need to respond to a situation viewed as threatening to quality patient care outcomes. Concerns may also be related to real or perceived institutional liabilities, patient satisfaction, or safety compromise, among others. Although education may be the correct remedy, it should not always be the *only* or even the first proposed solution to a concern of interest. Many times practice problems are unrelated to knowledge deficits, but rather are related to competing priorities, workload challenges, or an employee's free will (**EXEMPLAR 7-1**).

Wright (2015) reminds educators that when an educational strategy is proposed as the solution to a problem, it is important to bring the conversation back to discussion about the desired or intended outcome of the educational intervention. It may be that education is not the best response. It may be the most convenient response in terms of offering a straightforward action that demonstrates action in the face of a concerning problem; but, it may not be an approach that actually addresses the root of the practice problem. There are times when quality improvement strategies, including deeper digging, may be required to better understand the problem and potential solutions.

 EXEMPLAR 7-1 Free Will and Missed Opportunities: A Management Consideration

Jed Robinson, RN, has been employed on South Bay Hospital's telemetry unit for 6 years on 12-hour night shifts. Nurse Robinson is regarded as a competent nurse who works very well under pressure. He is well liked by his coworkers, but supervisors find that he can be a negative influence on the work group when he is dissatisfied with staffing levels or new policies and procedures.

South Bay Hospital has attracted a nationally known bariatric surgeon committed to developing a cutting-edge bariatric surgery service. Some nurses, including Nurse Robinson, are concerned about the impact that this service will have on the workload of the telemetry unit as many of the postoperative patients will require telemetry services. These concerns have been shared and discussed during a variety of unit and department meetings.

In preparation for this new program, the hospital purchased several new patient lifts and bariatric-specific beds. The equipment is not sophisticated but does require staff to learn how to adjust the equipment for emergency procedures and transports. In-services are arranged across all shifts. Educational posters are developed with posttest questions, and access to a Web-based educational module is purchased for a 4-week period. In lieu of the poster activity or Web-based program, staff may elect to read a continuing education article and complete its posttest.

Staff is required to select the teaching modality that is most convenient for them. Following this educational session, each nurse must demonstrate correct use of the lift and the specialty bed. The staff has 1 month to complete this educational module and to demonstrate competence with the equipment. By week 4, Nurse Robinson has failed to complete the education stating, "There is no way I'm coming in on my day off and the other times I've been too busy to leave my patients for an in-service on a bed!" Other nurses agree, resulting in a program completion rate of 60%.

During a meeting with the director of nursing education (DNE), the topic of the bariatric education program is raised. The nurse manager of the unit requests that the clinical nurse leader (CNL) responsible for the unit-based equipment roll-out schedule additional in-services to accommodate staff who had not elected to attend the previous programs. The bariatric program is progressing quickly, and staff will soon need to use the equipment. The CNL agrees to offer three more sessions. Again, turnout is poor.

Two days following the final education session, an obese woman suffers from respiratory distress. She is in a specialized bariatric bed. The emergency team arrives to intubate the patient but the nurse, Nurse Robinson, is unable to position the bed

(continues)

EXEMPLAR 7-1 Free Will and Missed Opportunities:
A Management Consideration   *(continued)*

flat. Other nurses come to the room to assist. After a period of 5 minutes, the patient is successfully intubated. As the team attempts to transport the patient to the intensive care unit, more difficulties arise when they realize that the bed will not fit through the door frame. After a lengthy discussion and several attempts, the nursing team successfully removes the bedrails and transports the patient.

The following morning, the DNE is contacted by the bariatric surgeon regarding the nurses' ineptitude with the bariatric equipment. Although the patient did not suffer harm, the potential for injury was high. He insists that the nursing staff require education.

The DNE meets with the CNL and nurse manager of the unit. The nurse manager's initial response is, "We'll have to set up more in-services right away. Staff have shared with me that they could not attend the in-services because they were too busy taking care of patients. You'll need to schedule additional education sessions immediately."

The CNL is asked to respond. After thoughtful consideration, the CNL summarizes the problem:

1. Education programs were offered over a 3-week period on a variety of shifts and a variety of days, including weekends. Attendance was poor.
2. Staff unable to attend the education sessions were encouraged to review the poster information and complete a posttest. Fifty percent of nurses who completed the skills demonstration acquired the necessary information via the poster opportunity. Each demonstrated hands-on competency.
3. Staff interested in a Web-based learning module were able to access the materials through the vendor's website. The posttest used for the poster session was available for these nurses. Forty percent of the nurses who completed the skills demonstration chose this education pathway. Each demonstrated hands-on competency.
4. Staff was permitted to read a continuing education article, self-study through the instruction booklet, and complete the posttest. Ten percent of staff who completed the skills demonstration acquired the necessary information using this selection and each demonstrated competency.

The CNL identified that the problem was no longer a knowledge deficit but rather a commitment issue. The CNL worked with the management team to design a strategy. Two nurses, both of whom had completed the education program, were asked for input. The action plan was as follows:

1. Staff who had completed the program and the skills assessment were recognized during a staff meeting.
2. Staff who had not completed the program and the skills assessment were identified as "not yet competent" (Wright, 2005) specific to the bariatric bed and lift. They were not permitted to use this equipment until competency was established. Charge nurses were notified as were the individual nurses.
3. Staff was given 1 week to complete the education program and the skills assessment. The only options for learning were numbers 2–4 noted earlier. No further in-service sessions were available. Self-study time was not paid beyond the shift pay.
4. Evaluative feedback was documented and placed in files to inform upcoming performance evaluations.
5. Staff choosing to not participate in the education opportunities was given the option to meet with the nurse manager to discuss other unit assignments that did not require bariatric equipment skills, given the hospital's decision to prioritize this particular program.

6. Staff discussions during meetings and individual conversations reinforced the new perspective on competency demonstrations. Staff participated in identifying convenient and effective teaching and learning strategies and were encouraged to contribute to competency identification for the upcoming year.

     Within the week, each nurse had completed the education program and demonstrated competence with the equipment. Nurse Robinson was reluctant to attend the program; however, alternate assignments within the hospital were unappealing. Nurse Robinson completed the program within the required time frame.

Staff Education: Influencing Staff via Educational Programming

Organizations are responsible for providing opportunities for education so that employees can achieve and maintain the skillset necessary for safe, quality practice. These educational opportunities are opportunities to learn. Employees are obliged to take advantage of these chances to meet their contractual obligation to provide safe care.

It is reasonable for employees to expect that educational programs will be offered on more than one occasion and in a scheduling pattern that accommodates more than one shift. It also makes sense for educational formats to vary and to include flexible options such as computer-assisted instruction, self-study modules, workshops, poster board formats, or Web-based instruction. These expectations are realistic and may even be obligatory on the part of the employing institution.

Employees have concurrent obligations. They are obligated to make themselves available to educational programs. Nurses are responsible for acquiring and maintaining the skills necessary for the level of practice expected of them by the employing institution and for which they accept compensation. Wright (2005) comments that the organization needs to recognize that employees may not be interested in the direction the organization is moving. If this is the case and the employee is not interested in availing himself or herself of the provided educational opportunities, then the employee should find a different organization in which to practice.

This stance is not threatening; rather, it is an honest appraisal of the situation. As noted by Wright (2005), "Employees should periodically reflect on their commitment to their organization's evolution, and if that commitment is not strong, find an organization to work for that is better aligned with his or her personal philosophies and goals" (p. 3). Wright (2015) also cautions that when education and remediation are inappropriately, sometimes automatically, applied, the problem may become blurred and cover up the real issue. During this period of confusion and ineffective action, patients may be harmed and outcomes may be adversely influenced.

Nursing administrators and advanced nurse leaders may find this position disconcerting. Anecdotal evidence suggests that when systems problems arise, education is often offered as a first-line response. When attendance is poor and nurses' skillsets remain amiss, advanced nurses or educators are frequently charged with providing additional teaching sessions. When low attendance rates persist, nurses are reminded of their responsibility to attend and then cajoled, implored, threatened, and perhaps penalized in some tangible fashion.

Advanced nurses may need to consider this loop and more carefully examine the linkages that reinforce the negative behaviors. Could it be that low attendance is the result of two or more influences: an incorrect assumption that education is needed to correct this particular clinical problem, and nurses' realizations that *mandatory* in-services are not truly mandated when there are no clear consequences associated with absences? In fact, employees may have become conditioned to believe that it is the responsibility of organizations to provide carte blanche programming and that this responsibility supersedes the obligation of the nurse to take advantage of the education.

The key point is that a root cause analysis is sometimes needed to identify whether the particular problem is actually related to a knowledge deficit. There are many times when nurses know the correct action or behavior but elect to not act as per policy stipulations or, in the case of equipment, per manufacturer's directions. Understanding the reasons why compromised practice standards or processes occur is important to correctly remedy the situation.

At times, the remedy *is* education. At other times, the solution relates to management interventions. This sort of analysis may be more time consuming than the typical "let's teach—that will fix the problem" reaction but will save money and needless effort by targeting interventions that will correct the underlying problem. The challenge may lie in changing the culture of nursing to one that views competence as radically different from education program attendance.

Developing Competence with Competencies

There is confusion surrounding the definition of competence (Tilley, 2008), and there are many problems with its measurement (Watson, Stimpson, Topping, & Porock, 2002; Wright, 2015). Smith (2012) observed that some of the greatest challenges in the nursing profession relate to developing, maintaining, and evaluating nurse competence. The root of competence confusion may relate to the lack of a conceptual definition of nursing competence, making it difficult to establish measurable operational definitions (Waddell, 2001).

Cowan, Norman, and Coopamah (2005) suggested that nursing requires complex combinations of knowledge, performance, skills, and attitudes, and this complexity necessitates consensus on a conceptual and operational definition. Tilley (2008) described the attributes of competency as the application of skills in all domains for the practice role, instruction focusing on select outcomes or competencies, allowances for increasing levels of competency, learner accountability, practice-based learning, self-assessment, and individually tailored learning experiences. Garside and Nhemachena (2013) suggested that competence is often easiest to define when viewed within the context of incompetence. This is similar to the frequently used colloquialism, "I know it when I see it." Unfortunately, assuring and promoting competence are critically important to contemporary nursing, and so advanced nurses are charged with determining the best ways to evaluate the many facets of nurse competence, particularly as related to direct care responsibilities.

Concept analyses of nurse competence provide useful insights that may be used to inform understanding of competence complexities. Smith (2012) explored the concept of nurse competence based on Rodgers' Evolutionary Concept Analysis Model. Smith investigated the published literature from 1990 to 2012 and conducted a thorough review of appropriate databases as well as hand-searching relevant reference lists. The literature revealed multiple attributes of the competence concept, including integrating knowledge into practice, experience, critical thinking, proficient skills, caring, communication, environment, motivation, and professionalism (Smith, 2012). Antecedents and consequences of nurse competence were also discerned. The consequences of competence attainment were identified as confidence, safe practice, and holistic care. Smith's work provides advanced nurses with an opportunity to review and reflect on the crux of nurse competence—what it is and how it should be supported and considered throughout the many education and evaluation endeavors that advanced nurses typically influence. The supportive environments necessary to promote competence need to encompass the many attributes and consequences of competence and recognize the importance of antecedents to competence (Smith, 2012).

Identifying domains of competence may be useful, as domains offer possibilities for practical evaluation strategies. Lyon and Boland (2002) suggested that competence domains may include knowledge, technical, cultural, and communication domains. Del Bueno, Barker, and Christmyer (1980) offered technical, critical thinking, and interpersonal domains as a model of competence. Smith's (2012) descriptions of attributes and consequences associated with the concept of competence also offer opportunities that might inform evaluation methods. These domain models may be useful to the advanced nurse when developing multifaceted strategies for developing nursing competencies and assessing nurse competence. In fact, measuring nursing students' competence is also a high-stakes endeavor that relies on a clear understanding of the concept of nurse competence. Whether evaluating competence of students or practicing nurses, valid and reliability assessment tools are imperative (Franklin & Melville, 2015).

Wright's (2015) Competency Assessment Model offers a unique and practical perspective on competencies (**FIGURE 7-6**). The model builds on four principles: (1) Selected competencies should matter to the people involved and to the organization. They should be realistic, partnered with quality improvement data, and collaboratively determined based on critical analysis; (2) competencies should be appropriately verified; (3) those involved in the process must have clearly articulated roles and responsibilities; and (4) when employee-centered competency verification is in play, a culture of engagement and commitment is promoted. Wright notes that the model is based on the principles of ownership, empowerment, and accountability.

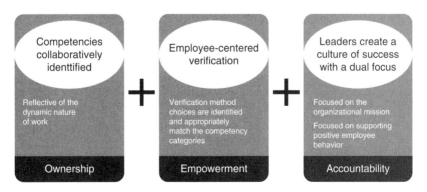

FIGURE 7-6 Wright Competency Model Elements of Success

Understanding the Nature of Competence and Competency

The terms *competence* and *competency* require definition, as they are often used interchangeably and may, in fact, be unique but related entities. Competence is often defined as a capacity to perform based on knowledge, whereas competency is the actual performance (Franklin & Melville, 2015; McConnell, 2001; Nolan, 1998; Smith, 2012). Confusion surrounding these definitions in professional practice is important to consider because the inaccurate interchangeability of terms worsens the challenge of crafting a clear definition.

Distinguishing competence from performance is challenging, and there is no clearly established link from these two concepts to capability and expertise (Watson et al., 2002). Although the notion of protecting the public by ensuring competent practitioners makes sense, the level of performance that actually demonstrates competence in practice has not been determined. An example of this concern is illustrated by a scenario in which an RN completes a medication administration examination for a critical care unit position. The RN scores a 90%. Does this score reflect medication administration competence, or is competence demonstrated only by a 100% score? If the RN scores an 85%, does this score indicate incompetence? Competence may seem simple, but it is a sophisticated issue. If the nurse earns a 50% score on this examination but demonstrates satisfactory medication delivery skills during practice or simulation, has the nurse demonstrated competency in this particular task while incompetent in the broader understanding of safe medication delivery?

Many health care agencies are investing time and money into systems to assess competency of nursing professionals. One example of such a system is the Performance-Based Development System (PBDS). This particular system uses video simulations, written out-of-context exercises, and visual out-of-context exercises to evaluate critical thinking manifested primarily as clinical judgment (del Bueno, 2005). PBDS may be provided in an online or hard-copy format. A review of literature did not yield published reliability or validity information on this system.

Advanced nurses must remember that attendance at an educational program does not ensure competence with the particular topic or skill. It is probably also true that demonstrating a performance in a controlled laboratory situation with a single skill in a simple environment as compared to a complex, stressful, real-world environment also does not signify competency. Of course, the more sophisticated and labor intensive the competency assessment, the more the activity costs. This is a legitimate concern that cannot be easily dismissed.

Competence assessment involves some form of evaluation by one person of another (Watson et al., 2002). When human interaction is involved in competence assessment, reliability is a potential concern due to the influence of social processes on the consistency of evaluative scores (McMullan et al., 2003; Watson et al., 2002). Validity is also a problem related to the lack of psychometrically established instruments used to determine competence. Reliability concerns are not often raised when nurses are planning skills labs assessments. Validity is discussed even less frequently. Both of these topics are critically important to the notion of competent practice (**EXEMPLAR 7-2**).

EXEMPLAR 7-2 Validity and Reliability as Applied to Competencies

A nurse manager identifies a need for professional nurses to improve their recognition of acute myocardial infarction (AMI) electrocardiogram (ECG) patterns after a potentially serious clinical event in the telemetry unit during which several nurses failed to recognize AMI ECG changes in a 52-year-old female patient. The manager consults with an education team composed of a Clinical Nurse Specialist (CNS), Clinical Nurse Leader (CNL), and department-based staff development educator. The team designs a program to develop competence in AMI ECG interpretations and creates outcomes measures to ascertain competency. The team selects a posttest and case study exercise as strategies for verifying competency. In addition, a mock clinical scenario using a simulation model is developed. This simulation experience will take place 2 weeks after the program and will be scored by the CNS and the CNL. The experience will consist of AMI ECG recognition and three associated scenarios: (1) acute destabilization with dysrhythmias, pulmonary edema, and hypotension; (2) preparation for and administration of thrombolytic therapy; and (3) immediate preparation for cardiac interventional therapy.

The CNS conducts literature and software searches to locate an infarct pattern test. None is located, and the CNS creates an examination. The case study exercises are actual 12-lead ECGs from patients who have had a variety of cardiac events and nonevents, including infarcts and angina episodes. Several staff nurses have agreed to supervise small groups of case study sessions and grade the tools.

Reflection Questions

1. Reliable measures are consistent measures. Where are the potential measurement problems specific to reliability?
2. Valid measures accurately reflect the true nature of what is being measured. A valid measure is a truthful measure. What validity concerns are associated with this competency program?
3. How might the education team improve the reliability and validity of this competency program?
4. Why do the posttest, case study, and clinical simulation work well together to evaluate competency with AMI ECG interpretation and treatment? What does each single evaluation strategy evaluate?

Skillful Nurses and Competency Assessment

Wright (2005, 2015) offers specific, practical suggestions for competency assessment. Wright asserts that competency assessment follows a continuum that evolves as the requirements of the nurses' jobs evolve (**FIGURE 7-7**). Competency assessment for the new hire should differ from that of the established RN. Wright (2005, 2015) suggests that competency assessment must be perceived by staff as a valuable process, or it will be perceived as a time waster.

One strategy for competency assessment is to engage staff in identifying the competencies that are required for safe and professional practice. Once the competency is determined, verification strategies should match the competency categories. Nurse leaders need to support and sustain a culture of success by promoting, nurturing, and rewarding positive employee performance related to competency assessment (Wright, 2005, 2015).

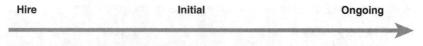

FIGURE 7-7 The Competency Continuum.

Reproduced from *The ultimate guide to competency assessment in health care* (3rd ed.) by Donna Wright. ©2005 Creative Health Care Management. Used with permission.

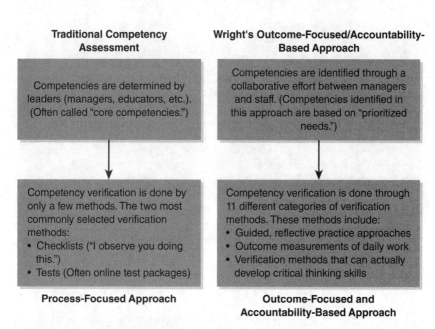

FIGURE 7-8 Traditional Assessment Versus Wright's Competency Assessment Model.

Reproduced from *The ultimate guide to competency assessment in health care* (3rd ed.) by Donna Wright. ©2005 Creative Health Care Management. Used with permission.

Wright's Competency Assessment Model (2015) is quite different from the traditional competency assessments used in many health care organizations, particularly given its outcome-driven focus that places accountability for competency verification on the employee (**FIGURE 7-8**).

Establish Organizational Policies Selectively and Judiciously

Advanced nurses are well advised to consider institutional policies as opportunities to reasonably and realistically guide nursing care processes and decision making. The goal of policies is to establish a required level of practice that the organization is obliged to satisfy. Wright (2005) cautions that when agencies develop policies that are unrealistic and not possible to meet given resources and opportunities, the organization sets itself up for accreditation deficiencies resulting from noncompliance with its own standards of care. For example, if a nursing department has a policy that requires a one-to-one sitter standard when a patient is admitted to a medical-surgical unit with a diagnosis that includes the potential for self-harm, then the institution is required to consistently provide this care ratio, regardless of circumstances. This is a self-selected, institutional policy that is now a hard and fast care expectation. If the department is unable to provide this level of supervision, even if other safe alternatives are available, the department is in a state of noncompliance with its policy. Accreditors take exception to this sort of practice standard violation, not because the accrediting agency requires the level and type of care that the policy dictates, but because the agency is noncompliant with its internally determined staffing requirement. Advanced nurses should reflect on this example when developing and approving policies. A tightly written, highly prescriptive policy designed to ensure certain processes, equipment, practices, and standards might read well but it is a policy with which the institution must consistently comply.

▶ Essentials for Educating with Excellence: Academic Teaching and the Advanced Nurse

Many advanced nurses are interested in teaching undergraduate nursing students, whereas others find that serving as a preceptor for graduate students is more to their liking. There are various opportunities to participate in nursing education, including doctoral studies. The nursing profession and the health care system are challenged by the shortage of professional nurses with advanced education and practice expertise. Faculty shortages are contributing to this problem because baccalaureate program enrollment figures cannot exceed the availability of nurse educators. APRN program enrollments are also constrained by an inadequate number of clinical sites and available preceptors.

The American Association of Colleges of Nursing (AACN, 2017) has identified that faculty shortages are limiting student capacity at a time when demand for professional registered nurses is high and increasing. In 2016, nursing schools in the United States turned away 64,067 qualified applicants from college/university undergraduate and graduate programs because of insufficient resources, including faculty, clinical sites, classroom space, clinical preceptors, and inadequate finances. A recent AACN report revealed that 1,567 faculty vacancies were identified in a survey of 821 nursing schools with baccalaureate and/or graduate programs (AACN, 2017). The response rate was 85.7%. Faculty availability is influenced by several factors: specifically, an aging workforce, increasing numbers of retiring faculty members, higher compensation packages in practice and private-sector settings that lure nurse educators away from academe, and an insufficient supply of master's and doctoral program students to meet the demand of downstream educational settings (AACN, 2017).

The shortage of formally prepared nurse educators coupled with the need for clinical experts puts nurses with advanced degrees and practice expertise in an ideal position to consider opportunities in clinical instruction, professorships, and part-time employment as adjunct faculty members. Advanced nurses need a clear understanding of the differences between these roles, the expectations of each, a general sense of the right questions to ask, and a handle on the responsibilities and challenges associated with the teaching role.

Adjunct and Part-Time Teaching Considerations

There are a number of ways for nurses to become involved in basic nursing education. In general, most nursing programs require a master's of science in nursing (MSN) degree of faculty members. Specialty certification is not usually required for clinical teaching, although it may be desirable to demonstrate expertise within a particular practice area. It is important to consider the content areas that might be available and contemplate the match or mismatch between the necessary content/practice expertise and the actual expertise and work to close this gap.

Some nurses prefer to work in a practice arrangement on a full-time or part-time basis and to teach as an adjunct faculty member for a university, 4-year college (baccalaureate program), or community college (associate of arts/science degree of nursing [ADN]). This type of teaching position is referred to as "adjunct" because the clinical instructor is a supplemental teaching resource who contributes to the overall education of the students and the quality of the program but does not have the responsibilities of a full-time faculty member. Usually adjunct faculty is hired on a semester basis or for a defined period of the academic year. Another consideration is that adjunct professors are not paid as full-time faculty, nor do they usually receive benefits. Advanced nurses interested in adjunct roles over a consistent, extended period of time might explore whether part-time faculty/instructor opportunities make more sense as compared to adjunct positions. The difference in status between adjuncts and part-time instructors varies by institution and is worth exploring when both options are available.

Other advanced nurses may elect to teach on a full-time basis while practicing clinically on a part-time basis. This clinical practice may be in the form of agency or per diem work, part-time employment, or in a joint appointment. A joint appointment is a combined position that links academic work to clinical practice. The nurse holding a joint appointment position typically straddles both worlds, academic and service, with varying accountabilities to administrators in each setting. This type of role can be challenging in its duality but is also stimulating. Challenges associated with joint positions may include a high workload, potential compensation deficiencies, and role conflicts. There are times when achieving work-life balance can be difficult when juggling multiple roles and having more than one supervisory reporting line can be frustrating; however, juggling an academic role, joint position, and practice arrangement also keeps things interesting and provides differing experiences that would likely not be found within the context of one employment role.

Adjunct or part-time clinical instructor positions are also available in basic nursing programs at the diploma (hospital-based) level. The more typical terminology in diploma education is *part-time* clinical instructor rather than *adjunct* faculty and probably relates to the historical differences between the hospital-based and university-based programs. There are fewer diploma programs in the United States than other types and, therefore, fewer teaching opportunities. For the purpose of this chapter, academic opportunities relate to college or university settings.

What Are Creative Teaching Strategies?

The descriptive phrase "creative teaching strategies" is commonly used by nurse educators. Some institutions of higher education use this phrase on evaluation forms as an aspect of teacher evaluations. In general, this phrase is a catchall term for a variety of teaching methods that are designed to engage the student in the process of learning as an active participant rather than as a passive receptacle of information.

Creative teaching or active learning strategies may include concept mapping, problem-based learning activities, case studies, simulation exercises, games, logs, journals, and role playing, as well as others. Education may be provided in the classroom (didactic teaching), laboratory (simulation or skills labs), clinical settings (also a type of laboratory setting), and via a teaching/learning online platform. Advanced nurses are well advised to explore how educational programs of interest provide instruction and investigate a bit about these resources, particularly if the applicant has little to no exposure to these sorts of tools and strategies.

Clinical Teaching Versus Clinical Practice: Duality and Harmony

Advanced nurses typically have some type of interest in nursing education and are generally committed to clinical practice excellence. Educators' clinical expertise advantages nursing students because the practice expertise contributes to the overall quality and relevance of the learning experience. Advanced nurses may find that their expertise is associated with unique challenges. It can be difficult to instruct students in settings that are challenged by a lack of experienced staff or a culture of mediocrity. Staff may approach the advanced nurse to ask for advice, assistance, or troubleshooting while the nurse is engaged in teaching students. Advanced nurses may feel inclined to participate in decision making and care provision that is not within their purview as nursing instructors but, rather, belongs with the employees of the host institution.

Advanced nurses may also find it difficult to teach at a rudimentary level when their usual practice is much more advanced. It can be tempting to launch into a discussion of abnormal physical assessment findings, complex pharmacology, or advanced pathology topics with students who are eager to learn and interested in everything and anything that the educator may be willing to share! At the same time, these students may not have had a pharmacology course or medical-surgical content or may not have practiced beyond providing fundamental care to a single patient assignment. Although the instructional conversations may be interesting, advanced nurses teaching as academic instructors need to stay focused on facilitating progression toward the final course objectives. This duality as educator and clinician can work in harmony if the instructor is clear about the responsibilities and focus of clinical teaching experiences.

Exploring the Possibilities of Teaching Beginning the Journey

Gathering information about clinical and classroom teaching is a good first step for those interested in nursing education. There is an array of potential questions that advanced nurses might want to consider when exploring classroom teaching (**BOX 7-11**) or clinical instruction opportunities (**BOX 7-12**). Consider these questions as jump-off points to assist in making certain that interviews are productive and informative.

The school of nursing's philosophy is an important consideration, as the philosophy should provide a context for educational experiences. The school's philosophy must be congruent with the philosophy of the larger university or college in which it exists. The university's philosophy and mission relate to the ways in which nursing education is provided.

BOX 7-11 Questions to Ask When Considering Classroom Teaching Opportunities

1. What is the mission of the school/university? How does this mission inform the nursing program? (This information is typically available on the organization's website and should be carefully reviewed.)
2. What is the strategic plan of the program/school/university?
3. What is the philosophy of the nursing education unit? How does this philosophy influence teaching expectations?
4. What are the student demographics?
5. How is inclusion of diverse students and faculty ensured and protected? Is diversity overtly and enthusiastically embraced, including sexual diversity and the broad range of other types of differences and how is this support for diversity manifested within the school/university?
6. What is the curriculum plan? How are courses sequenced?
7. Is there a faculty handbook that provides additional guidance and instruction?
8. How many varieties of student handbooks are available and are they organized by degree, program, or inclusive of all student programs? (Make certain to obtain a copy of the handbook relevant to the educational position of interest.)
9. How is faculty addressed by students? Is the dynamic formal or is the atmosphere informal?
10. How are course syllabi managed? May instructors change the course content? Must syllabi be consistent in all ways between course sections? Are there sections of syllabi that may only be changed by committee?
11. How are examinations provided? How are missed examinations addressed with students?
12. Is there a policy for assignments that are missed or submitted after the due date?
13. How are disciplinary issues handled? Are firearms permitted in the classroom? What are the security policies of the school/university?
14. What are the expectations surrounding office hours and faculty availability? Are personal cell phones permitted for student contact specific to academic concerns?
15. What are the rules around electronic mail?
16. How are final grades recorded into the academic system? Is there a formal requirement for midsemester grades or progress reports?
17. How are academically unsatisfactory students' needs addressed? What are the available student supports for tutoring or counseling?
18. Is there an academic integrity policy?
19. Are offices available for adjunct faculty? Is administrative support available for test construction, printing orders, and appointment management?
20. What is the accreditation cycle for this nursing program?
21. What educational platforms and distance learning tools are available to me?
22. Are virtual meeting systems available for use? Are faculty required to personally present to meetings or are virtual options available?

As an example, a Roman Catholic, private, urban university dedicated in the traditions of the Christian Brothers may have a different perspective on faculty obligations and student-to-faculty relationships than a large, publicly funded state university located in a rural region. Students may also have differing expectations of their selected program, depending on school type. The school of nursing exists within the confines of the university's mission. Advanced nurses need to consider the university's philosophy and make certain that it is compatible to their personal philosophy of education.

BOX 7-12   Sample Query Path for Fledgling Clinical Instructors

Questions to Ask:

1. How large is a typical clinical group?
2. How does the instructor become familiar with the clinical settings? Is there an orientation program, and if so, who arranges this orientation?
3. What is the name, job title, credentials, email, and telephone number of the clinical agency contact person?
4. How are the students oriented to the agency?
5. What is the appropriate dress, including identification, for clinical faculty?
6. Is there a student handbook that describes policies and procedures for medication administration, charting, student illness, absenteeism and lateness, dress code, and clinical preparation requirements?
7. How long is the clinical day? What is the typical schedule?
8. How are assignments shared with students? Are they posted at the clinical agency, and if so, when should they be posted?
9. What is the required student preparation for clinical, and when should this preparation occur?
10. How should an instructor respond to the poorly prepared student?
11. Secure a copy of the required clinical paperwork. What criteria are used to evaluate the preparatory work? When should the work be returned to the student? How does the clinical instructor respond to inadequately completed paperwork?
12. When are students evaluated? Secure a copy of the evaluation tool.
13. What resources are available to assist the student who is performing poorly or unsafely in the clinical setting?
14. What is the policy for office hours?
15. Is parking available at the clinical agency?
16. Is a preconference session required?
17. Is a postconference session required?
18. Are clinical activities scheduled solely at the clinical agency, or are there required activities that are scheduled for additional, outside sites?
19. How does inclement weather affect the clinical learning experience, and who makes decisions regarding early dismissal or clinical experience cancellations?
20. Are phone chains required? What is the expected mode of communication between the clinical instructor and the students?
21. What circumstances should be described and forwarded to the immediate course supervisor?
22. What are the clinical expectations for students specific to numbers of patients, intravenous and medication therapies, discharge planning, teaching, physical assessment, and charting?
23. How will course content and concerns be communicated to the clinical instructors to connect clinical and classroom learning activities?
24. How are instructors addressed in the clinical setting? Are formal titles required, or do instructors work with students on a first-name basis?

Reviewing the position's job description is important to understand the responsibilities of clinical instructors. Job descriptions may be written in broad terms to address the generic responsibilities associated with any type of nursing course. Be aware of the different responsibilities associated with the various teaching roles within the school.

For example, the responsibilities of a clinical instructor, classroom teacher working in a team, and course coordinator or single classroom professor are markedly different. These differences may not be clearly articulated in a job description. Advanced nurses should review the syllabi for course assignments and discuss the responsibilities of the course specific to clinical faculty or assistant classroom faculty. It may be helpful to network with other nurses who are engaged in employment as a part-time or adjunct instructor at the agency of interest. The perspectives of those in the field can be very useful.

Nurses considering an opportunity to take responsibility for coordinating and teaching a course may find that they have additional obligations including communicating with clinical instructors, arranging student experiences at affiliating agencies, and organizing paperwork, evaluations, and documentation specific to student performance issues. Differentiating between these roles and asking appropriate questions prior to accepting the position may help avoid problems or surprises during the semester. This information may also be useful for salary negotiation. Although there is often not much room for financial remuneration flexibility, a solid command of workload expectations certainly may tip the scales, particularly depending on the timing of the position start date and the availability or shortage of qualified instructors.

Many advanced nurses become initially involved in nursing education as part-time clinical instructors. Be aware that the responsibilities of clinical instructors can vary between schools and/or within schools. As an example, some programs require clinical instructors to participate in grading student assignments. Nurses need to seek information specific to the turnaround time for grading assignments as well as any opportunities for asking questions and seeking validation from more experienced colleagues that grades have been correctly assigned.

Difficulties associated with grading tend to relate to the clarity and detail of the assignment flyers. If grading activities rely on the subjective evaluation of the clinical instructor, the advanced nurse may find it helpful to ask that the instructor group meet to share insights and critiques prior to returning grades to students. This activity promotes interrater reliability and prevents the variability in grading that students perceive as unfair. Some programs do not require clinical instructors to grade assignments but may require paperwork evaluations using satisfactory versus unsatisfactory criteria. Again, this is an important area to explore before signing a contract.

Setting Limits: Focusing on the Educator Role During Instruction Time

New clinical instructors often find it difficult to establish boundaries with the staff on the assigned nursing unit. Advanced nurses are accustomed to serving as the practice expert and typically enjoy interacting with staff and troubleshooting patient care dilemmas. As a result, advanced nurses may feel conflicted when a situation develops on the assigned unit that appears to require their expertise.

Although it may be tempting to fully participate in the problem-solving activities of staff, the advanced nurse hired to teach is on the unit in the capacity of a nurse educator. Within this capacity, the instructor must attend to the learning needs of the students rather than the unit activities. Remember that each student is relying on the instructor to make certain that learning is occurring and that patients are safe. If the instructor becomes too involved in isolated patient care situations or practice dilemmas, students are left unsupervised, and patients are receiving care from individuals who are not licensed or prepared to practice with autonomy.

Another boundary challenge relates to complex patient care scenarios. There are times when patients' conditions deteriorate. Depending on the academic standing of the nursing student and the responsibilities and activities of the other students in the clinical group cohort, the instructor may be able to engage in prioritizing and intervening in the complex patient care situation with the intent of promoting student learning. However, the reality of this type of situation is that deteriorating patient circumstances demand time and attention. Acute instability may require medication orders, initiating a rapid response team consult, and, perhaps, verbal orders. These responsibilities are more appropriately met by the employed RN. It may be possible for a student to work closely with the RN and either assist or observe; however, the advanced nurse, while in the instructor role for multiple students, must step out and focus on the learning experiences of the remaining students.

Clinical instructors need to realize that they are not on the unit as direct care providers. Instructors are on the unit to teach. There are times when students will be unable to accomplish the tasks of patient care. These activities will need to be turned back to the staff. The clinical instructor cannot perform nursing care outside the purview of teaching students. It is difficult to acknowledge that total care has not been completed and to return these responsibilities to the staff; however, clear communication processes and ongoing updates assist in preventing misunderstandings.

Another potential problem area relates to the relationship between ancillary staff members and students. This relationship is a frequent "hot button" and has been known to create much stress for clinical instructors. It may be helpful to meet with the nurse manager and/or charge nurses before beginning the clinical experience to establish rules and procedures prior to the first day of clinical. If an advanced nurse is also employed as a part-time nursing student instructor on the same unit or in the same institution in which the advanced role is also held, proactive communication and boundary exploration becomes even more important to ensure a successful clinical learning experience.

In general, it is important to recognize that neither the students nor the instructor are agency employees. In fact, the clinical learning group is a guest to the institution. Ancillary staff members are paid employees. As such, certain responsibilities and tasks are assigned to them, for which they are paid. The employed RNs are responsible for assigning work to the ancillary staff members and for supervising this work.

Within this context, it is useful to explain to students and reinforce to staff that ancillary staff assigned to patients are required to meet the needs of the patients. If a student is also assigned to the patient, the student is responsible for completing assigned patient care activities as demanded by his or her learning needs. These needs are delineated on the course syllabus.

In other words, students are at the clinical agency to learn, whereas ancillary staff members are at the agency as employees. When a nursing assistant (NA) or other ancillary staff member receives a patient care assignment, the NA is responsible to the employed RN assigned to the particular patient. The NA is not accountable to the student; however, the student is also not accountable to the NA.

Rather, NAs should go about their work as they are paid to do within the confines of the usual practice patterns on the unit. If a nursing student is assigned to the same patient, the NA should not abdicate responsibility for patient care because "the patient has a student today." The student may or may not have responsibility for learning and practicing fundamental skills.

If a student is required to learn discharge teaching and planning, physical assessment, or other aspects of professional nursing care, the morning care routines of beds, baths, and weights may or may not be required of the student. Communication is absolutely critical in these scenarios. The clinical instructor needs to recognize that tact, kindness, and respect for others should be paramount in the interactions with staff members. Otherwise, issues with ancillary staff and professional staff may negatively affect student learning experiences. Instructors should view these interactions as opportunities to role model professional communication processes.

This same rationale explains why students should not be inappropriately used for patient transport, pharmacy pickups, and other routine tasks. When students spend too much time in these activities, they become resentful and frustrated because these activities take time away from critical experiences, thereby undermining the educational value of the day. Of course, in the event of a true patient care emergency, students may need to be flexible and assist as team members. It is important for the clinical instructor to recognize what sorts of situations are emergencies as compared to situations that are predictable and related to short staffing, sick calls, or poor planning.

Typically Atypical Nursing Students

Nurse demographics are changing, and the profession is welcoming and encouraging these changes. Society needs an increased number of nurses, and both society and the profession need these nurses to reflect the richly diverse cultural montage of the country. These needs are encouraging professional nursing organizations and foundations to increase recruitment efforts directed toward diverse students, including people from low socioeconomic backgrounds (Zuzelo, 2005).

The National Nursing Workforce survey is conducted every 2 years by the National Council of State Boards of Nursing (NCSBN) and the National Forum of State Nursing Workforce Centers to provide information about the U.S. nursing workforce. The most recent survey, conducted in 2017, is currently in the data analysis stage (NCSBN, 2018). The 2015 survey included invitations to randomly selected RNs (N = 140,154) and licensed practical/vocational nurses (N = 120,933) with a 30% total response rate across both categories (n = 78,700). Results specific to RNs revealed that 50% were age 50 years or older. An increasing proportion was male, up from 5.8% of those licensed prior to 2000 to 14.1% of those licensed between 2013 and 2015. Approximately 20% of RN respondents identified as racial/ethnic minorities and newly licensed RNs had a more diverse racial/ethnic profile than more experienced RN respondents (NCSBN, 2018).

The aging nursing workforce has been an ongoing concern within the profession and contributes to the prioritized emphasis on recruiting potential nurses from underrepresented groups. These concerns, coupled with the desires of disadvantaged and disenfranchised people to improve their quality of life and to contribute to the nursing profession, are changing the demographics of the nursing classroom. Advanced nurses working in academic nursing need to be prepared for the joys and challenges of a student body that includes people of all ages, even those near retirement age, races, religions, and socioeconomic backgrounds.

Zuzelo (2005) asserted that disadvantaged students present challenges to nurse educators who may be unprepared to identify and respond to the unique needs and characteristics of this group. Disadvantaged students come to higher education programs with different background experiences than do comparatively advantaged students. These past experiences may affect the ways that the student engages with classmates and faculty.

When an instructor values a consistent approach to students, there may be a tendency to use a one-size-fits-all teaching style. The problem with this approach is that it discounts the differences in the opportunities to learn. In other words, disadvantaged students may not have the same real-life opportunities to learn as a student who is academically and psychologically ready to learn at the college level. Educators need to keep these differences in mind as they work with clinical groups and classroom sections and strategize appropriately to meet the needs of these students, within reason. It is important for faculty to be fair and rigorous in expectations while simultaneously assisting students from all types of backgrounds to be as successful as their skills and abilities permit (**BOX 7-13**).

Handling the Angry Student

Advanced nurses may find it important to note that there is an increasing body of published literature suggesting that student incivility is a significant problem in nursing education (Rad & Moonaghi, 2016; Rawlins, 2017; Sauer, Hannon, & Beyer, 2017). Whether described as "attitude" (Zuzelo, 2005, p. 29) or categorized as incivility, aggression (Luparell, 2005), or "maladaptive anger behavior" (Thomas, 2003, p. 17), hostile and aggressive behaviors have been a long-standing concern over the past few decades of nursing and continue to be witnessed in nursing education. Incivility and threatening behaviors may be viewed as manifestations of a more aggressive society; however, nurse educators need to have a ready repertoire of strategies for dealing with student behaviors that may be unpredictable, uncivil, offensive, or even dangerous.

Although incivility is not a hallmark of nursing students in general, it is a phenomenon that is increasingly worrisome and should be not unexpected. There have been incidents of fatal violence directed at professors from students as well as stalking incidences and assault. Student anger may be triggered when students feel "different" or isolated from the normative group (Zuzelo, 2005), feel the perceived pressures

---

BOX 7-13 Strategies for Affirming Disadvantaged Students

1. Recognize the lack of role models for disadvantaged students and fill the void by personally reaching out.
2. Evaluate reading assignments, class activities, patient care assignments, and speakers to ensure that they reflect pluralism and diversity and are relevant to the experiences of students from a variety of backgrounds, including disadvantaged backgrounds.
3. Recognize that self-confidence, assertiveness, and teamwork are part of the hidden yet important curriculum of nursing education programs.
4. Counter student hostility with calm, quiet, and immediate discussion.
5. Offer additional supports to disadvantaged students, including students who are disadvantaged within the university setting because of minority status.
6. Consider joint projects between instructors and disadvantaged students, remembering that these particular students may be less likely to volunteer or ask for such experiences.

BOX 7-14 Anger Triggers for Students

1. Receiving only negative feedback without recognition of jobs well done.
2. Nonverbal expressions that are perceived as indicating disrespect, including sighing, eye-rolling, or other dismissive gestures.
3. Treating students differently based on sex. Avoid making sex-based requests such as, "I need one of the male students to assist with a transport."
4. Criticizing students for their opinions or feelings when honesty is requested.
5. Insulting or criticizing students in public forums including at nursing stations, in patient rooms, or during clinical conferences.
6. Making unexpected changes to clinical schedules, assignments, or locations and providing little to no notice.
7. Allowing perpetuation of stereotypical or prejudiced comments from other students without correction or redirection.
8. Tacit endorsement of bigotry by failing to immediately respond (e.g., tacitly endorsing disparaging comments about vulnerable or marginalized groups of people by failing to use the occasion as a teachable moment for equity and justice).

Data from Thomas, 2003.

---

associated with constructive criticism (Luparell, 2005), or experience common anger triggers (**BOX 7-14**). Thomas (2003) noted five common causes of nursing students' anger: (1) perceptions of teacher unfairness, discrimination, or rigidity; (2) unreasonable expectations of faculty; (3) overly critical instructors; (4) reactions to unanticipated changes; and (5) unresolved family issues that influence and inform reactions to situations in the educational setting. Nurses considering educator roles should think about these triggers and contemplate strategies to minimize the likelihood of evoking an unreasonably angry student response to an unreasonable teacher behavior.

Evaluating Students' Clinical Performance

Setting the tone for the clinical learning experience is important and should be carefully contemplated before the first day of clinical. The instructor should develop a loose script for the orientation day and make clear the behaviors required for satisfactory performance. The tone of the initial meeting and the clarity of shared information affect students' perceptions of the rigor associated with the clinical experience. Ultimately, these perceptions influence student behaviors and affect student performance evaluations.

A word of caution: Educators, particularly those new to the role, occasionally confuse rigor with meanness. Students should not feel threatened, bullied, or diminished by instructors. High expectations are able to coexist with warmth, friendliness, and genuine concern. Aggressively chastising students as a method of ensuring hard work and discipline is not an effective teaching method. Rather, it may perpetuate itself in practice when nurses "beat up" new colleagues or are intolerant of the needs of colleagues.

Clinical instructors are responsible for evaluating students' performance. This may be one of the more difficult aspects of academic nursing. Advanced nurses practicing as managers, staff development experts, preceptors, or staff leaders may have experience with evaluating the performance of new or established employees; however, evaluating students is somewhat different. The Clinical Instruction Algorithm© (**FIGURE 7-9**)

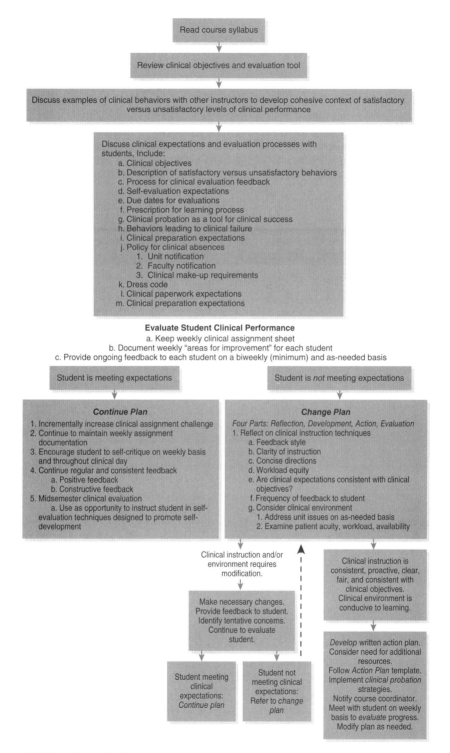

FIGURE 7-9 Clinical Performance Evaluation Algorithm.

© Patti R. Zuzelo.

is a useful pictorial representation of clinical instruction and evaluation processes. Instructor feedback suggests that it is easy to follow and a rapid way to understand the larger context of clinical instruction.

Students should be evaluated on an ongoing basis. The clinical instructor should be making conclusions based on patterns of behavior with the purpose of developing students and assisting them in their efforts to become proficient beginner clinicians. If a student is performing at an unsatisfactory level, inform the student immediately and follow an organized process for supporting the student in attempts to improve and develop competence (**EXEMPLAR 7-3**). There are strategies and guidelines available to assist the instructor with meeting the needs of the struggling student, including probationary processes, remedial support, or systematized warnings. Most higher education agencies have established processes to support at-risk and poorly performing students.

 EXEMPLAR 7-3 The Unprepared Student

Setting the Stage: Background Information

Suzanne Perkins is a 21-year-old junior nursing student entering her second semester of nursing courses. She has completed the Fundamentals of Nursing course as well as the Health Assessment and Health Promotion course. Suzanne is presently enrolled in a Medical-Surgical Nursing course that focuses on the adult client. Her clinical experience takes place at a local university hospital on a busy medical unit. The clinical instructor is responsible for a total of eight nursing students. The instructor reviewed the clinical objectives with the students during the first week of class. The evaluation tool was carefully reviewed with the students and questions were encouraged. Students were informed that the following week, they needed to be prepared to provide comprehensive nursing care to one patient. This assignment would include medication administration, with the exception of intermittent intravenous medications. Clinical paperwork would be collected at the end of the clinical day. Students who attended preconference without satisfactory evidence of clinical preparation would be sent off the clinical unit for the day. The instructor made certain that the students had her office phone number and email address. Policies for absences and lateness were reviewed.

Week 1

Suzanne presented to preconference on time and adequately discussed her general nursing plan of care for the day. She claimed to have had difficulty finding two of her assigned clients' medications and was unaware of the patient's bladder irrigation therapy required for hemorrhagic cystitis (she had not yet had this topic in nursing class). Her care provision for the day was organized, and she was professional and friendly on the unit. When dispensing medications, Suzanne was able to identify digoxin as a "cardiac glycoside" but was unable to relate the digoxin to the patient's long history of atrial fibrillation and congestive heart failure. Additionally, she identified Capoten as an "ACE inhibitor (angiotensin-coverting enzyme inhibitor)" but was unaware of the pharmacological action of this particular drug class. She identified that the drug was used for hypertension although her assigned patient had no documented history of hypertension. The instructor reviewed these concerns with Suzanne and related these issues to inadequate clinical preparation. The instructor noted that the content had been covered during a recent class session and that it was also included in recent required readings for class. Suzanne's comment to these concerns was, "I spent 4 hours getting ready for clinical! It's unrealistic to expect me to spend more time!" The instructor discussed strategies for clinical preparation

EXEMPLAR 7-3 The Unprepared Student   *(continued)*

with Suzanne and made certain that the student knew how to find information in the chart, how to prioritize multiple diagnoses, and how to fine-tune her medication preparation. The student expressed understanding and appreciation.

Week 2

Suzanne was assigned two patients; one patient required partial assistance with care, whereas the other required minimal assistance. The first patient was in the hospital with the diagnosis of deep vein thrombosis (DVT) and was receiving concurrent heparin and warfarin therapy. Suzanne was able to discuss DVT and the nursing care associated with such. She was unable to identify signs and symptoms of pulmonary embolus. Suzanne also was unable to explain why the patient was receiving both heparin and warfarin. Suzanne did adequately discuss the nursing care associated with anticoagulation therapy in general. After preconference, the instructor approached Suzanne about her preparation and the need to focus on the unique and specific needs of the patient and how these needs connect to the prescribed care and nursing care plan. Suzanne stated, "We haven't had any of this in class yet. You can't expect me to learn all of this the night before clinical. Besides, I think my preparation was as good as anyone else's!" After further discussion, Suzanne reluctantly acknowledged that she was behind in her readings and coursework. She vowed to be more focused the following week.

Week 3

Suzanne was assigned one patient with total complex care needs. The patient was alert and oriented to person and place with a diagnosis of hemiplegia secondary to an embolic cerebral vascular accident (CVA). Suzanne satisfactorily discussed the physical care needs of this patient. She was unable to relate the patient's CVA to her atrial fibrillation despite the fact that this information was noted in the chart on several occasions. Additionally, although she was aware of the patient's diarrhea, she was unaware of the patient's diagnosis of *Clostridium difficile* and treatment with Flagyl.

Reflection Questions

1. Was this student's clinical preparation satisfactory? How do you determine whether a student has sufficiently prepared for the clinical day? How much preparation time is reasonable to expect of a student?
2. Is information not yet covered in the classroom fair game for clinical?
3. How would you respond to Suzanne's comment, "Besides, I think my preparation was as good as anyone else's"?
4. In what ways could this performance issue with Suzanne affect the rest of the clinical group?
5. What types of documentation should the instructor maintain as she works with Suzanne?
6. Identify your concerns when you place yourself in this scenario as the instructor.
7. Identify your concerns when you place yourself in this scenario as the student.
8. Develop a possible action plan for Suzanne.

Most institutions require that students receive midsemester and end-semester clinical evaluations. A general guideline to consider is that students should not be surprised by the contents of their performance evaluation. Ideally, students should have an ongoing sense of how they are performing as measured against the clinical objectives (Zuzelo, 2000).

The Contractual Obligations of a Syllabus

Students should be evaluated against the clinical objectives of the course, and these objectives should be theoretically consistent with the course objectives delineated on the syllabus. The syllabus is a contract that instructors and students are obliged to follow. Changes in the syllabus should be immediately shared with students in writing.

Consider the syllabus as a static contract and avoid making unnecessary changes. It is important that students have a clear understanding of course expectations and activities at the start of the quarter; significant deviations from these plans could create situations that students find untenable, particularly given the number of students that are employed while attending school. Scheduling changes, for example, that may be seemingly innocuous may be perceived as significant barriers to students who need to provide available time for work schedules early in the semester or academic quarter or who have family responsibilities. Keep these issues in mind when considering syllabus changes and always keep students well informed. Advanced nurses need to appreciate the serious nature of contract obligations and rights established through school and course policies and procedures to avoid misunderstandings related to compromised due process requirements stemming from property rights.

Managing Student-Instructor Relationships and Communication

Many professors have experienced problems with students lacking a clear understanding of boundaries and telephoning faculty at inappropriate times of day, calling about minutiae, or to engage in general conversation. Clinical instructors subjected to these demanding telephone conversations need to set immediate limits and expeditiously end the call with a reminder to the student that email may be a more reasonable mode of communication for nonessential concerns.

In addition to inappropriate student calls, clinical instructors may also experience students' family members calling to inquire about grades or performance. It is not unheard of for unsatisfactorily performing students to share the instructor's cell phone number with family members, including parents. Not only are these particular calls uncomfortable and surprising, they also place the instructor in an awkward position. Students over the age of 18 are entitled to privacy and the academic institution is required to protect this privacy right. Their scholastic performance is considered private information, regardless of who is paying the tuition bills.

Parents are occasionally frustrated by the privacy restriction, but instructors cannot share information about a student's performance with family, friends, or acquaintances unless the student has granted written permission or accompanies the family member to an in-person meeting with educators or administrators. In general, it may be wise to provide students with contact numbers and addresses that are solely work related rather than home phone numbers, addresses, or personal email addresses.

Fitting into the Academic Environment

Many faculty organizations encourage adjunct faculty members to attend meetings and contribute verbally to discussions while restricting voting to the full-time professoriate.

If an advanced nurse is working as an adjunct or part-time instructor, it is important to share the "adjunct point of view" during faculty meetings. Today's educator shortage frequently creates a dichotomy of classroom faculty and clinical faculty. At times, this relationship is cantankerous as educators struggle with resource and workload challenges that are not much different from those experienced in service settings. Full-time faculty members regard highly those clinical instructors who attend meetings, communicate regularly with course faculty, offer well-written and organized evaluation data, and exert positive influences on students. Highly regarded instructors usually enjoy long-term relationships with professor colleagues and have opportunities for participating in academic research, mentoring, and other types of support.

▶ Conclusion

Many advanced nurses enjoy teaching and serve as effective educators. There are multiple opportunities to teach in nursing, and it is not uncommon to find many advanced nurses participating in educational activities across a variety of venues, including hospitals, universities, and public agencies. First teaching occasions can be nerve-wracking as the nurse attempts to learn the ropes and develop a teaching plan that is appropriate for the particular learner.

Teaching can be an exciting enterprise, and excellent educators are needed in so many areas within and outside health care organizations that nurses with advanced degrees and practice expertise can often have their pick of opportunities. It is rewarding to facilitate growth in others, and the teaching role is usually satisfying, both personally and professionally.

References

Agency for Healthcare Research and Quality. (2015a). Introduction. Retrieved November 26, 2017, from http://www.ahrq.gov/professionals/quality-patient-safety/quality-resources/tools/literacy-toolkit/healthlittoolkit2-intro.html.

Agency for Healthcare Research and Quality. (2015b). Use the teach-back method: Tool #5. Retrieved November 26, 2017, from http://www.ahrq.gov/professionals/quality-patient-safety/quality-resources/tools/literacy-toolkit/healthlittoolkit2-tool5.html.

Agency for Healthcare Research and Quality. (2015c). Tip 6. Be cautious about using readability formulas. Retrieved January 24, 2018, from https://www.ahrq.gov/professionals/quality-patient-safety/talkingquality/resources/writing/tip6.html.

Agency for Healthcare Research and Quality. (2016). Health literacy measurement tools. Revised. Retrieved January 24, 2018, from https://www.ahrq.gov/professionals/quality-patient-safety/quality-resources/tools/literacy/index.html#rapid.

Agency for Healthcare Research and Quality. (2017a). Health literacy. Retrieved November 26, 2017, from https://www.ahrq.gov/professionals/clinicians-providers/resources/health-literacy.html#tools.

Agency for Healthcare Research and Quality. (2017b). The patient education materials assessment tool (PEMAT) and user's guide. Retrieved November 30, 2017, from http://www.ahrq.gov/professionals/prevention-chronic-care/improve/self-mgmt/pemat/index.html.

Almkuist, K. D. (2017). Using teach-back method to prevent 30-day readmissions to patients with heart failure. A systematic review. *MedSurg Nursing, 26,* 309+. Retrieved January 24, 2018, from http://link.galegroup.com.ezproxy2.library.drexel.edu/apps/doc/A514512710/AONE?u=drexel_main&sid=AONE&xid=f70d40e7.

American Association of Colleges of Nursing. (2017). Nursing faculty shortage fact sheet. Retrieved January 26, 2018, from http://www.aacnnursing.org/Portals/42/News/Factsheets/Faculty-Shortage-Factsheet-2017.pdf.

Arozullah, A. M., Yarnold, P. R., Bennett, C. L., Soltysik, R. C., Wolf, M. S., Ferreira, R. M., . . . , Davis, T. (2007). Development and validation of a short-form, rapid estimate of adult literacy in medicine. *Medical Care, 45*(11), 1026–1033.

Bastable, S. B. (2013). *Nurse as educator: Principles of teaching and learning for nursing practice* (4th ed.). Sudbury, MA: Jones & Bartlett Learning.

Centrella-Nigro, A., & Alexander, C. (2017). Using the teach-back method in patient education to improve patient satisfaction. *The Journal of Continuing Education in Nursing, 48*, 47–52.

CommunicateHealth, Inc., Boston University, & RTI International. (2018). *Health literacy tool shed.* Retrieved January 24, 2018, from https://healthliteracy.bu.edu/.

Cowan, D., Norman, I., & Coopamah, V. (2005). Competence in nursing practice: A controversial concept. A focused review of the literature. *Nurse Education Today, 25*, 355–362.

Davis, T. C., Crouch, M. A., Long, S. W., Jackson, R. H., Bates, P., George, R. B., & Bairnsfather, L. E. (1991). Rapid assessment of literacy levels of adult primary care patients. *Family Medicine, 23*(6), 433–435.

Davis, T. C., Long, S. W., Jackson, R. H., Mayeaux, E. J., George, R. B., Murphy, P. W., & Crouch, M. A. (1993). Rapid estimate of adult literacy in medicine: A shortened screening instrument. *Family Medicine, 25*(6), 391–395.

del Bueno, D. (2005). A crisis in critical thinking. *Nursing Education Perspectives, 26*(5), 278–282.

del Bueno, D., Barker, F., & Christmyer, C. (1980). Implementing a competency-based orientation program. *Nurse Educator, 5*(3), 16–20.

DeWalt, D. A., Callahan, L. F., Hawk, V. H., Broucksou, K. A., Hink, A., Rudd, R., & Brach, C. (2010). Health literacy universal precautions toolkit. (Prepared by North Carolina Network Consortium, The Cecil G. Sheps Center for Health Services Research, The University of North Carolina at Chapel Hill, under Contract No. HHSA290200710014.) AHRQ Publication No. 10-0046-EF. Rockville, MD: Agency for Healthcare Research and Quality. Retrieved November 26, 2017, from https://www.ahrq.gov/sites/default/files/wysiwyg/chain/practice-tools/toolkit-with-appendix.pdf.

Doak, L. G., & Doak, C. C. (Eds). (2004). Pfizer principles for clear health communication (2nd ed.). Retrieved November 30, 2017, from https://www.pfizer.com/files/health/PfizerPrinciples.pdf.

Dumenci, L., Matsuyama, R. K., Kuhn, L., Perera, R. A., & Siminoff, L. A. (2013). On the validity of the rapid estimate of adult literacy in medicine (REALM) scale as a measure of health literacy. *Communication Methods Measurement, 7*(2), 134–143. doi: 10.1080/19312458.2013.789839

Franklin, N., & Melville, P. (2015). Competency assessment tools: An exploration of the pedagogical issues facing competency assessment for nurses in the clinical environment. *Collegian, 22*, 25–31.

Garside, J. R., & Nhemachena, J. (2013). A concept analysis of competence and its transition in nursing. *Nurse Education Today, 33*, 541–545. doi:10.1016//j.nedt.2011.12.007

Harvard T. H. Chan School of Public Health. (2018). Heath literacy. Retrieved January 24, 2018, from https://www.hsph.harvard.edu/healthliteracy/plain-language-resources/.

Harvard T. H. Chan School of Public Health, Health Literacy Studies. (2015). Welcome. Retrieved November 26, 2017, from https://www.hsph.harvard.edu/healthliteracy/.

Hedman, A. (2008). Using the SMOG formula to revise a health-related document. *American Journal of Health Education, 39*, 61–64.

Institute for Healthcare Improvement. (2018). Ask me 3. Good questions for your health. Retrieved January 24, 2018, from http://www.npsf.org/page/askme3.

Institute of Medicine. (2004). *Health literacy: A prescription to end confusion.* Washington, DC: The National Academies Press. Retrieved from https://doi.org/10.17226/10883.

Jacobson, T. A., Thomas, D. M., Morton, F. J., Offutt, G., Shevlin, G., & Ray, S. (1999). Use of a low-literacy patient education tool to enhance pneumococcal vaccination rates. A randomized controlled trial. *Journal of the American Medical Association, 282*(7), 646–650.

Jordan, L. M. (2016). Health literacy made simple [pdf]. Retrieved January 24, 2018, from https://www.jointcommission.org/assets/1/18/health-literacy-pcmh.pdf.

Luparell, S. (2005). Why and how we should address student incivility in nursing programs. In M. H. Oermann & K. T. Heinrich (Eds.), *Annual review of nursing education: Strategies for teaching, assessment, and program planning* (pp. 23–36). New York, NY: Springer.

Lyon, B. L., & Boland, D. L. (2002). Demonstration of continued competence: A complex challenge. *Clinical Nurse Specialist, 16*(3), 155–156.

Mahadevan, R., Center for Health Care Strategies. (2013). Health literacy fact sheets. Retrieved January 24, 2018, from https://www.chcs.org/resource/health-literacy-fact-sheets/.

McConnell, E. (2001). Competence vs. competency. *Nursing Management, 32*(5), 14–15.

McMullan, M., Endacott, R., Gray, M. A., Jasper, M., Miller, C., Scholes, J., & Webb, C. (2003). Portfolios and assessment of competence: A review of the literature. *Journal of Advanced Nursing, 41*(3), 283–294.

National Center for Education Statistics. (n.d.[a]). National assessment of adult literacy. What is NAAL? Retrieved January 23, 2018, from https://nces.ed.gov/naal/.

National Center for Education Statistics. (n.d.[b]). 1992 national adult literacy survey. Retrieved January 23, 2018, from http://nces.ed.gov/pubsearch/pubsinfo.asp?pubid=199909.

National Center for Education Statistics. (n.d.[c]). Performance levels. Overview of the literacy levels. Retrieved January 23, 2018, from http://nces.ed.gov/naal/perf_levels.asp.

National Center for Education Statistics. (n.d.[d]). National assessment of adult literacy—demographics. Overall. Retrieved November 30, 2017, from https://nces.ed.gov/naal/kf_demographics.asp.

National Council of State Boards of Nursing. (2018). National nursing workforce study. Retrieved January 26, 2018, from https://www.ncsbn.org/workforce.htm.

National Institutes of Health. (n.d.). *Clear communication.* Retrieved January 23, 2018, from https://www.nih.gov/institutes-nih/nih-office-director/office-communications-public-liaison/clear-communication.

Nolan, P. (1998). Competencies drive decision making. *Nursing Management, 29*(3), 27–29.

Office of Disease Prevention and Health Promotion. (2010). National action plan to improve health literacy. Retrieved January 23, 2018, from https://health.gov/communication/HLActionPlan/pdf/Health_Lit_Action_Plan_Summary.pdf.

Office of Disease Prevention and Health Promotion. Healthfinder.gov. (2013). Partnership for clear health communication—PCHC. Retrieved January 24, 2018, from https://healthfinder.gov/FindServices/Organizations/Organization.aspx?code=HR3761.

Office of Disease Prevention and Health Promotion. Healthfinder.gov. (2018). Health communication and health information technology. Retrieved January 24, 2018, from https://www.healthypeople.gov/2020/topics-objectives/topic/health-communication-and-health-information-technology/objectives.

Parker, R. M., Baker, D. W., Williams, M. V., & Nurss, J. R. (1995). The test of functional health literacy in adults: A new instrument for measuring patients' literacy skills. *Journal of General Internal Medicine, 10,* 537–541.

Pfizer, Inc. (2018a). Your health is our purpose. Retrieved January 24, 2018, from https://www.pfizer.com/health-wellness.

Pfizer, Inc. (2018b). Health literacy. Retrieved January 24, 2018, from https://www.pfizer.com/health/literacy.

Pfizer, Inc. (2018c). Your health. Managing your health. Health literacy. Health professionals. Retrieved January 24, 2018, from https://www.pfizer.com/health/literacy/healthcare-professionals.

Pfizer, Inc. (2018d). Universal precautions for health communications. Retrieved January 24, 2018, from https://www.pfizer.com/health/literacy/healthcare-professionals/precautions.

Plain Language Action and Information Network. (n.d.[a]). Home. Retrieved January 24, 2018, from https://www.plainlanguage.gov/.

Plain Language Action and Information Network. (n.d.[b]). Checklist for plain language. Retrieved January 24, 2018, from https://plainlanguage.gov/resources/checklists/checklist/

Plain Language Action and Information Network. (n.d.[c]). Document checklist for plain language on the web. Retrieved November 25, 2017, from https://plainlanguage.gov/resources/checklists/web-checklist/.

Plain Language Action and Information Network. (n.d.[d]). *Reasons why the English language is hard to learn.* Retrieved January 24, 2018, from https://plainlanguage.gov/resources/humor/why-english-is-hard-to-learn/.

Plain Language Action and Information Network. (n.d.[e]). Before and after: Losing weight HHS brochure. Accessed November 25, 2017, from https://plainlanguage.gov/examples/brochures/hhs-brochure/

Rad, M., & Moonaghi, H. K. (2016). Strategies for managing nursing students' incivility as experienced by nursing educators: A qualitative study. *Journal of Caring Sciences, 5,* 23–32.

Rawlins, L. (2017). Faculty and student incivility in undergraduate nursing education: An integrative review. *Journal of Nursing Education, 56*, 709–716.

Rudd, R. E. (2007). Health literacy skills of U.S. adults. *American Journal of Health Behavior, 31*(1), S8–S18.

Rudd, R. E. (2015). The evolving concept of health literacy: New directions for health literacy studies. *Journal of Communication in Healthcare, 8*, 7–9. doi:10.1179/1753806815Z

Sauer, P., Hannon, A., & Beyer, K. (2017). Peer incivility among prelicensure nursing students: A call to action for nursing faculty. *Nurse Educator, 42*, 281–285. doi: 10.1097/NNE.0000000000000375

Schwartzberg, J., Cowett, A., VanGeest, J., & Wolf, M. (2007). Communication techniques for patients with low health literacy: A survey of physicians, nurses, and pharmacists. *American Journal of Health Behavior, 31*(1), S96–S104.

Shoemaker, S. J., Wolf, M. S., & Brach, C. (2014). Development of the patient education materials assessment tool (PEMAT): A new measure of understandability and actionability for print and audiovisual patient information. *Patient Education and Counseling, 96*, 395– 403. doi:10.1016/j.pec.2014.05.027

Smith, S. A. (2012). Nurse competence: A concept analysis. *International Journal of Nursing Knowledge, 23*(3), 172–182.

Thomas, S. P. (2003). Handling anger in the teacher–student relationship. *Nursing Education Perspectives, 24*(1), 17.

Tilley, D. (2008). Competency in nursing: A concept analysis. *Journal of Continuing Education in Nursing, 39*(2), 58–64.

University of Washington, Harborview Medical Center. (2018). EthnoMed home page. Retrieved January 24, 2018, from http://ethnomed.org/ethnomed.

Waddell, D. (2001). Measurement issues in promoting continued competence. *Journal of Continuing Education in Nursing, 32*(3), 102–106.

Watson, R., Stimpson, A., Topping, A., & Porock, D. (2002). Clinical competence assessment in nursing: A systematic review of the literature. *Journal of Advanced Nursing, 39*(5), 421– 431.

Weiss, B. D. (2007). *Health literacy and patient safety: Help patients understand. Manual for clinicians* (2nd ed.). Chicago, IL: American Medical Association Foundation. Retrieved January 24, 2018, from https://med.fsu.edu/userFiles/file/ahec_health_clinicians_manual.pdf.

Wikipedia. (2017). Readability test. Retrieved January 24, 2018, from https://en.wikipedia.org/wiki/Readability_test.

Wolf, M., Davis, T., & Parker, R. (2007). The emerging field of health literacy research. *American Journal of Health Behavior, 31*(1), S3–S5.

Wright, D. (2005). *The ultimate guide to competency assessment in health care* (3rd ed.). Minneapolis, MN: Creative Health Care Management.

Wright, D. (2015). *Competency assessment field guide. A real world guide for implementation and application.* Minneapolis, MN: Creative Health Care Management.

Zuzelo, P. (1999). Professional practice and the NCLEX examination. A bottom-line approach. *Nurse Educator, 24*(3), 11–12, 28.

Zuzelo, P. (2000). Clinical probation: A supportive process for the at-risk student. *Nurse Educator, 25*, 216–218.

Zuzelo, P. (2005). Affirming the disadvantaged student. *Nurse Educator, 30*, 27–31.

CHAPTER 8

Keeping Patients Safe: Preventing Unintended Adverse Consequences and Reducing Errors

Patti Rager Zuzelo, EdD, RN, ACNS-BC, ANP-BC, CRNP, FAAN

The patient safety movement was galvanized in 1999 by the Institute of Medicine (IOM) report, *To Err Is Human: Building a Safer Health System* (Kohn, Corrigan, & Donaldson, 2000). This report fundamentally changed how providers, policy makers, and the public view health care safety and focused national attention on the mistakes and errors occurring in a deficient system that, at the time, permitted 44,000 to 98,000 needless patient deaths each year due to medical error (Kohn et al., 2000). Although certainly one of the most highly recognized initiatives, the IOM report was not the first attempt to address health care safety concerns. White (2004) noted that the earliest safety and quality efforts can be traced to 1955, although this work was not specific to patient safety initiatives but to patient outcomes, complications, and strategies for establishing measures to monitor outcomes.

Approximately 40 years later, in the mid-1990s, interest in medical errors and patient safety peaked with the convening of the first Annenberg Conference on Patient Safety, the establishment of the National Patient Safety Foundation (NPSF), and President Clinton's formation of the Advisory Commission on Consumer Protection and Quality in the Health Care Industry. In 1996, the Joint Commission (TJC) launched its Sentinel Event Policy for the voluntary reporting of sentinel events. By 2000, continued momentum in the patient safety and quality movement led the Agency for Health Care Policy and Research (AHCPR) to change its name to the Agency for Healthcare Research and Quality (AHRQ) and become a funding powerhouse for research focused on patient safety, error reduction, strategic planning specific to patient safety, and technology utilization in the interest of enhancing quality of care (White, 2004).

Within this same period of time, the Business Roundtable established the Leapfrog Group, a national nonprofit organization with the mission of triggering "giant leaps forward in the safety, quality and affordability of U.S. health care by using transparency to support informed health care decisions and promote high-value care" (Leapfrog Group, n.d.). Leapfrog Group works toward health care transparency. The organization has invested almost two decades in collecting, analyzing, and publishing hospital data on safety, quality, and resource utilization so that purchasers can make good decisions as they search for high-value care (Leapfrog Group, n.d.).

Despite the efforts of private and public organizations and policy initiatives, errors have increased in number with Leapfrog Group (n.d.) currently estimating that 400,000 lives are annually lost because of preventable medical errors. Avoidable errors are recognized as the third leading cause of death in the United States (Makary & Daniel, 2016). Preventable medical errors are not a uniquely American problem. The Care Quality Commission (CQC) of the National Health Service (NHS) actively addresses patient safety and care service quality. Recently, the CQC noted that 11% of NHS acute, nonspecialist trusts were rated as inadequate for safety (Tingle & Minford, 2017). An NHS trust is an organization or agency set up to deliver a particular specialized service or to provide care within a particular geographical area. A review of published literature reveals the international scope of patient safety concerns. One recent publication describes a safety culture training program implemented in China and focused on the attitudes of nurse managers toward patient safety (Xie et al., 2017).

Advanced nurses have been involved in workplace safety initiatives throughout this trajectory and are uniquely positioned to serve as patient safety experts across a variety of care settings. As patient safety is indistinguishable from quality care (Aspden, Corrigan, Wolcott, & Erickson, 2004), the goal of delivering quality patient care is in concert with, and contributes to, creating and sustaining an environment of safety. This chapter introduces advanced nurses to current patient safety perspectives and opportunities while sharing suggestions for websites, tools, and resources that may be used to create and sustain a culture of safety through the integration of evidence-based practice with patient safety practices.

▶ Human Error and Types of Error

Most practicing nurses are well aware of the high rates of errors and near misses that occur on a daily basis across the health care system. The number of actual errors and prevented errors is staggering. Appreciating the various types of errors and their triggers may assist advanced nurses in planning and implementing targeted strategies that minimize error likelihood and improve patient outcomes. Reason's work (1990) on human error provides interesting theoretical and practice perspectives on basic error mechanisms, types and consequences of errors, and techniques for assessing and reducing the risks of errors.

Human error theory (HET) (Reason, 1990) suggests that organization failures in complex systems cause accidents. Reason (1990) asserts that the term *error* denotes an intentional act. Other error types depend upon two kinds of failure—slips and lapses—and mistakes. Errors may be active or latent. Latent errors lie dormant for a long period of time until they align with enough other factors to breech the system's defenses.

The alignment of latent failures and a variety of triggering events is referred to as the dynamics of accident causation, or the Swiss cheese model of accident causation (**FIGURE 8-1**). The figure illustrates a trajectory of accident opportunity that penetrates several defensive systems and is the result of complex interactions between latent failures and triggering events. In this model, latent failures at the managerial levels combine with psychological precursors, and unsafe acts within a context of local triggering events lead to an accident opportunity. When these factors and influences align, accidents are more likely to occur, characterized by the holes of a Swiss cheese wedge aligning to allow for unimpeded passage through the cheese wedge. A few examples of organizational failures include lack of administrative commitment to safety, blurred safety responsibilities, poor training, inconsistent application of policies and procedures, and punitive work environments.

Reason (1990) points out that very few unsafe acts actually result in damage or injury, even in systems that are unprotected. Findings from a focus group study exploring the influence of technologies on registered nurses' work illustrate the many ways that nurses work around and bypass technology-related rules and routines in efforts to meet patient care needs, save time, or minimize frustrations. Rarely do these system breeches lead to patient harm (Zuzelo, Gettis, Hansell, & Thomas, 2008). However, when mistakes do occur, they may be catastrophic.

Reason (1990) pessimistically observes that while engineered safety devices offer barriers against most single errors, human and mechanical, there are no guaranteed

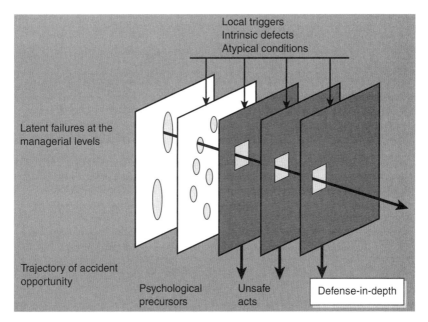

FIGURE 8-1 The Dynamics of Accident Causation. The diagram shows a trajectory of accident opportunity penetrating several defensive systems. This results from a complex interaction between latent failures and a variety of local triggering events. It is clear from this figure, however, that the chances of such a trajectory of opportunity finding loopholes in all of the defenses at any one time is very small.

technological defenses against the accumulation of latent failures that provide opportunities for errors within organizations, including high-risk health care systems (**EXEMPLAR 8-1**). Reducing the likelihood of errors by minimizing latent failures, scrutinizing and improving systems, and rapidly evaluating the effectiveness of process changes are requisite activities to promote safety and certainly fall within the purview of nursing practice whether this practice occurs within the context of an advanced role or at the sharp point of direct patient care delivery.

Accident causation theory is very relevant to nurses' practice and is applicable to health care organizations as well as to specific types of clinical care areas. As an example, critical care poses great risk for patients related to (1) increased patient

 EXEMPLAR 8-1 The Unsafe Act: The Case of the Infusion Pump

Tim Bradley, RN, is a new intensive care unit nurse with 1 year of experience. One evening, Tim is presented with a newly admitted, critically ill patient requiring intravenous antibiotics, high-volume fluid resuscitation, and vasopressor and inotropic support therapy to treat progressive shock. The patient is deteriorating, and Tim is rapidly responding to each ailing system.

This particular shift, there had been a registered nurse sick call. This individual was not replaced. The remaining nurses were very busy providing care to unstable patients. As a result, Tim was independently handling his patient's care needs.

Tim's patient was prescribed dopamine 400 mg/250 mL at 7 µg/kg/minute. The patient weighed 80 kg.

Unit policy required high-risk medication infusions via Smart Pump devices capable of identifying and preventing adverse drug events (ADEs) when used as designed. Tim was familiar with the correct use of the Smart Pump infusion devices and had been correctlyeducated; however, during his orientation, his preceptor had also encouraged Tim to bypass the pump technology. Tim's colleagues shared with him a variety of ways to avoid "dealing with the drug library and all those alerts!" The rationale was to "save time" by "bypassing" the information required when setting up the infusion device alerts.

Tim was in a hurry. His patient required many medications. Tim felt rushed and pressured. When he saw the dopamine infusion order, he decided to hang the medication without the use of the Guardrails alerts. His intent was to go back after hanging the remaining medications and set up the dopamine infusion as per policy.

Tim calculated the dopamine infusion rate. He set the infusion pump as per his calculation. Tim did not realize that he had mistakenly calculated an infusion rate of 70 µg/kg/minute. Within a short period of time, the patient exhibited tachycardia and ventricular irritability with increased blood pressure significantly above the desired mean arterial pressure. Scared that he had made an error, Tim immediately rechecked the dopamine dosage and quickly discovered his error. The patient did not suffer apparent untoward effects once the dose was corrected; however, certainly the error could have resulted in a fatal outcome.

This exemplar provides an overview of an unsafe act that violated an established rule because the rule violation was perceived as a routine, common act. Nurses had violated this particular rule on many occasions but the preconditions of nurse inexperience, high acuity, and inadequate supports in combination with established workarounds or shortcuts contributed to the actual adverse drug event.

acuity, (2) high frequency of invasive interventions, (3) high medication volume, (4) need for speedy decision-making processes and associated intervention, and (5) other factors, including patient characteristics. In one study, researchers found that critical care patients experienced 1.7 errors per day, 29% with the potential to cause significant harm or death (Pronovost, Thompson, Holzmueller, Lubomski, & Morlock, 2005). Across the United States, that data extrapolate to 85,000 errors every day, of which 24,650 are potentially life threatening. Nursing homes and ambulatory care settings are also not immune from error. In fact, because the number of outpatient visits each year far exceeds the number of inpatient visits, the opportunity for error in that setting is also considerable (Aspden et al., 2004). Errors are also expensive with significant fiscal implications. Stopping errors saves thousands of dollars per intercepted event (Bravo & Cochran, 2016).

Medication errors experienced in intensive care units (ICUs) are of international concern. A recent study in Spain, the SYREC study (named from an acronym referring to a Spanish title meaning "safety and risk in critical care patients") was conducted over a 24-hour observational period across all adult Spanish ICUs for a final sample size of 79 units (Merino et al., 2012). Physicians, nurses, and nurse's aides shared details about near-miss incidents, actual incidents that did not cause discernible patient harm, and adverse incidents that did harm a patient in some sort of way. Findings revealed that many patients (N = 591) were affected by one or more incidents during the observation period. Those who experienced adverse events sustained temporary damage in 29% of cases while those who sustained severe compromise or resulted in death occurred in 4% of such events. The majority of incidents of all types were categorized as avoidable (Merino et al., 2012).

Advanced nurses need to consider that most health care settings are associated with risks for errors. Operating rooms are notoriously risk settings for wrong-site, wrong-procedure, wrong-patient errors (WSPEs). These types of errors are considered *never events* that should never occur and, if they do, it is likely that serious underlying safety problems are in play (Patient Safety Network [PSNet], 2017). These sorts of errors often make headlines and contribute to the anxiety and fear that many experience when preparing for a surgical event. Adverse experiences are rare when counted within operating room settings; however, rates increase when the operating room setting is broadened to include other settings like ambulatory surgical facilities or interventional radiology (PSNet, 2017). The Leapfrog Group (2017a) noted that its Fall 2013 *Hospital Safety Score* system assigned grades to more than 2,500 general hospitals in the United States with earned scores of A (n = 813), B (n = 661), C (n = 893), D (n = 150), and F (n = 22). Advanced nurses should view this data with concern and determination. Certainly there are opportunities for immediate and significant improvements. The Leapfrog Group (2017b) has 2017 survey results available that may be viewed by location or by hospital name.

Healthgrades (2017a) is an organization that provides consumers and providers with trustworthy information that assists consumers to find and schedule appointments with providers. It also provides information that may be used by providers to improve the quality of services. Healthgrades integrates three factors into the data that it provides to consumers: patient satisfaction, experience match, and hospital quality. Patient satisfaction is measured using nine questions that have been adapted from the CMS Clinician and Group Consumer Assessment of Healthcare Providers and Systems (CG CAHPS) survey. The goal is to provide data to prospective patients that relate to multiple aspects of patient satisfaction, including (1) likelihood of recommending the provider to others; (2) office and staff; (3) convenience of arranging urgent appointments; (4) practice environment; (5) friendliness; (6) wait time; (7) experience with physician; (8) quality of explanations of medical conditions; (9) provider communication; and (10) provider time spent with patients (Healthgrades, 2017b).

Healthgrades (2017c) is equally focused on providing experience and hospital quality data to consumers via its search engine. The experience match category responds to how well the providers match the consumers' search requirements. The match percentage is an aggregated score based on up to 9 aspects of a provider's experiences relative to the search parameters, including the provider's experience with the specific condition of concern, procedure history, patient volume specific to the condition/procedure of concern, total patient volume, board certification, specialization, board actions, sanctions, malpractice claims, and education/degree.

The Healthgrades hospital quality data are informed by Medicare claims from approximately 4,500 hospitals across the country over the most recent 3-year period (Healthgrades, 2017d). Quality reports are based on clinical outcomes for the most frequent in-hospital procedures and conditions. Data are adjusted depending on patient risk factors. Analyses inform other reports as well including multiple award categories (**TABLE 8-1**). These consumer tools are data driven and highly influential.

TABLE 8-1 Healthgrades, Awards

Award	Description	Web Address
Women's Care Excellence		
Gynecologic Surgery Excellence Award™	Superior outcomes in surgeries of female reproductive system and some urinary tract and rectum conditions	https://www.healthgrades.com/quality/gynecologic-surgery-excellence-award-recipients-2017
Labor and Delivery Excellence Award™	Superior care of women during and after childbirth	https://www.healthgrades.com/quality/labor-and-delivery-excellence-award-recipients-2017
Obstetrics and Gynecology Excellence Award™	Superior outcomes during and after childbirth and in surgeries that treat disease and conditions of female reproductive system	https://www.healthgrades.com/quality/obstetrics-and-gynecology-award-excellence-recipients-2017

Award	Description	Web Address
Patient Safety, Outstanding Patient Experience, Distinguished Hospital for Clinical Excellence		
Patient Safety Excellence Award™	Recognizes hospitals that have the lowest occurrences of 14 preventable patient safety events. Award winners are in the nation's top 10% for patient safety	https://www.healthgrades.com/quality/patient-safety-excellence-award-recipients-2017
Outstanding Patient Experience Award™	Overall outstanding patient experience	https://www.healthgrades.com/quality/outstanding-patient-experience-award-recipients-2017
Distinguished Hospital Award for Clinical Excellence™	Rated in the nation's top 5% of hospitals with the lowest risk-adjusted mortality and complication rates across a minimum of 21 of 32 common diagnoses and procedures	https://www.healthgrades.com/quality/distinguished-hospital-award-for-clinical-excellence-recipients-2017
America's Best Hospitals		
America's 50 Best Hospitals Award™	Top 1% of hospitals in the nation for overall clinical excellence for at least 6 consecutive years. Based solely on clinical outcomes	https://www.healthgrades.com/quality/top-hospitals-2017
America's 100 Best Hospitals Award™	Top 2% of hospitals in the nation for overall clinical excellence for at least 6 consecutive years. Based solely on clinical outcomes	https://www.healthgrades.com/quality/top-hospitals-2017

As transparency increases and consumers concurrently improve their data retrieval sophistication, there will likely be more pressure on providers and health care systems to work on improving performance indicator scores across the Healthgrades categories platform. Advanced nurses need to think about the relationship between patient satisfaction, health encounter experiences, and care quality to perceptions of safety. It seems reasonable for consumers to perceive satisfying and high-quality care experiences as safe care. For this reason, advanced nurses may want to consider safety as having a reciprocal relationship with quality and satisfaction.

Since the release of the IOM report (Kohn et al., 2000), there has been an abundance of published patient safety–focused literature. Multiple recommending and regulatory agencies offer guidelines and mandates. Many organizations provide evidence-based practice guidelines to assist clinicians in providing standardized evidence-based care.

The volume of materials and ever-changing safety standards and best practices may be overwhelming to advanced nurses, particularly those who are new to putting patient safety principles into practice. The advanced nurse, whether in direct or indirect care roles, is absolutely pivotal in assessing clinical environments for accident and error opportunities, collaborating with appropriate team members to proactively improve systems or to meaningfully react to occurrences, and rapidly evaluating the outcomes of purposefully designed system changes. Actively engaging in this work requires a preliminary review of the definitions of terms commonly used in patient safety projects and publications (**TABLE 8-2**).

TABLE 8-2 Definitions of Selected Key Terms in Patient Safety

Term	Definition
Adverse event	An event that results in *unintended* harm related to a health care intervention rather than the underlying disease.
Error	A planned action is not completed as intended; the wrong plan is used to achieve a desired goal; or an action has not been taken or has been incompletely/inadequately provided (omission).
Near miss or close call	A close call or near miss is an event or situation that could have resulted in an accident, injury or illness, but did not, possibly by chance or by deliberate intervention.
Incident	A patient safety event that reached the patient whether or not harm was incurred.
Safety	Being free from harm or risk as a result of prevention and mitigation strategies.

For a comprehensive and standardized list of patient safety terms and definitions refer to: National Quality Forum. (2009). NQF patient safety terms and definitions. Retrieved July 8, 2018 from, www.qualityforum.org/Topics/**Safety**_Definitions.aspx

▶ Creating a Just Culture for Patient Safety

Achieving and sustaining a culture of safety requires an understanding of the values and beliefs within a particular organization. AHRQ (2017a) describes a patient safety culture as the degree to which an organization's culture supports and nurtures patient safety. Patient safety culture refers to the beliefs, values, and norms that are shared by health care practitioners and other staff throughout the organization that influences their actions and behaviors. AHRQ (2017a) asserts that patient safety culture can be measured by uncovering what is rewarded, supported, required, and accepted in an organization as it connects to patient safety.

The notion of a "just culture" denotes a culture where people can report mistakes, errors, accidents, or waste without negative repercussions (AHRQ, 2013). In a just culture, individuals remain accountable for their actions but they are not held responsible for flawed systems that permit earnest, trained people to err. Sharing and disclosure are prominent features of a just culture because efficiencies and quality improvement processes depend on the frontline staff to drive improvements, and such drive requires a sense of safety. Staff must feel empowered to point out errors, defects, and system failures that could cause patient harm (AHRQ, 2013). A just culture is not an "anything goes" culture. In other words, individuals may be held personally accountable for intended actions that are unsafe and violate rules. But, in highly protected systems with established defense systems, such unsafe acts are more likely in a highly specific, often atypical, set of circumstances (Reason, 1990).

AHRQ's Comprehensive Unit-based Safety Program (CUSP) (2013) provides an online training video that describes just culture. Content includes discussion about three categories of behaviors that are expected and need to be managed. The first category is to understand that humans will make mistakes and will drift into risky places. The key point is that these mistakes are inadvertent and are considered a slip, lapse, or mistake. A significant idea is that these actions were not intentional; they were inadvertent. The second behavior category is at-risk behaviors. Rather than an inadvertent action, these behaviors are the result of a choice and these choices increase risk. The risk is either unrecognized or mistakenly believed to be acceptable because of the circumstances. The third behavioral category is reckless behavior. This behavior type is also a choice but it is selected with a conscious disregard for substantial and inexcusable risk.

In the just culture, each of these behavior types should be associated with a different response (AHRQ, 2013). The individual who has made a mistake should be consoled and then the system should be examined for possible changes that would reduce or eliminate future opportunities for similar mistakes. The at-risk behaviors generally happen more frequently than human error and need to be carefully reviewed and considered. Many times, these risky behaviors end with positive results rather than negative outcomes and so the risky choice is reinforced. The appropriate response to these sorts of behaviors is to assist the person in understanding the potential risk and coaching them to make safe choices while also scrutinizing the incentive system around the individual so as to modify the system and reduce the positive incentives that support the risky choice. The third category, reckless behaviors, needs to be managed through remediation or a punitive response. Making the determination of what is a risky choice versus a reckless behavior may be challenging and advanced nurses need to partner with other leaders and with staff to make certain that the line of demarcation between the two behavior types is clearly understood within any given situation.

Highly Reliable Organizations

Organizations with a just culture have characteristics in common. These organizations have leaders who support bidirectional communications founded on mutual trust, with the ability for all employees to speak up and raise concerns, as well as the willingness to listen when others have a concern. In addition, there are shared perceptions of the importance of safety, coupled with a systems approach to analysis of safety issues. Patient safety permeates the culture, and there is an emphasis on continuous improvement (Clements, 2017; Vogus & Singer, 2016).

Highly reliable organizations (HROs) tend to be exceptionally consistent and are particularly good at avoiding error (Hines et al., 2008). They rarely have significant accidents and value opportunities to consider near-missed errors so that they can learn from the context of the near-miss event and analyze potential remediation strategies to prevent the possibility of future failures (Chassin & Loeb, 2013). HROs are characterized by several organizing concepts: sensitivity to operations with staff maintaining an ongoing organizational awareness, reluctance to simplify, preoccupation with failure, deference to expertise, and resilience (Clements, 2017; Hines et al., 2008; Vogus & Singer, 2016). Chassin and Loeb (2013) observe that rather than a preoccupation with *avoiding* failure, health care organizations act as if failure is an inevitable aspect of daily work. They offer that the evidence of this fatalistic view lies in the thousands of health care–associated infections, wrong-site/person/procedure (WSPP) errors in operating rooms, fires in surgical suites, poor handwashing routines, and other errors that are, unfortunately, commonplace.

One telling example of risk oversimplification is evidenced in application of TJC's universal protocol (Chassin & Loeb, 2013). This process was designed to stop WSPP surgical interventions by requiring a simple three-step approach: (1) verify patient identify and planned procedure, (2) mark the surgical site, and (3) conduct a timeout prior to initiating the surgery and reconfirm that the patient, procedure, and operative site are correctly established (TJC, 2017a). In fact, the American periOperative Registered Nurses (AORN) in partnership with TJC has sponsored a "National Time Out Day," first initiated in 2016, to increase awareness of the importance of the universal protocol (TJC, 2017b). However, despite this simple and seemingly appropriate safety process, wrong-site surgeries persist. Chassin and Loeb (2013) suggest that this simple procedure does not take into account the complexities of surgical processes and operational issues. One such intervening influence is poor communication between health care professionals, particularly including intimidating behaviors and other occasions of lateral violence and bullying.

Progress toward creating a culture of patient safety requires honest, routine error reporting. Errors and near misses are reported in organizations in which staff feels safe reporting errors. In organizations with a culture of patient safety, the emphasis is on *why* the error occurred, versus *who* made the error (**FIGURE 8-2**). The Institute for Safe Medication Practices (ISMP) content validated tool (Zuzelo, Inverso, & Linkewich, 2001), *ASSESS-ERR™ Medication System Worksheet*, provides an excellent exemplar of the sorts of questions and analyses that should be included

---

✓ ASSESS - ERR™
MEDICATION SYSTEM Worksheet

Patient MR# _____   Incident # _____
(if error reached patient)   if no callback identified: ❏

Date of error: _____   Date information obtained: _____   Patient age: _____

Drug(s) involved in error: _____

Non-formulary drug(s)?	❏ Yes	❏ No
Drug sample(s)?	❏ Yes	❏ No
Drug(s) packaged in unit dose/unit of use?	❏ Yes	❏ No
Drug(s) dispensed from pharmacy?	❏ Yes	❏ No
Error within 24 hours of admission, transfer, or after discharge?	❏ Yes	❏ No
Did the error reach the patient?	❏ Yes	❏ No

Source of IV solution:
❏ Manufacturer premixed solution   ❏ Pharmacy IV admixture   ❏ Nursing IV admixture

Brief description of the event: (what, when, and why) _____
_____
_____
_____

Possible causes	Y/N	Comments
Critical patient information missing? (age, weight, allergies, VS, lab values, pregnancy, patient identity, location, renal/liver impairment, diagnoses, etc.)		
Critical drug information missing? (outdated/absent references, inadequate computer screening, inaccessible pharmacist, uncontrolled drug formulary, etc.)		
Miscommunication of drug order? (illegible, ambiguous, incomplete, misheard, or misunderstood orders, intimidation/faulty interaction, etc.)		
Drug name, label, packaging problem? (look/sound-alike names, look-alike packaging, unclear/absent labeling, faulty drug identification, etc.)		
Drug storage or delivery problem? (slow turn around time, inaccurate delivery, doses missing or expired, multiple concentrations, placed in wrong bin, etc.)		
Drug delivery device problem? (poor device design, misprogramming, free-flow, mixed up lines, IV administration of oral syringe contents, etc.)		

FIGURE 8-2 Assess-ERR™ Medication System Worksheet *(Continues)*

Possible causes	Y/N	Comments
Environmental, staffing, or workflow problems? (lighting, noise, clutter, interruptions, staffing deficiencies, workload, inefficient workflow, employee safety, etc.)		
Lack of staff education? (competency validation, new or unfamiliar drugs/devices, orientation process, feedback about errors/prevention, etc.)		
Patient education problem? (lack of information, noncompliance, not encouraged to ask questions, lack of investigating patient inquiries, etc.)		
Lack of quality control or independent check systems? (equipment quality control checks, independent checks for high alert drugs/high risk patient population drugs etc.)		

Did the patient require any of the following actions after the error that you would not have done if the event had not occurred?

❑ Testing ❑ Additional observation ❑ Gave antidote

❑ Care escalated (transferred, etc.) ❑ Additional LOS ❑ Other _____

Patient outcome:

FIGURE 8-2 *(Continued)*

in a root-cause analysis review. Advanced nurses should note that the questions are not driven by "*who* did what" but by the causes of error related to the overall work context and medication use systems. Leaders use errors to help staff evaluate processes and learn how to prevent a recurrence of an error, rather than to blame. Two encouraged strategies that can assist with error analysis and risk assessments are failure mode and effects analysis (FMEA) (American Society for Quality [ASQ], 2018a; TJC, 2017c) and root cause analysis strategies (RCA) (ASQ, 2018b; Duwe, Fuchs, & Hansen-Flashen, 2005; TJC, 2017d).

Measuring Safe Culture

Building on the premise that patient safety culture is measurable, AHRQ (2017a) has developed a Surveys on Patient Safety Culture (SOPS™) program that allows health care agencies to assess staff perceptions of patient safety culture in five settings: hospital, medical office, nursing home, community pharmacy, and ambulatory surgery center. These surveys are publicly available and free to anyone in the United States. Permission is required to use the survey internationally (AHRQ, 2017a).

Results of AHRQ surveys may assist advanced nurses and other members of the leadership team to assess the perception of patient safety within their organizations, whether errors are reported and discussed in an appropriate forum, and whether there is an atmosphere of continuous learning based on the principles of patient safety. Each health care institution can use the completed survey data to calculate its percentage of positive responses on each item. Those data can be submitted to AHRQ for entry into a national database. The AHRQ Hospital Survey on Patient Safety Culture allows comparisons between the submitting hospital and other similar hospitals. This report enables each hospital to compare itself to benchmark hospitals (AHRQ, 2017a).

Safety culture assessments are useful tools for measuring organizational conditions that lead to adverse events and patient harm in hospitals. The assessment is the starting point from which action planning begins and patient safety changes evolve (Institute for Healthcare Improvement [IHI], 2018a). Reassessments serve as barometers to measure the success of improvement interventions. Once the cultural assessment is complete, the advanced nurse can use the data to integrate evidence-based guidelines into everyday practice for patient care. Advanced practice nurses working in office practices, nursing homes, or ambulatory surgery centers, in addition to hospitals, might find value in initiating an interprofessional effort to examine how staff perceive patient safety and to develop a planned response, perhaps using an established quality improvement method such as Plan-Do-Check-Act, to positively influence aspects of the culture that require attention.

Each unique survey has an associated toolkit that includes frequently asked questions (FAQs), the survey form in English and Spanish and available in alternate file formats. A survey user's guide is provided for each survey (AHRQ, 2017a). The guide provides an overview of key concerns and major decisions concerning administration and reporting. Sampling guidance is provided as is direction for report construction. Comparative database reports are available and information for those agencies interested in submitting their data to AHRQ. There are action planning tools, a research reference list, and a webcast from AHRQ that offers strategies for implementing "just culture" within a health care system (AHRQ, 2017a).

Creating a Safe Environment

Patient safety tools include those that measure the impact of bundled interventions designed to improve processes and outcomes (AHRQ, 2017b). As a result of various projects and studies, safety scholars recognize that variables contributing to errors include factors associated with (1) communication, (2) inadequate flow of information, (3) human problems, (4) patient-related issues, (5) organizational transfer of knowledge, (6) staffing patterns and work flow, (7) technical failures, and (8) inadequate policies and procedures (AHRQ, 2018; Carayon & Wood, 2010; Phillips, 2005).

Identified factors provide opportunities for constructing a typology that categorizes types of error influences that may be collectively or individually considered. Clustering error influences assists in designing and studying targeted interventions. For example, interruptions during medication administration may compromise patient safety by contributing to errors, similar to distracted driving and its relationship to motor vehicle crashes and other injury types (D'Esmond, 2017). This particular phenomenon is directly related to work flow concerns and inadequate policies and procedures implemented during medication administration practice. Nurse burnout is associated with patient safety (Johnson et al., 2016) and falls within the category of human problems.

Workaround Triggers as Maladaptive Responses to Care Barriers

Workarounds are nonstandard strategies for accomplishing work that needs to be done but is obstructed by dysfunction processes and obstacles (Tucker, 2009). Workarounds demonstrate organizational resilience (Tucker, 2009). Advanced nurses should ascertain how staff has adapted practice by working around systematic or episodic care process obstructions. The typology of error factors provides possible insights into care delivery barriers that may trigger workarounds. Nurses have unparalleled skill at developing workarounds to solve problems. These workarounds may be risky and increase the possibility of patient safety compromise. Workarounds may remediate problems in the short term but often contribute to long-term problems.

As a simple example, if a nurse does not have a patient's medications and solves this problem by borrowing medications from another patient, this exemplifies first-order problem solving (Spear, n.d.; Tucker & Edmondson, 2002). The nurse has met the needs of the patient in the immediate period by securing the needed medications. But, medications are now no longer available for the patient for whom they were intended and there has been no scrutiny as to the root of the problem. This analysis is second-order problem solving (Tucker & Edmondson, 2002). Busy nurses working to provide essential direct care do not have opportunity to engage in second-order problem solving. Frankly, they do not have the time to do so and may not have access to the interprofessional input likely needed for this sort of problem solving.

Advanced nurses are well suited to leading second-order problem-solving analyses. Second-order problem solving involves a system analysis of why the error occurred—what part of the system failed the nurse and the patient (Tucker & Edmondson, 2002). Root cause analysis is needed to understand and permanently fix the problem. It is often easier to work around problems, especially when the staff nurses believe that they have reported this issue previously and no action has been taken. Advanced nurses must partner with staff to investigate concerns and to craft reasonable, efficient solutions to the clinical problems. Partnering facilitates staff buy-in, because the nurses helped to broker the solution. Nurses with advanced responsibilities must make it easier for staff to do the right thing while making it more difficult to do a workaround.

These first-order and second-order problem-solving concerns are not unique to the direct care areas. Health care departments of all sorts are challenged by problems that directly or indirectly influence patient care outcomes and many of these problems affect safety. Advanced nurses typically have many opportunities to identify and address direct and indirect care processes that potentially put patients and staff at risk.

Technologies that become episodically or chronically problematic in direct care service areas are often ripe for intervention using first-order problem solving (Zuzelo, Gettis, Hansell, & Thomas, 2008). For example, in the direct care environment when a nurse needs to administer a heparin infusion and is unable to locate an intravenous infusion pump during a busy shift, the nurse might consider options that are not best practice, including retrieving a pump that was hidden in the dirty utility room as an "emergency" option given the staff perception that pump availability is limited in the practice setting. Alternatively, the nurse could make a decision that an antibiotic infusing via a controller is less risky than continuous heparin infusion and so discontinue the controller on the potentially dangerous antibiotic to have it available for the heparin dosing. Both circumstances use first-order problem solving and increase risk of patient harm and both require examination using second-order problem solving.

Technologies have certainly influenced the RN's work and nurses in advanced roles need to consider these technologies and their potential impact on safety. A qualitative study used focus groups to collect data about nurses' concerns as they work with technologies in practice (Zuzelo et al., 2008). Findings revealed many opportunities for second-order problem solving within the practice domain of advanced nurses. Participants identified improvements in practice related to technological efficiencies. Patient outcomes were enhanced by technologies that improved assessment accuracy and protected patients from harm, including alarm capabilities and wound devices that supported healing. Participants also noted negative aspects of technology that had deleterious influences on nursing routines and, at times, patient safety outcomes. Many of these concerns required timely investigation and responses based on careful analysis—the work of advanced nurses.

Zuzelo et al. (2008) reported that equipment use system gaps, failing or compromised equipment, and education deficiencies were problematic. Equipment was often scarce and locating, setting up, and, at times, hiding equipment consumed a good bit of nursing time. Nurses often mixed equipment components in an effort to jury-rig systems that could satisfy an immediate need, although not in the long term. Crashing computer systems were particularly frustrating given the reliance on computers for most documentation, ordering, and tracking responsibilities. Advanced nurses working in informatics, quality improvement, and safety departments might provide good insights into addressing these sorts of systems issues, including establishing a common, systemwide, and shared nomenclature for equipment and parts.

Advanced nurses in education roles should consider opportunities to hardwire accurate instruction on safe equipment use into orientation programs and regularly scheduled updates. Participants recognized concerning inaccuracies that were perpetuated by staff when teaching new hires or other types of professional or ancillary staff. Misinformation about policies and procedures specific to new technologies were sustained by the lack of convenient, regularly scheduled teaching sessions that were viewed as necessary so that staff feedback, recommendations, and critique could be elicited and addressed (Zuzelo et al., 2008). Participants commented that there were extensive new product rollouts and introductory, mandatory inservice expectations. However, rarely did advanced nurses return to staff to conduct needs assessments or elicit feedback. As a result, nurses felt subject to technology changes rather than experiencing a sense of ownership over efforts to make these technologies work as intended.

Staff shared that complicated, inefficient, and scarce technologies encouraged workarounds. Participants learned risky ways to circumvent safety systems that often contributed to interpersonal strife between nurses who were infuriated by these high-risk practices and those who utilized such strategies as timesavers (Zuzelo et al., 2008). Nurses noted that some manufacturers designed features that prevented equipment workarounds and these technologies were typically used in exacting fashion.

Keeping Staff Safe

Participants shared one example of a particularly important safety consideration related to ergonomically unfriendly technology features (Zuzelo et al., 2008). Nurses reported that equipment weight, including monitoring systems, contributed to challenging patient transports with significant potential for staff injury (Zuzelo et al., 2008). Transport monitors, including cardiac equipment, are heavy and transports that involved lifting monitors onto beds and moving the system with the patient also on board created opportunities for strain injuries.

Mobile medication delivery systems were viewed as convenient for bedside medication administration but required nurses to maintain a prolonged standing position; custom seats are often available but not always purchased. Physical ailments reportedly occurred as a direct result of this prolonged standing, including lower leg edema, plantar fasciitis, and other musculoskeletal and vascular complaints. Advanced nurses need to consider these employee safety concerns when making decisions about product purchasing.

There are times when patient rooms are not safe for staff or for patients and families. Opportunities for slips, falls, and trips as a result of dirty or cluttered floors, inconvenient and hazardous positioning of personal belongings, and power cord and furniture placements need to be considered and corrected. Stichler (2017) shared ideas for a safe patient room design following an interprofessional team workshop. These ideas included technology-centric smart room capabilities, voice-activated equipment and devices to reduce the need for reaching and touching, bedside medication and supply provision that utilizes barcode technology, misters and lights designed to reduce transmission of *Clostridium difficile*, nonskid flooring, and other key features (Stichler, 2017). It is particularly interesting to consider how patient rooms might look if advanced nurses had the opportunity to recreate care environments!

Healthy Work Environments Require Skilled Communication

Nurses must be as proficient in communication skills as they are in clinical skills. The concept of communication is complex, encompassing verbal, written, and nonverbal skills. Advanced nurses must role model expert communication techniques and offer constructive feedback to staff nurses as they develop their communication skillsets. Excellent communication is open, respectful, clear, and includes effective listening skills that convey empathy and promote dialogue.

One strategy that has been effective in facilitating clear, direct communication among caregivers is the SBAR strategy. SBAR is an acronym for *situation, background, assessment,* and *recommendation.* SBAR is a situational briefing model characterized by appropriate assertion, critical language, and awareness and education. It is a vital model designed to address the different communication styles used and valued by nurses, physicians, and other clinicians. Published literature reveals that SBAR is being utilized internationally as a framework to enhance, particularly, nurse-physician communication but also interprofessional communication involving a variety of health care professionals (Lee, Dong, Lim, Poh, & Lim, 2016; Randmaa, Mårtensson, Swenne, & Engström, 2014; Ting, Peng, Lin, & Hsiao, 2017). Research findings support that SBAR provides an effective strategy to improving safe communication exchanges between health care providers. Advanced nurses may want to consider the best way to implement SBAR communication and involve interprofessional team members in this initiative (**TABLE 8-3**).

Advanced nurses practicing in the clinical setting can assist staff with developing a template that guides communications with physicians and other team members using the SBAR strategy and incorporating the consistent use of particular elements that relate to the specific patient population. For example, if caring for patients admitted to a cardiopulmonary specialty unit, the cardiac rhythm would be consistently included in every communication. Additional strategies to improve communication include conducting briefings, being assertive, developing situational awareness, understanding the differences in expert and novice decision making, and conducting debriefings (Volker & Clark, 2004). Communication successes will develop over time and will assuredly occur with practice, repetition, and constructive feedback to staff.

TABLE 8-3 SBAR

Short (30- to 60-Second) Communication Exemplar

Situation	**What is happening with the patient?** "Hello, Dr. Jones, this is Peter Franklin. I am calling from 2 West. I am taking care of Mr. Green in room 212, a patient of Dr. Johnson who went to the OR today for a colectomy. He has been back from the PACU for 4 hours. I have just reassessed him."
Background	**What is the important clinical information?** "Over the past 4 hours, his BP has dropped from 120/78 to 98/58, his heart rate has increased from 70 to 96 beats per minute, his respiratory rate is 24, and his urine output was 60 mL/hour for the first 2 hours and has dropped to 30 mL each hour for the past 2 hours. He is receiving IV fluids, D5.45NS + 20 meq KCL at 125 mL/hour. His postop labs were unremarkable, his hemoglobin was 10.2. His estimated blood loss was 450 mL."
Assessment	**What do you think the problem is?** "I think he is dry; hypovolemic."
Recommendation	**What do you think he needs? If you think the patient needs to be seen by the physician or nurse practitioner, do not be afraid to say so.** "I think his intravenous fluid rate needs to be increased or he needs a normal saline intravenous fluid challenge. If his urine output does not increase or his vital signs do not normalize within the hour after starting more fluids, I will let you know so that he can be evaluated by you or the nurse practitioner."

Data from Leonard et al., 2004; Phillips, 2005.

Paying Attention to Handovers and Handoffs

Handoffs, also referred to as handovers, occur when nurses or other direct care providers hand over responsibility and accountability for care of a patient to another health professional. This transition requires communication of key information necessary for care continuity and safe care delivery. The point of care transition is well recognized as a potentially unsafe juncture, depending on the quality of communication and accuracy of reported data. The inconsistent nature of handoffs contributes to its potential risk for mismanagement (Bakon, Wirihana, Christensen, & Craft, 2017; Croos, 2014).

Bakon et al. (2017) conducted an integrative review of the literature pertaining to differing handover models and processes and their efficacious effects on handover communication quality. The review used an inductive exploratory design. Cumulative Index of Nursing and Allied Health Literature (CINAHL), PubMed, and Science Direct databases plus a manual citation search of the reference lists of retrieved publications from the database searches were utilized in the literature exploration. The literature yield (N = 16) was appraised using the Critical Appraisal Skills Program (CASP, 2017). Findings suggest that while there are various handover/handoff models currently used in practice, there is no evidence that any one model is superior.

The Bakon et al. (2017) review is particularly interesting because it illuminates the current state of handoff processes based on the English-language literature published over the past 10 years. Bakon et al. (2017) point out that there are four types of handoffs: verbal bedside, tape-recorded, verbal, and written. One mixed method study used a pretest/posttest design and found that patients preferred a bedside handover so that they could be kept apprised of their treatment plan and engage with nursing staff members (Bradley & Mott, 2014). This particular study aligns with the current emphasis on rounding and bedside reporting as strategies to enhance patient engagement in care and to avoid errors and miscommunications.

The Joint Commission Center for Transforming Healthcare (2018a) was created in 2008 with the goal of solving the most critical of safety and quality problems in health care by using a systematic approach to analyze and correct delineated breakdowns in care. Its focus is to transform health care into a high reliability industry (The Joint Commission Center for Transforming Healthcare, 2018a). The Center has several targeted initiatives, including handoff communications; and, specific to this particular concern, it created the Targeted Solutions Tool® (TST®) for Hand-off Communications (The Joint Commission Center for Transforming Healthcare, 2018b). This tool eases examination of hospitals' and systems' current handoff processes and provides a measurement system that produces the data necessary for handoff process improvements. The TST® for Hand-off Communications identifies areas of focus, provides customizable data collection forms, and provides guidelines (Joint Commission Center for Transforming Healthcare, 2018b).

Huddling is another strategy designed to improve interprofessional and intraprofessional communication related to safety topics (Kylor, Napier, Rephann, & Spence, 2016), team efforts (IHI, 2018b), and patient care needs (Lubinensky, Kratzer, & Bergstol, 2015). Leadership huddles may be used to enhance situational awareness that informs subsequent problem-solving discussions. Sikka, Kovich, and Sacks (2014) report that one health care system experienced an increased safety events reporting rate of 40%, indicating better detection of safety compromises as well as enhanced organizational transparency. IHI (2018b) describes huddles as very brief meetings or exchanges that support full participation of bedside and frontline staff by limiting the time and keeping the topic in clear focus. IHI (2018b) provides a *Huddles* pdf tool that provides advanced nurses and others with huddle implementation guidance.

Advanced nurses may want to consider implementing huddles as a strategy to improve safety. Successful huddle programs require planning, training, practice, and a culture change that will take time, persistence, and a consistent leadership approach. These same efforts and influences are needed when creating a standardized handoff system and initiating SBAR communication. Evidence supports that these communication strategies do improve safety culture and contribute to high organizational reliability.

▶ Quality and Safety Education in Nursing

Patient safety as a discipline is a relatively new phenomenon. Many nurses, as well as other health care providers, did not explore the science of safety and error reduction or the relationship of culture to patient safety during formal nursing education experiences. Nurses may be inclined to consider patient safety as closely aligned with the traditional five rights of medication administration. These five "rights" include right patient, right drug, right dose, right route, and right time (Institute for Safe Medication Practices [ISMP], 2007); and although they have been universally taught in all types of basic nursing education programs, the mantra is woefully ineffective as a primary strategy for preventing medication errors, particularly when contrasted to the far more systems-based, comprehensive strategies (IHI, 2018c; ISMP, 2007).

Many nurses will recall learning these rights by rote as students, and new graduate nurses were often drilled about these rules during clinical experiences involving medication or treatment deliveries. Nurses may continue to view these five rights as the gold standard of error prevention; however, these five rights are best viewed as the intended goals of safe medication practices. They do not offer strategies for nurses interested in achieving these goals other than a rather overwhelming perception that error is the result of individual performance and good nurses do not make mistakes. Given that nurses do not come to work intending to commit errors, opportunities for error and accident reduction must be more broadly based than relying on drilled processes.

ISMP (2007) asserts that nurses and other providers are often cited as deficiently following the five rights when medication errors occur; however, nurses cannot be held accountable for achieving the five rights when procedural rules cannot be followed because of systems issues. The idea that if nurses follow the five rights errors will be averted is contrary to the new systems perspectives on medication use safety and human error.

Advanced nurses interested in using creative, evidence-based resources for educating new-to-practice nurses as well as more experienced staff without much formal exposure to health safety and quality topics will appreciate the opportunities available through the Quality and Safety Education for Nurses (QSEN) (2017a) project, a comprehensive resource devoted to addressing the "challenge of preparing future nurses with the knowledge, skills, and attitudes (KSAs) necessary to continuously improve the quality and safety of the healthcare systems within which they work."

The QSEN project (2017a) was initiated in 2005 with funding from the Robert Wood Johnson Foundation. Originally focused on nursing prelicensure programs, in 2012 the QSEN initiative extended to graduate education programs by providing educational resources and training to support the ability of faculty in graduate programs, master's and doctoral, to teach quality and safety competencies (QSEN, 2017b). QSEN competencies for prelicensure and graduate nurses are available at http://qsen. org/education/. There is also a Spanish version of the competencies. QSEN (2017b) competencies are organized in six domains: patient-centered care, teamwork and collaboration, evidence-based practice, quality improvement, safety, and informatics. Each competency domain has a unique definition and associated KSAs. Definitions are consistent between prelicensure and graduate competencies but KSAs differ in response to the demands of graduate level advanced nursing practice.

Nurses in advanced roles need to be aware of the QSEN competencies and QSEN education endeavors, resources, and expectations. QSEN has the support of many professional organizations (QSEN, 2017c) and has international influence in nursing education and practice. Advanced nurses should recognize that for approximately one decade, nursing students have been educated in programs that have integrated QSEN competencies and learning resources. Nurses leave their prelicensure program with good understanding of safety and quality and recognize the features of safety science that should inform practice. Once these nurses begin practice, they may become disillusioned and disappointed when experienced colleagues express skepticism or naiveté' about processes designed to improve and enhance quality and safety.

The faculty learning modules available on QSEN's website are rich resources (http://qsen.org/faculty-resources/courses/learning-modules/) that could benefit advanced practice nurses, nurse educators, staff development professionals, nurse preceptors, and managers who are interested in tools and strategies for enhancing quality and safety outcomes. Module topics are designed to assist faculty with integrating QSEN competencies into nursing curricula (QSEN, 2017d). There are 18 available modules and while some likely have more relevance to nursing education settings than to practice environments, there are many modules that would serve to enhance advanced nurses' and staff nurses' expertise (**BOX 8-1**).

Advanced nurses may want to consider opportunities to establish academic-practice partnerships as a way to generate interest in and commitment to QSEN competencies (Koffel, Burke, McGuinn, & Miltner, 2017). QSEN competences are consistent with TJC and Magnet standards and this alignment may be beneficial to health care organizations, and the reciprocal benefits to nursing education programs is that students would learn to apply the theory of quality improvement and safety science to the real world of health care.

Safety and Quality Organizations

The complexity of overlapping and unique regulatory versus recommending agencies within health care is extraordinary. Advanced nurses practicing in a variety of roles are often held accountable for compliance with multitudes of guidelines, competencies, rules, and regulations. TJC accreditation is a nationwide seal of approval indicating that organizations meet high performance standards. The Joint Commission International (JCI) is considered the gold standard accreditation for global health care (JCI,

BOX 8-1 QSEN Learning Modules

Title

1. Appreciating the Complexity of Nursing Work: Implications for Nursing Education
2. Managing the Complexity of Nursing Work: Cognitive Stacking
3. Mindfulness: Implications for Safety, Self-Care and Empathy in Nursing Education
4. Informatics
5. Embedding QSEN Competencies in Beginning Clinical Courses
6. Teaching Patient-Centered Care Using Narrative and Reflective Pedagogies
7. Nursing, Nursing Information Management, and Nursing Informatics
8. Strategies for Making Assessment of QSEN Competencies Efficient and Conducive to Learning
9. Managing Curricular Change for QSEN Integration
10. Interprofessional Education (IPE): Learning for Practice
11. Integrating QSEN in to the Intermediate Nursing Curriculum. Working with Courses that Focus on Specialty Populations
12. Integrating QEN into the Advanced Nursing Curriculum
13. Cultivating a Culture of Justice in Nursing Education and Healthcare
14. Strategies for Incorporating Rubrics in Assessment of QSEN Competencies
15. Using Simulation in Leadership Courses: Providing a Means for Application of Core Concepts
16. Preparing Students to Think Through the Complexities of Practice in Post-clinical Conferences
17. Patient Safety: Our intent is to do no harm—so why do errors happen?
18. Embedding QSEN Competencies in Prelicensure Curricula: Fostering Continuous Improvement

Data from QSEN Institute, Case Western Reserve University. Faculty Learning Modules. Retrived from http://qsen.org/faculty-resources/courses/learning-modules/.

n.d.[a]). JCI has initiated and partnered on many efforts to improve safety within the international health care system (JCI, n.d.[b]).

There are numerous regulatory and recommending agencies within the United States and across the world that address health care safety and quality; many of their recommendations overlap given their shared evidence base. Key U.S. organizations include, but are not limited to, the Center for Medicare and Medicaid (CMS), IHI, AHRQ, National Patient Safety Goals® (NPSG), TJC, and National Quality Foundation (NQF).

Tools of the Trade

The World Wide Web has dramatically influenced patient care delivery. The safety component of advanced practice and its many associated responsibilities are inextricably linked to the use of electronically available tools in the form of assessment tools, guidelines, and other references, many of which can be downloaded without charge (**TABLE 8-4**). A majority of professional associations offer information about patient safety topics, particularly those relevant to the area of practice or to the role represented by the organization. Advanced nurses are encouraged to take full advantage of the many resources and build their safety skills repertoire in ways that are advantageous to the patients and systems that they serve.

TABLE 8-4 Select Examples of Patient Safety Websites

Name	Website	Limited content description
Institute for Safe Medication Practices (ISMP)	www.ismp.org	Nonprofit education organization that addresses medication safety
		Medication safety tools and resources: high-alert medication list, confused drug list, error-prone abbreviation list, do-not-crush list
		USP – ISMP Medication Error reporting system
		Links to numerous patient safety sites
		Consultation opportunities
		Federal Drug Administration and ISMP Tall Man Letters for look-alike drugs (http://www.ismp.org/Tools/tallmanletters.pdf)
		Extensive education resources for professionals and public
Agency for Healthcare Research and Quality (AHRQ)	www.ahrq.gov	■ Invests in research and evidence to make health care safer and improve quality
		■ Creates materials to teach and train health care systems and professionals to help them improve care for their patients
		■ Generates measures and data used to track and improve performance and evaluate progress of the U.S. health system
		■ Uses and shares evidence-based tools and resources to improve the quality, safety, effectiveness, and efficiency of health care
		■ Offers 47 unique programs with toolkits, additional resource connections, and other related assessments, documents, and multimedia opportunities
		■ Newsletters, online journals
		■ Funding opportunities
		■ Big data accessibility
		■ Web morbidity and mortality presentations and resources categorized by prioritized populations

Name	Website	Limited content description
Federal Drug Administration	www.fda.gov	■ Product recalls, product safety ■ MAUDE data base and medical device reporting ■ Programs include: Program Alignment, Innovation, Globalization, Food Safety Modernization Act, Regulatory Science, Tobacco, Transparency, Medical Countermeasures, Sentinel Initiative
National Guideline Clearinghouse	http://www .guidelines.gov	■ AHRQ's public resource for evidence-based clinical guidelines
Institute for Healthcare Improvement	www.ihi.org	■ Vision: Everyone has the best care and health possible ■ Mission: Improve health and health care worldwide ■ Uses the science of improvement to improve quality, safety, and value in health care ■ IHI Open School offers many online classes, and a video library online and opportunities for practicum experiences

References

Agency for Healthcare Research and Quality. (2013). Understand just culture. Retrieved January 27, 2018, from https://www.ahrq.gov/professionals/education/curriculum-tools/cusptoolkit /videos/07a_just_culture/index.html.

Agency for Healthcare Research and Quality. (2017a). Surveys on patient safety culture™. Retrieved November 12, 2017, from https://www.ahrq.gov/professionals/quality-patient-safety/patient safetyculture/index.html.

Agency for Health Research and Quality. (2017b). Patient safety measure tools and resources. Retrieved January 27, 2018, from https://www.ahrq.gov/professionals/quality-patient-safety/patient -safety-resources/index.html.

Agency for Healthcare Research and Quality. (2018). CUSP. Retrieved January 27, 2018, from https:// www.ahrq.gov/professionals/education/curriculum-tools/cusptoolkit/index.html.

American Society for Quality. (2018a). Failure model effects analysis (FMEA). Retrieved November 13, 2017, from http://asq.org/learn-about-quality/process-analysis-tools/overview/fmea.html.

American Society for Quality. (2018b). What is root cause analysis (RCA?). Retrieved January 27, 2018, from http://asq.org/learn-about-quality/root-cause-analysis/overview/overview.html.

Aspden, P., Corrigan, J. M., Wolcott, J., & Erickson, S. M. (Eds.). (2004). *Committee on data s standards for patient safety. Patient safety: Achieving a new standard for care.* Washington, DC: National Academies Press.

Bakon, S., Wirihana, L., Christensen, M., & Craft, J. (2017). Nursing handovers: An integrative review of the different models and processes available. *International Journal of Nursing Practice, 23*, e12520. doi:10.1111/ijn.12520

Bradley, S., & Mott, S. (2014). Adopting a patient-centred approach: an investigation into the introduction of bedside handover to three rural hospitals. *Journal of Clinical Nursing, 23*, 1927–1936. doi:10.1111/jocn.12403

Bravo, K., & Cochran, G. (2016). Nursing strategies to increase medication safety in inpatient settings. *Journal of Nursing Care Quality, 31,* 335–341. doi: 10.1097/NCQ.0000000000000181

Carayon, P., & Wood, K. E. (2010). Patient safety. The role of human factors and systems engineering. *Studies in Health Technology and Informatics, 153,* 23–46.

Chassin, M. R., & Loeb, J. M. (2013). High-reliability health care: Getting there from here. *The Milbank Quarterly, 91,* 459–490.

Clements, K. (2017). High-reliability and the I-PASS communication tool. *Nursing Management, 48,* 12–13. doi:10.1097/01.NUMA.0000512897.68425.e5

Critical Appraisal Skills Programme (CASP). (2017). Home. Retrieved January 27, 2018, from http://www.casp-uk.net/

Croos, S. (2014). The practice of clinical handover: A respite perspective. *British Journal of Nursing, 23,* 733–737.

D'Esmond, L. K. (2017). Distracted practice and patient safety: The healthcare team experience. *Nursing Forum, 52,* 149–164.

Duwe, B., Fuchs, B., & Hansen-Flashen, J. (2005). Failure mode and effects analysis application to critical care medicine. *Critical Care Medicine, 21,* 21–30.

Healthgrades. (2017a). About us. Retrieved November 11, 2017, from https://www.healthgrades.com/about/.

Healthgrades. (2017b). Patient satisfaction. Retrieved November 11, 2017, from https://www.healthgrades.com/quality/patient-satisfaction.

Healthgrades. (2017c). Experience match. Retrieved November 11, 2017, from https://www.healthgrades.com/quality/experience-match.

Healthgrades. (2017d). Hospital quality. Retrieved November 11, 2017, from https://www.healthgrades.com/quality/hospital-ratings-awards.

Hines S, Luna, K, Lofthus J, et al. (April, 2008). Becoming a high reliability organization: Operational advice for hospital leaders. (Prepared by the Lewin Group under Contract No. 290-04-0011.) AHRQ Publication No. 08-0022. Rockville, MD: Agency for Healthcare Research and Quality. Retrieved January 27, 2018, from https://archive.ahrq.gov/professionals/quality-patient-safety/quality-resources/tools/hroadvice/hroadvice.pdf.

Institute for Healthcare Improvement. (2018a). Develop a culture of safety. Retrieved January 27, 2018, from http://www.ihi.org/resources/Pages/Changes/DevelopaCultureofSafety.aspx.

Institute for Healthcare Improvement. (2018b). Tools. Huddles. Retrieved January 27, 2018, from http://www.ihi.org/resources/Pages/Tools/Huddles.aspx.

Institute for Healthcare Improvement. (2018c). Improve core processes for administering medications. Retrieved January 27, 2018, from http://www.ihi.org/resources/Pages/Changes/ImproveCoreProcessesforAdministeringMedications.aspx.

Institute for Safe Medication Practices. (2007, January 25). The five rights: A destination without a map. Acute Care ISMP Medication Safety Alert! Retrieved November 20, 2017, from http://www.ismp.org/newsletters/acutecare/articles/20070125.asp.

Institute for Safe Medication Practices. (2012). ASSESS-ERR™ medication system worksheet. Retrieved November 13, 2017, from http://www.ismp.org/Tools/AssessERR.pdf.

Johnson, J., Louch, G., Dunning, A., Johnson, O., Grange, A., Reynolds, C., . . . O'Hara, J. (2016). Burnout mediates the association between depression and patient safety perceptions: A cross-sectional study in hospital nurses. *Journal of Advanced Nursing, 73,* 1667–1680. doi:10.1111/jan.13251

Koffel, C., Burke, K., McGuinn, K., & Miltner, R. (2017). Integration of quality and safety education for nurses into practice. Academic-practice partnership's role. *Nurse Educator, 42,* 549–552. doi:10.1097/NNE.0000000000000424

Kohn, L., Corrigan, J., & Donaldson, M. (Eds.). (2000). *To err is human: Building a safer health system.* Washington, DC: National Academies Press.

Kylor, C., Napier, T., Rephann, A., & Spence, A. (2016). Implementation of the safety huddle. *Critical Care Nurse, 36,* 80–82.

Leapfrog Group. (n.d.). Mission and vision. Retrieved January 26, 2018, from http://www.leapfroggroup.org/about/mission-and-vision.

Leapfrog Group. (2017a). Hospital errors are the third leading cause of death in U.S., and new hospital safety scores show improvements are too slow. Retrieved November 11, 2017, from http://www.hospitalsafetygrade.org/newsroom/display/hospitalerrors-thirdleading-causeofdeathinus-improvementstooslow.

Leapfrog Group. (2017b). Compare hospitals. 2017 survey results are now available. Search for hospitals in your area. Retrieved November 11, 2017, from http://www.leapfroggroup.org/compare -hospitals.

Lee, S. Y., Dong, L., Lim, Y. H., Poh, C. L., & Lim, W. S. (2016). SBAR: Towards a common interprofessional team-based communication tool. *Medical Education, 50,* 1145–1172. doi:10.1111/medu.13171

Lubinensky, M., Kratzer, R., & Bergstol, J. (2015). Huddle up for patient safety. *American Nurse Today, 10*(2). Retrieved November 20, 2017, from https://www.americannursetoday.com/huddle -patient-safety/.

Makary, M. A., & Daniel, M. (2016). Medical error—the third leading cause of death in the US. *BMJ, 353,* i2139. doi:10.1136/bmj.i2139

Merino, P., Álvarez, J., Martin, M. C., Alonso, Á., Gutiérrez, I., & SYREC Study Investigators. (2012). Adverse events in Spanish intensive care units: The SYREC study. *International Journal for Quality in Health Care, 24,* 105–113. doi:10.1093/intqhc/mzr083

Patient Safety Network. (2017). Patient safety primer. Wrong-site, wrong-procedure, and wrong-patient surgery. Retrieved November 11, 2017, from https://psnet.ahrq.gov/primers/primer /18/wrong-site-wrong-procedure-and-wrong-patient-surgery.

Phillips, J. (2005). Neuroscience CC: The role of the APN in patient safety. *AACN Clinical Issues, 16,* 580–591.

Pronovost, P. J., Thompson, D. A., Holzmueller, C. G., Lubomski, L. H., & Morlock, L. L. (2005). Defining and measuring patient safety. *Critical Care Clinics, 21,* 1–19.

Quality and Safety Education for Nurses. (2018a). About. QSEN. Retrieved January 27, 2018, http:// qsen.org/about-qsen/.

Quality and Safety Education for Nurses. (2018b). Project overview. The evolution of the Quality and Safety Education for Nurses (QSEN) initiative. Retrieved January 27, 2018, from http://qsen.org /about-qsen/project-overview/.

Quality and Safety Education for Nurses. (2018c). Professional organizations. Retrieved January 27, 2018, from http://qsen.org/faculty-resources/organizations/.

Quality and Safety Education for Nurses. (2018d). Faculty learning modules. Retrieved January 27, 2018, from http://qsen.org/faculty-resources/courses/learning-modules/.

Randmaa, M., Mårtensson, G., Swenne, C., & Engström, M. (2014). SBAR improves communication and safety climate and decreases incident reports due to communication errors in an anaesthetic clinic: A prospective intervention study. *BMJ Open, 4,* e004268. doi:10.1136/bmjopen-2013-004268

Reason, J. (1990). *Human error.* New York: Cambridge University Press.

Sikka, R., Kovich, K., & Sacks, L. (2014, December 5). How every hospital should start the day. *Harvard Business Review.* Retrieved November 20, 2017, from https://hbr.org/2014/12 /how-every-hospital-should-start-the-day.

Spear. S. (n.d.). How can you identify and confront workarounds? Institute for Healthcare Improvement. Open School. Retrieved January 27, 2018, from http://www.ihi.org/education/IHIOpenSchool /resources/Pages/Activities/SteveSpearSolvingWorkarounds.aspx.

Stichler, J. (2017). Designing safe patient rooms. *Health Environments Research & Design Journal, 10*(5), 7–11.

The Joint Commission. (2017a). Universal protocol. Retrieved November 13, 2017, from https://www .jointcommission.org/standards_information/up.aspx.

The Joint Commission. (2017b). National time out day. Retrieved November 13, 2017, from https://www .jointcommission.org/national_time_out_day_2017/.

The Joint Commission. (2017c). Standards. Risk assessments—how and when. Retrieved November 13, 2017, from https://www.jointcommission.org/standards_information/jcfaqdetails.aspx?Standards FaqId=1267&ProgramId=46.

The Joint Commission. (2017d). Framework for conducting a root cause analysis. Retrieved November 13, 2017, from https://www.jointcommission.org/framework_for_conducting_a_root_cause_analysis_and _action_plan/.

The Joint Commission Center for Transforming Healthcare. (2018a). About us. Retrieved January 27, 2018, from https://www.centerfortransforminghealthcare.org/about_us.aspx

The Joint Commission Center for Transforming Healthcare. (2018b). Targeted Solutions Tool® for hand-off communications. Retrieved January 27, 2018, from http://www.centerfortransforminghealthcare .org/tst_hoc.aspx.

The Joint Commission International. (n.d.[a]). About JCI. Retrieved January 27, 2018, from https://www.jointcommissioninternational.org/about/.

The Joint Commission International. (n.d.[b]). Projects supporting our mission. Retrieved January 27, 2018, from https://www.jointcommissioninternational.org/about-jci/projects-supporting-our-mission/.

Ting, W. H., Peng, F. S., Lin, H. H., & Hsiao, S. M. (2017). The impact of situation-background-assessment-recommendation (SBAR) on safety attitudes in the obstetrics department. *Taiwanese Journal of Obstetrics & Gynecology, 56,* 171–174. doi:10.1016/j.tjog.2016.06.021

Tingle, J., & Minford, J. (2017). Improving patient safety in the NHS: The culture change agents. *British Journal of Nursing, 26,* 708–709.

Tucker, A. L. (2009). Workarounds and resiliency on the front lines of health care. *Perspectives on Safety.* Retrieved January 27, 2018, from https://psnet.ahrq.gov/perspectives/perspective/78.

Tucker, A. L., & Edmondson, A. C. (2002). When problem solving prevents organizational learning. *Journal of Organizational Change Management, 15,* 122–138.

Vogus, T. J., & Singer, S. J. (2016). Creating highly reliable accountable care organizations. *Medical Care Research and Review, 73,* 660–672. doi:10.1177/1077558716640413

Volker, D. L., & Clark, A. P. (2004). Taking the high road: What should you do when an adverse event occurs, Part II. *Clinical Nurse Specialist, 18,* 180–182.

White, S. V. (2004). Patient safety issues. In J. Byers & S. White (Eds.), *Patient safety: Principles and practice.* New York: Springer.

Xie, J., Ding, S., Zhong, Z, Zeng, S., Qin, C., Qi-feng, Y., . . . Zhou, J. (2017). A safety culture training program enhanced the perceptions of patient safety culture of nurse managers. *Nurse Education in Practice, 27,* 128–133. doi:10.1016/j.nepr.2017.08.003

Zuzelo, P., Gettis, C., Hansell, A., & Thomas, L. (2008). Describing the influence of technologies on registered nurses' work. *Clinical Nurse Specialist, 22*(3), 132–240.

Zuzelo, P., Inverso, T., & Linkewich, K. (2001). Content validation of the Medication Error Worksheet©. *Clinical Nurse Specialist, 15,* 253–259.

CHAPTER 9

Influencing Outcomes: Improving the Quality of Care Delivery

Patti Rager Zuzelo, EdD, RN, ACNS-BC, ANP-BC, CRNP, FAAN

The contributions of all types of advanced nurses, including advanced practice registered nurses (APRNs), are under scrutiny within and outside the profession as health care delivery models change and systems react to uncertainties related to the Patient Protection and Affordable Care Act (Obama Care or the Affordable Care Act [ACA]) and recent legislative efforts to modify its central and defining components and requirements. Interprofessional education (IPE) and new care models are increasingly emphasized as opportunities to improve communication among team members and, ultimately, to provide better and safer care that yields improved health outcomes. Conflict persists between organized medicine and advanced nurse providers while grassroots efforts intensify to develop partnerships that challenge status quo power structures in efforts to support just cultures, safe care, and teams that rely on collaborative problem solving.

Uncertainties persist within health care systems secondary to unclear roles, overlapping responsibilities, and competition. Some advanced roles face unique challenges including the Clinical Nurse Specialist (CNS) and Clinical Nurse Leader (CNL) roles. The CNL role, an advanced generalist role originally conceived as an opportunity for people with college degrees interested in changing careers and entering nursing with a master's degree in nursing, presents potential challenges to the CNS as the delineation between CNL and CNS job responsibilities and skillsets appear occasionally murky, overlapping, and poorly articulated in real-world practice environments. In states without CNS title protection, nurse practitioners (NPs) and other RNs with or without graduate degrees in nursing view CNS opportunities as appropriate career options, while administrators, confronted with shortages of CNS applicants and confused by the unique skills each APRN role offers, may hire an assortment of nurses into CNS positions, including those prepared as nurse educators.

It is noteworthy that there has been some progress at the state level in CNS title protection; for example, the General Assembly of Pennsylvania has passed House Bill Number 1238, amending the Professional Nursing Law and providing for the definition of CNS (Pennsylvania General Assembly, 2015). CNSs continue to face state-specific practice barriers, including four states that either do not recognize the CNS as an advanced practice nurse or have no available data regarding CNS recognition; three states that do not provide the CNS with advanced practice authority; and 14 states that require the CNS to have a collaborative agreement for practice. Twenty-eight states provide the CNS with full scope of practice and 17 states permit the CNS to independently prescribe (National Council of State Boards of Nursing [NCSBN], 2017a, 2017b). Variability across states related to dependent or independent practice, advanced practice status, and pharmaceutical/durable goods prescription authorities create additional challenges for the CNS and resulting barriers to people who would benefit from CNS expertise.

NPs are also experiencing regulatory challenges largely in response to push-back from the medical establishment related to competition and independent practice opportunities. The American Medical Association (AMA) recently continued its vigorous resistance to allowing independent practice for physician's assistants and advanced practice nurses, seeking to protect a physician-led team model (AMA, 2017; American Urological Association [AUA], 2017). The AMA House of Delegates debated and voted on a number of resolutions including those specific to oppose nonphysician practitioners' independent practice efforts (**BOX 9-1**). The American Association of

---

BOX 9-1   AMA House of Delegates Interim Meeting, November 14, 2017 Adopted Resolutions

American Medical Association (AMA) Resolution 214: ADVANCED PRACTICE REGISTERED NURSE COMPACT

Resolved to create a consistent national strategy to oppose nationwide efforts to grant independent practice to non-physician practitioners; effectively educate the public, legislators, regulators, and healthcare administrators; and "effectively oppose state and national level legislative efforts aimed at inappropriate scope of practice expansion of non-physician healthcare practitioners… (AMA, 2017, p. 306)."

AMA Resolution 229: OPPOSITION TO LICENSING FOR INDIVIDUALS HOLDING DEGREE OF DOCTOR OF MEDICAL SCIENCE

Resolved to "oppose the holders of the degree of Doctor of Medical Science from being recognized as a new category of health care practitioners licensed for the independent practice of medicine (AMA 2017. p. 309)" and the AMA will "work with interested state medical associations and national medical specialty societies to oppose legislation to create a Doctor of Medical Science license (AMA, 2017, p. 309)."

AMA Resolution 230: OPPOSE PHYSICIAN ASSISTANT INDEPENDENT PRACTICE

Resolved to "adopt policy to oppose legislation or regulation that allows physician assistant independent practice (AMA, 2017. p. 301)."

Nurse Practitioners (AANP) responded in vigorous fashion and offered a presidential rebuttal that included, "Every major study over the last 50 years has found care provided by nurse practitioners to be safe, effective and similar in outcome to care provided by physicians. There is no study that suggests that care provided in states with more restrictive licensure is safer than states with independent licensure" (AANP, 2017).

Nurse anesthetists (NAs) are currently able to practice independently, without anesthesiologist supervision, in 17 states (Santiago, 2017). The American Society of Anesthesiologists (ASA) argues for physician anesthesiologists to continue to lead anesthesia care and asserts that a 2014 Cochrane Collaboration literature review was unable to find science that supports the premise that NA care is equivalent to anesthesiology-driven care (ASA, 2017). The organization calls for more study on this issue and reiterates its position that anesthesia care delivery must be physician led (ASA, 2017).

These scenarios serve as powerful examples of concerns that directly affect advanced nurses and the public. Each stakeholder group, whether driven by nurses or physicians, offers outcomes data to support its regulatory and policy recommendations. Outcomes data are critical to the position's defense and its success or persuasiveness. Other variables do influence the discussion, including financial ramifications, provider availability, and legislative/regulatory motivating factors. APRNs and other advanced nurses need to maintain a vigilant focus on the importance of health outcomes and the ways that nurses influence these outcomes. Rigorous approaches to research, including valid and reliable data collection and analysis, must be assured so that policy decisions are based on reputable and true scientific findings.

▶ The Impact of the Doctor of Nursing Practice Degree on Advanced Nurses

The proposed requirement by the American Association of Colleges of Nursing (AACN, 2004) of a doctorate in nursing practice (DNP) as the minimum level of entry into advanced nursing practice initially triggered polarized reactions that influenced organizational discussions and contributed to many task force charges, white papers, and planning activities throughout all aspects of the profession. Although the AACN position on the DNP has not been consistently embraced in full by professional organizations that serve and represent APRNs, the number of nurses interested in practice doctorates has increased in a fashion that is consistent with recommendations proffered by *The Future of Nursing* report (Institute of Medicine [IOM], 2010). Some APRN organizations have offered time frames for practice doctorate requirements; the National Association of Clinical Nurse Specialists (2017) calls for a DNP for entry into CNS practice by 2030 and those interested in the National Certification Exam offered by National Board for Certification and Recertification of Nurse Anesthetists will require a DNP or Doctor of Nurse Anesthesia Practice (DNAP) degree by 2025 to sit for the initial NA credentialing examination. Other professional groups, including the AANP, American College of Nurse-Midwives (ACNM), and the American Organization of Nurse Executives (AONE), are supportive of the DNP degree and recognize its value but do not endorse it as a mandatory minimum educational requirement for those nurses or roles represented by the particular organization (AANP, 2013; ACNM, 2012; AONE, 2007).

There is confusion surrounding the *mandatory* nature of the DNP, and many advanced nurses and APRNs anecdotally share concerns and mistaken information about the necessity of the degree. A quick Web-based search reveals many nursing-focused blogs with postings concerning questions about whether the DNP is mandatory for movement into more advanced roles. The DNP is not required for practice by any state board of nursing. There certainly are benefits to doctoral preparation and some students may find it cost effective to move directly from a bachelor of science in nursing (BSN) degree through to a DNP degree; however, others may prefer to complete a master of science in nursing (MSN) degree and delay, avoid, or progress slowly through a DNP plan of study.

The degree discussion is important because it illustrates the importance of and preference for robust outcomes data. Some organizations suggest that there are no outcomes data supporting the premise that DNP preparation improves nurse-provided care outcomes. DNP students do develop scholarly projects that may be referred to as doctoral, scholarly, or capstone projects. There are potential opportunities for this vast array of work to be examined for outcomes data that could be compiled and used to provide support for the positive impact of the DNP-prepared nurse on health or practice outcomes compared to the master's prepared nurse; however, perhaps these projects represent required isolated academic efforts rather than sustained evidence-based practice (EBP) improvements directly influenced by the DNP degree. The challenge lies in determining whether DNP-prepared nurses influence outcomes in ways that differ from those with MSN preparation. To date, this sort of comparison is not available and, perhaps, might not be the best approach. The critical point is that *outcomes management* and *outcomes measurement* are frequently raised as important to this education and practice discussion, just as outcomes are particularly important to conversations about health care quality, including effectiveness and costs.

In addition to the *unique* role challenges confronting the wide variety of advanced nurses, there are also shared challenges related to regulatory and legislative initiatives; for example, the Centers for Medicare & Medicaid Services (CMS, 2015) lengthened its list of noncovered hospital-acquired conditions (HACs) and the Hospital Consumer Assessment of Healthcare Providers and Systems (HCAHPS) survey results are having profound ramifications on health care systems. Advanced nurses work to address differing aspects of these and other challenges and while doing so, are challenged to consider, "What differences in care processes and outcomes are amenable to improvement through the individual and collective efforts of nurses, particularly nurses with advanced skills and education?" Nurses with advanced preparation, including and not limited to APRNs, need to collect, analyze, and share outcome data advancing the premise that nurses make unique contributions to positive patient outcomes and that these outcomes are measurable, meaningful, and important. This chapter introduces some important ideas about outcomes, discusses trends, describes resources and tools, identifies challenges, and offers suggestions.

▶ What Is an Outcome?

An outcome is the end result of particular health care practices and interventions. The paramount need for outcomes research was made obvious in the early 1980s when studies confirmed that surgical procedures and medical practices varied in frequency and type based upon geography rather than disease rates. In addition, there was no established way to compare the results of differing treatment approaches (Agency for Healthcare Research and Quality [AHRQ], 2000). These early discussions focused on patient outcomes related to prescribed medical therapies and interventions and stimulated outcomes discussions related to nursing practice as well as other types of clinical services.

Kleinpell and Gawlinski (2005) define outcomes as a "measure of healthcare quality, and often, effectiveness is measured by the outcomes that are produced" (p. 43). Nursing-sensitive outcomes are influenced by nurses' care practices. Nursing-sensitive patient outcomes (NSPOs) are best understood as "patient outcomes that are amenable to nursing intervention" (Given & Sherwood, 2005, p. 773). There is a need for increased research on the leadership outcomes of advanced practitioners given that the current state of evaluation research focuses on a limited range of patient, care, and performance-related outcomes (Elliott, Begley, Kleinpell, & Higgins, 2014). Nurses in advanced roles of all sorts should consider opportunities to measure their influence on outcomes that are meaningful whether specific to patient care or not. Certainly indirect care responsibilities are integral to high-quality health care delivery systems and a keen eye on goals and measures is important, particularly given scarce resources.

Nurses do not influence all patient outcomes, but many outcomes are responsive to nursing interventions. Outcomes that are influenced by nurses in collaboration with other health care providers are important, but these particular outcomes, while affected by nurses, do not reflect nursing's *unique* contributions to health care structures and processes. Identifying the unique contributions of nurses, including those directly attributable to nurses' influence, is key to the future of nursing practice. It is imperative that advanced nurses collect and analyze carefully considered data sets that quantify the impact that nurses have on health outcomes. Nurses recognizing and marketing the differences that they make in direct care patient outcomes and indirect care outcomes is critical to improving the health care system. Indirect care outcomes might be considered as outcomes that relate to policy efforts, administrative processes and policies, leadership responsibilities, educational endeavors, informatics and the influence on care outcomes that are affected by changes in information management systems, and other non-patient care activities.

If advanced nurses are able to discern which end results of patient care are directly affected by nursing interventions, then they will be able to determine better ways to intervene, and thus contribute to improving health care system and patient outcomes. This linkage between nursing care and NSPOs provides justification for the current emphasis on evidence-based nursing (EBN). While there is ambiguity in the definition of EBN and continued discussion as to what EBN should and should not be, the synergy is clear between outcomes and evidence.

Evidence in all its forms, qualitative and quantitative, should inform nursing interventions (Zuzelo, 2006) and should assist in the measurement of nurses' effect on outcomes as well as on improvements in the structures and processes of health care systems. NSPOs should be evaluated and future interventions should be revised or maintained depending upon the outcomes. Quality of care is determined by outcomes (**FIGURE 9-1**). Measuring advanced nurses' influence on outcomes and

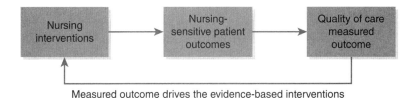

Measured outcome drives the evidence-based interventions

FIGURE 9-1 The Feedback Loop: Evidence-Based Practice, Outcomes Management, and Quality.

quality of care is important to marketing advanced nursing practice, justifying the fixed costs associated with competitive compensation, and securing the full-time equivalents necessary for hiring nurses with advanced preparation and skills.

▶ Outcomes Measures: Key Players and Driving Forces

Advanced nurses need to be familiar with the organizations and databases commonly used to ascertain health care quality and necessary to inform high-stakes decisions related to credentialing, benefits purchasing,

The National Database of Nursing Quality Indicators

Advanced nurses must become well informed about the National Database of Nursing Quality Indicators (NDNQI®), a program developed by the American Nurses Association (ANA) and managed by the University of Kansas School of Nursing. NDNQI was acquired by Press Ganey in 2014 (Press Ganey, 2015). NDNQI is a national database that collects data at the nursing unit level. Indicators are regularly added and new projects are developed and implemented regularly. The database is dynamic and offers a variety of reports that enable institutions to compare their outcomes to those of other similar institutions across the country (ANA, 2002). Over 2,000 hospitals nationwide use the NDNQI program to track and improve nursing-sensitive quality measures (Press Ganey, 2015). Press Ganey (2017) provides a searchable resource library that includes many resources, including reports, articles, webinars, case studies, videos, and other multimedia informational sources that are available immediately or via download after receipt of basic demographic information.

The best way to appreciate the importance of NDNQI is to understand its history (Montalvo, 2007). The ANA launched the Safety and Quality Initiative in 1994 to investigate and describe the empirical linkages between nursing care and patient outcomes. This project was early in the outcomes measurement movement and served to guide and support discussions about the connection between nurse staffing patterns and nurse preparation to patient care outcomes. Other organizations had called for outcomes measurement as early as the 1970s, including the Joint Commission (TJC), the Visiting Nursing Association (VNA) of Omaha, and the National League for Nursing (NLN). The ANA's initiative was the first report card–style report specific to acute care hospital nursing (ANA, 1995).

The outcome of the Safety and Quality Initiative was a report entitled, *The nursing care report card for acute care* (ANA, 1995). This report card identified 21 measures of hospital performance with a conceptual or quantifiable link to nursing services in acute care. The report card also established 10 nursing quality indicators that had a direct relationship to nursing services within acute care settings. Each indicator was operationally defined in careful terms to promote consistency in data collection and analysis. It is worthwhile to go back to this original ANA report and review the complexity and detail of the measures used to establish reliable and valid indicators.

One of the most reliable predictors of outcome indicators was the percentage of RNs of the total staff (Moore, Lynn, McMillen, & Evans, 1999). Staff mix, nurse education, and the numbers of available RNs continue to be an important indicator with a direct effect on patient mortality in the hospital setting (Aiken, Clarke, Sloane, Sochalski, & Silber, 2002; Aiken et al., 2011). Hours per patient day (HPPD) is another important metric used to compare staffing levels within and between health care organizations; however, there is mounting criticism concerning the adequacy of HPPD related to appropriate nurse staffing levels (Kirby, 2015). There is a need to consider staffing and skill mix within the context of achieved outcomes. Kirby (2015) asserts that it is important to quantify the savings associated with positive outcomes and to determine the staffing numbers and patterns that contribute to these outcomes. Advanced nurses need to consider this point as it directly relates to maximizing the utility of NDNQI data. Appreciating the import of NDNQI requires understanding about the quality indicators and its potential contributions to outcomes research and comparative effectiveness research.

Moore et al. (1999) cautioned that findings of the ANA report card, as well as summative evaluations compiled by other outcomes studies, should be considered within the framework of several contextual concerns. First, Moore et al. noted that there was no clear agreement about the indicators that should have been included in a report card. Second, the availability, reliability, and validity of these indicators had not always been demonstrated. Third, once indicators had been consensually selected, there was no consensus about how long it will take to have valid and reliable measures for the indicators. Fourth, many databases contained compromised data from which report cards are generated; and, fifth, report card data may have been meaningful to one stakeholder group to the exclusion of others that are also important (Moore et al., 1999). Similar concerns were identified by Burston, Chaboyer, and Gillespie (2013) following a review and synthesis of the published literature using an explicit methodology that included a rigorous search strategy. Despite these early and ongoing concerns, the ANA report card is acknowledged as an important and significant beginning to developing formalized, nursing-specific outcomes measurement. This foundational effort continues to inform quality determinations specific to nursing care delivery.

The NDNQI evolved from this early nursing care report card effort. In 1997, ANA issued a request for development and maintenance of the national database. The University of Kansas School of Nursing housed this initiative (Owens & Koch, 2015). For the next 3 years, a series of ANA-funded pilot studies established the selected indicators and developed operational definitions and data collection methodologies for each indicator. In 1998, NDNQI began accepting data from participating hospitals and providing fee-based reports. ANA identified 10 nursing-sensitive quality indicators for acute care; each had a recommended definition (**BOX 9-2**).

The ANA's organizational intent was to provide opportunities for hospitals to collect and report on indicators to make clear the difference that RNs make in the provision of safe, high-quality patient care. NDNQI is dynamic and collaborative, working to further define quality improvement (QI) indicators with the National Quality Forum (NQF), a membership-based nonprofit, nonpartisan organization that strives to improve health care (NQF, 2017), as well as collaborating with TJC (Owens & Koch, 2015). The NDNQI efforts have broadened to include various patient populations, hospital and unit types, institutional bed numbers, and structure indicators related to RN characteristics. Quality indicators (N = 19) continue to reflect structure, process, and outcomes of nursing care (Owens & Koch, 2015). NDNQI is also integral to Magnet nursing data requirements (Press Ganey, n.d.).

Many advanced nurses practice in acute care institutions that are interested in pursuing Magnet status through the American Nurses Credentialing Center (ANCC).

> **BOX 9-2** Nursing-Sensitive Quality Indicators for Acute Care Settings
>
> 1. *Skill mix caring for patients; Registered Nurses, Licensed Practical/Vocational Nurses, and Unlicensed staff*
> 2. *Total nursing care hours provided per patient day*
> 3. *Pressure ulcer prevalence*
> 4. *Patient falls*
> 5. *Patient falls with injury*
> 6. Patient satisfaction with pain management
> 7. Patient satisfaction with educational information
> 8. Patient satisfaction with overall care
> 9. Patient satisfaction with nursing care
> 10. *Nosocomial infection rate (Central line catheter-associated bloodstream infection)*
> 11. Registered nurse satisfaction

Data from Owens & Koch, 2015 with original indicators italicized Montalvo, 2007.

To seek accreditation, health care agencies' leadership may elect to participate in NDNQI to assist with data collection and quality tracking necessary for the Magnet Recognition Program®. Magnet certification achievement recognizes and celebrates exceptional nursing departments. NDNQI reports provide one view of quality evaluation that is nursing specific and offer opportunities for benchmarking or comparisons. Additional information related to joining NDNQI may be accessed via Press Ganey's (2017) *Nursing Excellence Solution*.

Measuring outcomes is important but should not be performed independent of outcomes management. Unless measurement is conducted and results are managed as components of QI, problems arise related to data collection activities that are not valued as meaningful and meaning making. This potential problem is similar to the issues that arise when research studies are conducted but findings are not used to inform and improve practice. Advanced nurses should identify and measure outcomes that are important to their particular institution or type of clinical practice and then manage these outcomes to improve quality using available evidence.

When nurses in advanced roles consider Magnet accreditation processes, NDNQI and its historical roots in ANA's *The nursing care report card for acute care*, and outcomes mandate from public and private foundations, organizations, and accreditors, then linkages between QI, EBP, and outcomes become evident and fairly simple to explain to nursing colleagues who may not have an understanding of the connecting relationships (**FIGURE 9-2**).

Leaders and Partners in Outcomes Measurement and Management

There are a number of organizations focusing efforts on improving health care outcomes and quality, in addition to ANA's landmark efforts and the subsequent efforts of Press Ganey partnered with ANA. Some organizations have a multidisciplinary focus while others predominately serve a particular stakeholder group. Overall, there are many stakeholders with significant vested interest in the outcomes measurement and management movement (**FIGURE 9-3**).

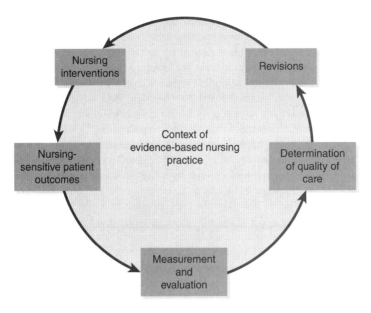

FIGURE 9-2 Nursing-Sensitive Quality Loop.

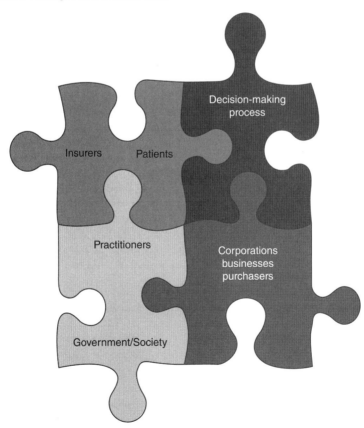

FIGURE 9-3 Stakeholders in Health Care Outcomes.

Corporations and smaller businesses have vital interest in outcomes measures as a data source to facilitate decision making about which plans and services provide employees with the best care (as measured by outcomes) in the most cost-effective manner (a fiscal outcome). For example, the Leapfrog Group (n.d.) describes itself as a "nonprofit watchdog organization that serves as a voice for health care purchasers, using their collective influence to foster positive change in U.S. health care. Leapfrog is the nation's premier advocate of hospital transparency—collecting, analyzing and disseminating hospital data to inform value-based purchasing." This organization has had important influence on data-driven outcome management and measurement, particularly related to choosing hospitals for care based on comparison data.

Leapfrog Group is involved in other initiatives that may not appear to be outcomes centric at first glance but are, in fact, very related to end results or the bottom line of safe care delivery—for example, providing access to the CANDOR Toolkit, developed by AHRQ (2017) to assist hospital providers and leaders with honest responses to adverse events including honest communication and effective resolution processes. Leapfrog's efforts particularly focus on outcomes related to value and safety, including never events. Advanced nurses will find helpful its Web-based resources and tools but should keep in mind that much of the focus is on risk, adverse events, and value-based purchasing. While this is critically important summarized data, it does not provide information about potential savings and benefits associated with positive outcomes (Kirby, 2015), a more difficult metric to measure than frequencies of harmful events or costs.

Health care consumers, including individual or organizational purchasers, benefit from the increasing access to outcomes-driven data necessary to make informed decisions as to where to seek general or specialty care services. TJC's Quality Check® and Quality Reports® provide consumers with access to information about how well accredited and certified organizations perform and, when appropriate, how this performance stacks up against National Quality Improvement Goals (TJC, 2016a). As an example, potential "customers" can ascertain the percentage of patients with a suspected cardiac event who receive aspirin therapy upon arrival to local emergency departments (EDs) and make informed decisions as to which provides better care, based upon this criterion. The Quality Reports and Quality Check build upon the data submitted to the TJC database, ORYX, from health care organizations.

Pioneers in Quality is a TJC program that focuses on offering assistance to hospitals as they work toward adopting electronic clinical quality measures (TJC, 2017a). Available supports include educational programs, electronic resources, advisory council, speaker's bureau opportunities, and other resources. It is also a recognition program that acknowledges three hospital contribution categories: expert, solution, and data (TJC, 2017b).

Another resource for helping consumers and employers choose between competing health maintenance organization (HMO) and preferred provider organization (PPO) plans is the Health Plan Employer Data and Information Set (HEDIS®). HEDIS is a program of the National Committee for Quality Assurance (NCQA) that facilitates decision making based upon value and cost of service. HEDIS consists of standardized performance measures that are related to many significant public health issues. NCQA provides a State of Health Care Quality Report that offers consumers access to viewing HEDIS measures online and also provides archived report. This annual report focuses on major quality issues by providing data-based performance trends for each measure (**TABLE 9-1**). More than 90% of American

TABLE 9-1 Selected HEDIS Measures of Care (NCQA, 2016)

HEDIS Measures of Care

1.	Overuse and Appropriateness	a.	Avoidance of antibiotic treatment in adults with acute bronchitis
		b.	Use of imaging studies for low back pain
		c.	Nonrecommended prostate-specific antigen (PSA) screening in older men
2.	Screening, Prevention, and Wellness	a.	Adult body mass index (BMI) screening
		b.	Colorectal cancer screening
		c.	Flu vaccinations
		d.	Diabetes and cardiovascular disease screening and monitoring for people with schizophrenia and bipolar disorder
3.	Chronic Condition Management	a.	Use of spirometry testing in the assessment and diagnosis of chronic obstructive pulmonary disease (COPD)
		b.	Controlling high blood pressure
		c.	Statin therapy for patients with cardiovascular disease and diabetes
		d.	Antidepressant medication management
		e.	Annual monitoring for patients on persistent medications
4.	Measures Targeted Toward Children and Adolescents	a.	Lead screening in children
		b.	Appropriate treatment for children with upper respiratory infection
		c.	Metabolic monitoring for children and adolescents on antipsychotics
5.	Measures Targeted Toward Older Adults	a.	Fall risk management
		b.	Osteoporosis testing and management in older women
		c.	Medication management in the elderly
6.	Measures of Value and Utilization	a.	Emergency Department utilization
7.	Consumer and Patient Engagement and Experience	a.	About CAHPS
		b.	Rating of health plan
		c.	Rating of health care
		d.	How well doctors communicate
		e.	Rating of specialist
		f.	Customer service

Data from from National Committee for Quality Assurance. (2017). 2017 State of health care quality table of contents. Retrieved from http://www.ncqa.org/report-cards/health-plans/state-of-health-care-quality/2017-table-of-contents

health plans use HEDIS to measure performance outcomes related to care and service (NCQA, n.d.), and these data may then be used by stakeholders to select the best health plan for their particular needs. Data are audited to protect validity (NCQA, n.d.). HEDIS also includes Consumer Assessment of Healthcare Providers and Systems (CAHPS) survey results to provide measures of members' satisfaction with plans' service provision, including claims processing, customer service, and responsiveness (NCQA, n.d.).

Web-accessible HEDIS measures of care are available via NCQA's annually provided *The State of Health Care Quality Report*. Advanced nurses will be interested in HEDIS measures of care that pertain to their particular area of direct practice or to those areas in which they have influence based on education or administrative responsibilities. Each measure is linked to its definition and an explanation as to why the measure is important and relevant, based on evidence. References are provided in a "bottom line" format (NCQA, 2016). Summary data are organized by year and compared across commercial insurance plans (HMO and PPO), Medicaid (HMO), and Medicare (HMO and PPO).

Other stakeholders in health care outcomes include practitioners and the public. Practitioners are affected by outcomes-driven data in a variety of ways. They need to compile and submit data, and these data collection processes require time and effort. Practitioners' records are available for public review: specifically, malpractice cases and complaints through the National Practitioner Data Bank (NPDB, n.d.[a]); and indirectly, through publicly available outcomes data related to the practitioners' employing institution or the National Provider Identifier (NPI) Database (NPIdb) from the NPI Registry (2017).

The NPDB (n.d.[a]), housed within the U.S. Department of Health and Human Services, is a federal repository of reports accessible only to registered entities (**FIGURE 9-4**). This database has been in existence since 1986 with the signing of the Health Care Quality Improvement Act (HCQIA) by President Reagan (NPDB, n.d.[b]). From 1990 to 1998, the NPDB was queried more than 15 million times by state licensing boards, hospitals, and other health care entities. The NPDB had originally worked separately from the Healthcare Integrity and Protection Data Bank (HIPDB) that had been authorized in 1996 by the Health Insurance Portability and Accountability Act of 1996 as an effort to combat fraud and abuse in health insurance and delivery. Initially the HIPDB and NPDB operations were managed as separate entities but by 2013, the two systems merged into one database (NPDB, n.d.[b]). The general public does not have right of access to NPDB reports; however, many health care organizations, including state licensing and certification authorities, are required to report, query, or do both to the NPDB. The available information is a form of outcome data that is provided to protect the public and its health care system from practitioners who would, perhaps, otherwise move state-to-state without offering full disclosure of malpractice or other previously damaging performance (see Figure 9-4).

Some established organizations and foundations are directly partnered with nursing while others do not have a formal relationship with nursing organizations but do provide a variety of supports in the form of electronic resources, conferences, database information, benchmarking, public education initiatives, or printed materials. Advanced nurses need to become familiar with some of the critical contributors to the outcomes movement (**TABLE 9-2**), particularly since these

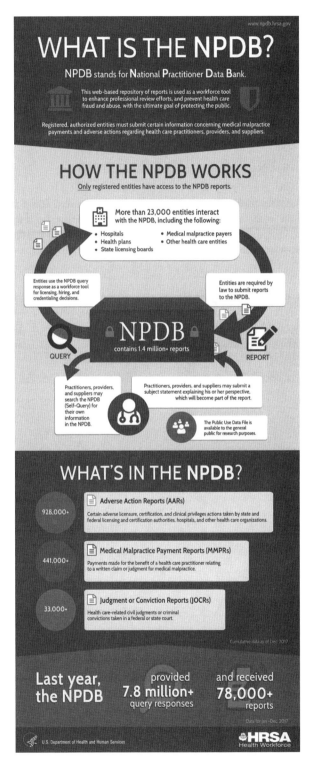

FIGURE 9-4 What is the National Practitioner Data Bank?

Reproduced from National Practitioner Data Bank. (n.d. 1). About us. Retrieved December 27, 2017, from https://www.npdb.hrsa.gov/resources/whatIsTheNPDB.jsp

organizations often offer a variety of materials that are useful to nurses responsible for evaluating clinically based patient care operations and for identifying opportunities to positively influence patient outcomes. At times advanced nurses are directed to investigate and solve specific clinical issues. These directives may be driven by complaints, benchmarking analyses that reveal room for improvement, new programs, or other types of critical incidents. Other times, advanced nurses identify problems and opportunities that are apparent to them because of their expertise and experiences.

Take Advantage of Available Resources

Advanced nurses should investigate available resources for QI before planning interventions or before putting effort into "home-grown" resources. It is not uncommon for nurses to brainstorm and problem-solve practice issues without first reviewing tools, reports, and guidance documents that are established as valid, reliable, and accessible. Many organizations have readily available, relevant, free materials that are

TABLE 9-2 Select Partners in Health Care Outcomes Measurement, Management, and Quality Improvement

Partner	Website	Description
National Quality Forum (NQF)	http://www.qualityforum.org/Home.aspx	Nonprofit, nonpartisan, membership-based organization working to catalyze health care improvements (NQF, 2018a). Excellent resource for uniform, evidence-based measures necessary for health care quality measurement. NQF does not create measures. It uses an endorsement process that involves diverse public and private sector stakeholders to support quality improvement. A Consensus Standards Approval Committee (CSAC) considers all measures recommended for NQF endorsement (NQF, 2018b).
National Patient Safety Foundation (NPSF)	http://www.npsf.org/ http://www.ihi.org/Topics/PatientSafety/Pages/default.aspx	NPSF partnered with the IHI in May 2017 to form a new entity focused on patient safety and improved outcomes (IHI, 2017a).

Partner	Website	Description
Institute for Healthcare Improvement (IHI)	http://www.ihi .org/resources /Pages/default .aspx	Provides extensive resources for quality improvement. Website offers white papers, multimedia content, instructional materials, and popular tools that provide measurement guidance (IHI, 2017b).
Patient-Centered Outcomes Research (PCOR) at Agency for Healthcare Research and Quality (AHRQ)	https://www .ahrq.gov/pcor /index.html	AHRQ invests in disseminating and supporting implementation of PCOR findings into practice using the PCOR Cycle that involves: delivering health care, identifying evidence gaps, researching answers, and disseminating evidence (AHRQ, 2016). AHRQ contributes to this work by creating evidence syntheses from PCOR findings and designing understandable tools and education. AHRQ distributes this evidence and supports those entities and professionals that use the evidence for practice improvement (AHRQ, 2016).
American Society for Quality (ASQ)	https://asq.org/	ASQ works to support a global knowledge network that works to improve quality improvement. It offers 18 certifications and provides many quality-related learning tools and products. ASQ has individual and organizational members (ASQ, 2017).

very user friendly and well organized. Using established resources can also ensure that networking opportunities are more relevant.

For example, central line infection is a significant clinical concern across a variety of care settings but particularly in high-acuity nursing practice. Preventing central line–associated bloodstream infection (CLABI) was one of the six outcomes initiatives of the Institute for Healthcare Improvement (IHI) established as part of the early 100,000 Lives Campaign and continued as a priority in the 5 Million Lives Campaign (IHI, n.d.). A search of IHI's website reveals a free, downloadable how-to-guide, *Prevent Central Line-Associated Bloodstream Infection* (IHI, 2012) that includes evidence-based care components of the IHI Central Line Bundle. A bundle is a group of evidence-based interventions that when used concurrently results in better outcomes than when followed individually. This guide provides clear instructions, defined outcomes, and supporting data for interventions that promote teamwork and reduce infection rates. An advanced nurse confronted with a need to prevent or reduce the prevalence of central line infections would be wise to begin by reviewing the IHI resources, available for public use, before attempting to develop a policy, procedure, or program based upon a literature review. As with most IHI resources, free registration is necessary to access materials.

Establishing an Outcomes Project of Interest

Advanced nurses may have difficulty focusing on any one particular project that pertains to an outcome of interest. At times, nurses feel pulled in multiple directions and may be tackling multiple outcomes simultaneously thereby contributing to burnout. Nurses in many types of advanced roles, including practice roles and indirect care roles, often have some responsibility for engaging staff in meaningful work designed to enhance care quality or specific outcomes. Working on projects with staff and colleagues is an ideal way for advanced nurses to accomplish necessary QIs while also building colleagues' expertise and supporting interprofessional team relationships. Identifying and selecting one outcome of interest may be the most difficult aspect of the improvement project.

Search for Gaps Between the Actual Versus the Desired State of Practice

There are a number of ways to identify a pertinent outcome measure that may be amenable to nursing practice changes and that will positively affect the quality of care delivery. It is important to solicit input from nursing staff members if their participation is needed for project success, including data collection and implementing practice changes. Advanced nurses should consider available outcomes measurement data, including benchmarking results from NDNQI, TJC, HCAHPS, and other high-stakes reports, as potential opportunities for gap analyses and subsequent improvement efforts.

There may be opportunities for outcomes improvement revealed through careful review of patient, physician, or staff complaints. Nurses often recognize systems problems that negatively affect outcomes, and these staff worries may provide insight into possible topics for project development. Incident reports offer opportunities for measuring and managing significant outcomes including but not limited to falls, medication errors, needlestick injuries, workplace violence, communication processes, transfusion errors, or compromised patient safety. Many times, staff members have ideas for projects but need encouragement and support before they will attempt to address the issue in an organized, formal process (**BOX 9-3**).

Another strategy that may be useful when searching for outcomes improvement projects is a "waste walk" (Lean Enterprise Institute, 2012). This approach involves a planned visit of team members who begin with a huddle to review the purpose of the activity and to ensure that all team members are consistent in their understanding and approach. The team members then make physical walking rounds on the units of interest and observe for occasions of wastefulness that, if removed, would benefit the institution. This may be a useful preliminary exercise for those interested in involving staff in projects that improve efficiencies by eliminating waste and that may

BOX 9-3 Solicitation for Staff Input on Projects

Wanted: Unit-Based Projects

Have a great idea for a unit-based problem? Thinking about a better way of doing things? Recognize a problem just waiting to be solved or an outcome that you know requires improvement? Interested in participating in a unit-based workshop on literature searches?

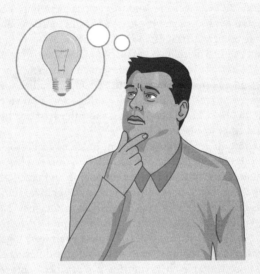

I am looking for RNs who are interested in developing and initiating unit-based projects related to clinical practice. Leadership and enthusiasm are "must-haves"! Technical skills and research expertise are not required.

Talk with your colleagues. Consider developing a simple project that might be of interest to other nurses or other interprofessional team members. Think about the possibility of presenting your work at a local, regional, or national conference as either a poster or podium presentation. I will help you throughout the process. Guarantee it!

If you have an idea and are willing to assist in guiding a project, please contact me via email: jones@hospital.edu. I'd enjoy sitting down with you and chatting over a cup of coffee. The coffee is my treat!

serve as catalyst projects for encouraging staff on a trajectory of process improvement projects. These sorts of activities are concrete, practical, have real-world benefits, and may facilitate staff engagement in QI initiatives.

Collaboratively Select a Project of Shared Interest

Once gaps in a system of care provision have been identified, it is often productive to elicit staff input via group discussion. Staff meetings, informal chats, and electronic discussions are good methods for soliciting input and garnering ideas. It may be useful to collectively develop a list of outcomes that staff believe may be better managed. This list should be prioritized and reduced to a reasonable number of projects. The nurse leader should facilitate the prioritization process by using some type of sensible procedure including casting votes, assigning numeric values to projects and rank ordering based upon collective scores, Q-sort methodology, or Delphi technique to reduce the number of projects and to include only the most valued. The decision-making group may also find that the priorities are clearly evident after discussion.

Advanced nurses may want to consider competitions or contests to elicit QI ideas or EBP projects from staff (**EXEMPLAR 9-1**). Involving nurses in the identification of outcomes projects can accomplish several goals. Active involvement in project selection facilitates staff engagement, and this engagement improves participation. Outcomes projects provide opportunities to teach staff about outcomes management, measurement, and resources. For staff who have been practicing for more than 10 years and who have not been involved in formal academic programs, an outcomes project may be the first exposure to the outcomes movement. Advanced nurses should keep in mind that outcomes projects do not have to be complex; rather, simple and elegant design is ideal for a first-time venture. Keeping things simple provides opportunities for relatively fast successes that can encourage staff enthusiasm and hardwire a feeling of confidence and empowerment.

Another important opportunity inherent in staff-based projects is the likely possibility of interprofessional collaboration between nurses, physicians, and other professional counterparts. Interprofessional education and practice are essential to team building and, ultimately, to improving the collaborative communication and practice patterns that are necessary to positive patient outcomes (Nester, 2016; The Josiah Macy Jr. Foundation, 2015). Interprofessional projects help to break down communication barriers. As various types of professionals work together, they get to know each other as colleagues and learn to appreciate the differing perspectives and areas of expertise that team members contribute to practice improvements.

There are many resources available to advanced nurses who are interested in joining the well-established IPE movement in health care (NLN, 2018; The Interprofessional Education Collaborative [IPEC], 2017). The Josiah Macy Jr. Foundation (2015) is an excellent place to begin self-directed IPE learning, and it is likely that opportunities and ideas will come to mind as advanced nurses explore project exemplars, writings, links, and opportunities related to IPE and its goal of meeting the IHI (2018) Triple Aim: (1) improving the patient experience of care, including quality and satisfaction; (2) improving populations' health; and (3) reducing per capita health care costs.

Crafting the Outcomes Project

As mentioned, advanced nurses may become involved in outcomes management through interest in improving a clinical outcome or through assignation by the chief nurse executive or other administrator. For example, if urinary tract infection (UTI) rates increase within the surgical service line, the advanced nurse may be asked to participate in a multidisciplinary ad hoc committee exploring strategies for reducing nosocomial UTI rates, or assigned responsibility to lead a nursing project exploring EBP changes that might improve this concerning UTI outcome measure. The current emphasis on outcomes management and measures fits nicely with the EBP movement as the interventions that may be used to improve outcomes should be consistent with or based upon current EBP recommendations.

EXEMPLAR 9-1 Competitions as Opportunities to Trigger Evidence-Based Outcomes Projects

One example of a mechanism to elicit an evidence-based outcomes project from nursing professionals is the *Unearthing the Evidence* contest that was regularly sponsored by a large, urban health care network's department of nursing (**FIGURE 9-5**). The contest had its origins in a research utilization competition that had been known as the Sacred Cow competition, designed to encourage nurses to submit fully developed research projects proposing simple but elegant research questions that had relevance to nursing practice within the organization. The organization's nurse researcher was available to support applicants in crafting their applications, if requested. The selected project was funded with a small grants award. The winning nurse, often a novice first-time researcher, was required to present the study findings during a subsequent nursing grand rounds poster session.

After a number of years of dwindling submissions, the Sacred Cow competition was stopped. The *Unearthing the Evidence* competition was created to encourage nurses to consider nursing and medical practices and offer suggestions for improvement based upon available evidence. The required format was narrative but also succinct with less of an academic structure. One winning submission addressed bladder catheterization practices and offered recommendations for change based upon a compelling need to reduce urinary tract infections. This project stimulated interest and was well received. Some recommendations were implemented by nursing in partnership with physicians. The following year's winning project explored the frequency and type of saline lock use on a telemetry care unit in an effort to preliminarily explore the possibility of changing unit policy. This project served as the catalyst for a staff nurse to begin his journey as a beginning researcher and author (Szablewski, Zuzelo, Morales, & Thomas, 2009). This exemplar illustrates the positive effect that these sorts of competitions can have on nurses' professional development, providing that the necessary supports are made available.

The "Unearthing the Evidence" Contest

Identify a nursing or medical practice that is used on a fairly regular basis BUT that should be changed based upon published evidence.
Example: Saline lavage with suctioning is not supported in the literature for adult patients requiring airway suctioning. The evidence is clear. NO SALINE! And yet . . . the practice continues in some institutions on some units or by some nurses . . . .

Submit a description of the current practice and offer a recommendation for change. Include copies of references

Entries will be judged on:

1. Commonness of the nursing or medical practice. Think about the things that we do every day in practice . . . are they really grounded in evidence? Are there alternative strategies we should be using? How do nurses accomplish these interventions in other countries?

2. Relevance to direct patient care

3. Quality of literature support

4. Realism of practice change suggestion (including fiscal reality)

Prize: $100 American Express Gift Certificate

Recognition in upcoming E^3 Newsletter

Admiration of nursing colleagues

FIGURE 9-5 *Unearthing the Evidence* Competition Announcement.

The CMS policy to ensure safe, high-quality care by designating select HACs as nonreimbursed expenses has also triggered the need for outcome management and QI efforts (CMS, 2015). In 2008, CMS designated 10 HAC categories as compared to 14 categories in 2017, excluding International Classifications of Diseases–Revision 10 (ICD-10) subdiagnoses. The most recent list is 13 pages in length (https://www .cms.gov/ICD10Manual/version33-fullcode-cms/fullcode_cms/P1059.html) (CMS, 2017a) (**TABLE 9-3**).

It is worth noting that there is much administrative consternation about publicly reported outcomes as well as adverse patient outcomes that reflect poor quality. HACs have serious financial ramifications and quality of care implications. The worrisome HACs, important indicators collected through the NDNQI, and measures from other established quality audits offer advanced nurses meaningful opportunities to "show their stuff" and demonstrate their impact on improving quality metrics. Nurses should design useful continuous QI projects using established methodologies and data sets to change processes that affect patients at the point of care. Seize the opportunities offered by HACs and nurse-sensitive indicators!

Selecting Indicators That Measure Improvement

There are major limitations in the management and measurement of nursing outcomes (Jones, 2016). Lack of solid data that measures nursing processes and patient outcomes hinders nurses in their efforts to improve quality of care. Jones's (2016) discussion of outcomes measures in nursing provides an excellent overview of historical and contemporary challenges in outcomes measurement. Nursing has a social contract with the public that requires the nursing profession to self-monitor so as to assure the public that it is providing quality performance (Jones, 2016). To this end, advanced nurses need to have a good understanding of quality measures and systems of management. Many advanced nurses are likely new to this work and may be hesitant about critiquing and selecting instruments for outcomes measurement. Seeking expert consultation is always a good idea and continuing to build personal expertise is certainly an option, particularly through doctoral studies.

When advanced nurses design a project, including the data collection plan, they need to consider the validity, reliability, and feasibility associated with the instruments that will be used in outcomes measurement. It is often better to use a preexisting well-established instrument or a portion of an instrument rather than creating a new one. Creating a valid and reliable instrument requires careful processes that often involve quantitative methodologies, expert input, and pilot testing. Too often, surveys, Likert scales, and other tools and instruments are casually developed by nurses in an effort to quantify a measure of interest. These sorts of tools may or may not provide valid and reliable measures. As a result, persistent skepticism will likely result when the advanced nurse claims that a QI initiative was successful as evidenced by analysis of data collected via an untested tool.

If no instrument is available that examines the outcome or process of interest and constructing a tool is the only option, advanced nurses should make certain to establish content validity, interrater/observer reliability, test-retest, and internal consistency. Establishing the reliability of the tool and its usability are important activities. It may be necessary to confer with a nurse scientist or other colleague who has established instrumentation expertise. Choosing to use a tool that does not have

TABLE 9-3 Nonreimbursed Hospital-Acquired Condition (HAC) Categories (Secondary Diagnoses Not Included), Organized by Year

2008 HAC Categories (CMS, 2008)	2017 HAC Categories (CMS, 2017a)
1. Foreign object retained after surgery	1. Foreign object retained after surgery
2. Air embolism	2. Air embolism
3. Blood incompatibility	3. Blood incompatibility
4. Stage III and IV pressure ulcers	4. Stage III and IV pressure ulcers
5. Falls and trauma	5. Falls and trauma
6. Manifestations of poor glycemic control	6. Catheter-associated urinary tract infection
7. Catheter-associated urinary tract infection	7. Vascular catheter-associated infection
8. Vascular catheter-associated infection	8. Surgical site infection—mediastinitis after coronary artery bypass graft procedures
9. Surgical site infection following: coronary artery bypass graft, bariatric surgery, orthopedic procedures (spine, neck, shoulder, elbow)	9. Manifestations of poor glycemic control
10. Deep vein thrombosis (DVT)/pulmonary embolism (PE) following total knee replacement; hip replacement	10. DVT/PE with total knee or hip replacement procedures
	11. Surgical site infection—bariatric surgery procedures
	12. Surgical site infection—certain orthopedic procures of spine, shoulder, and elbow procedures
	13. Surgical site infection following cardiac implantable electronic device procedures
	14. Iatrogenic pneumothorax with venous catheterization procedures

established validity and reliability undermines the believability and worth of the entire outcomes project.

At the start of project planning, advanced nurses should establish a measurement plan. When working with colleagues or interprofessional teams, make certain to solicit input from those who have expertise in the measures of interest and familiarity with associated processes. In consultation with the project improvement team, achieve consensus on the following key items: (1) name of the measure of interest, (2) the type of measure, (3) rationale for the selected measure, (4) operational definition to ensure consistency, (5) methodology including data collection and sampling plan, (6) data display, (7) evaluation of data availability, (8) baseline data opportunity and acquisition, (9) target or end goal, and (10) data sources (Health Quality Ontario [HQO], 2013). Consider several measures and varying types so as to capture a complete picture (HQO, 2013).

Outcomes measures address end results and they evaluate system performance. Process measures relate to the steps or inputs that lead to the systems outcomes. Detailing steps in the process of interest can be challenging, and it is useful to engage the people who actually participate in the various process components to ensure accurate and comprehensive understanding of the inputs. It can be quite helpful to put effort into designing a flowchart that accurately depicts the process of interest. Make certain to include the hands-on experts in the construction of this detailed flowsheet since those participating in the work process are the ones who best know what is actually done versus what might be described in a policy or procedures. Balancing measures examine unintended effects of the newly applied changes. In other words, advanced nurses need to determine whether a change to one input creates unanticipated effects downstream.

Once an appropriate measure and/or instrument has been selected, keep in mind that data collection activities have associated expenses related to personnel, data storage, printing, purchasing, among other types of costs. The budgetary impact of data collection and outcomes tracking should be considered before beginning the project. In addition, data collection requires proactive planning. Advanced nurses need to determine who will collect the data and what processes will be followed. Ensuring a consistent, reliable process of data collection, particularly if there is more than one data collector, is essential. It is also important to decide how missing data will be managed during the project.

Keep in mind that data are worthless if clinicians believe they are inaccurate in its measurement, collection, or analyses. To protect data integrity, HQO (2013) offers a few suggestions such as using a flowchart to graphically depict the data collection process, verifying that data entry processes have integrity, considering data analysis prior to actual data collection, and reporting on the data in a regular and timely fashion. Data reporting may include quarterly reports for staff review, updates during staff meetings, signage, or electronic messages.

▶ Systematically Examining and Managing Outcomes to Improve Quality

QI is an important component of nursing practice. This indirect care responsibility is a critical skill that advanced nurses need to develop so that they are able to adeptly utilize a systems approach to QI that correctly ascertains the effects of practice changes on outcomes. There are often a variety of possible ways to influence outcomes, and discerning whether the selected interventions have yielded maximum positive effects given committed resources is an important question.

Another important consideration when planning QI activities is accessibility of organized data. There is a great amount of collected data in health care institutions, but it is often in disarray. Data collection activities may be episodic, inconsistently reported, and superficially reviewed. Establishing organized systems of data collection, storage, and retrieval processes is important to QI initiatives.

HQO (2013) notes that there are differences between research and QI measurements (**TABLE 9-4**). Many advanced nurses are familiar with the research process and have experience with traditional measurement concerns through graduate research studies or clinical research projects. A key difference between research and QI measurements is that measurement for improvement occurs frequently and is often performed rapidly in small batches so as to accelerate the implementation of desirable changes.

Advanced nurses must be able to compare the costs to benefits of practice changes; and this analysis requires a systematic, scientific approach. There are a number of approaches to QI that may be useful, including plan-do-study-act (PDSA), Six Sigma, rapid cycle improvement, positive deviance (PD), failure mode and effects analysis (FMEA), root cause analysis (RCA), and flowcharting. The American Society for Quality (ASQ) provides overviews of these commonly used QI techniques. ASQ (2017a) offers individual and organizational memberships with opportunities for networking and support. A brief overview of each methodology may be useful to stimulate further exploration or activity.

TABLE 9-4 Contrasting Measurement for Improvement to Measurement for Research

	Measurement for Research	Measurement for Learning and Process Improvement
Purpose	To discover new knowledge	To bring new knowledge into daily practice
Tests	One large "blind" test	Many sequential, observable tests
Biases	Control for as many biases as possible	Stabilize the biases from test to test
Data	Gather as much data as possible, "just in case"	Gather "just enough" data to learn and complete another cycle
Duration	Can take long periods of time to obtain results	"Small tests of significant changes" accelerates the rate of improvement

© Queen's Printer for Ontario, 2013. Reproduced with permission. Health Quality Ontario. (April 2013). Quality improvement primers. Measurement for quality improvement. Page 4. Retrieved December 28, 2017, from http://www.hqontario.ca/Portals/0/documents/qi/qi-measurement-primer-en.pdf

Plan-Do-Check Act

Plan-do-check-act (PDCA) is the fundamental process of Total Quality Management (TQM) developed by W. Edwards Deming in the 1950s. PDCA is also referred to as PDSA, the Deming cycle, Shewhart cycle, or Deming wheel (ASQ, 2017b). Regardless of its title, the process consists of four steps: plan, do, study (check), and act (**TABLE 9-5**). These steps should be viewed as circular and continuous. PDSA quality improvement uses the scientific method to implement and test the effects of changes on the performance of the health care system based on outcomes of interest. When used in TQM or continuous quality improvement (CQI) projects, PDCA is user friendly and may be useful when working with multidisciplinary groups or staff nurses unfamiliar with CQI processes. It is a cyclical and iterative process that requires an ongoing assessment of needs and effects (Peterson, Adlard, Hayakawa, McClean, & Feidner, 2015) (**FIGURE 9-6**).

PDCA may be used to accomplish a number of goals. It was originally designed as a model for CQI and is successfully used for such activities in the private and public sector and in all types of ventures, including health care (Williams & Fallone, 2008). One example of the application of the PDCA process is provided by a collaborative effort of CNSs to recognize, prevent, and treat pediatric pressure ulcers (Peterson et al., 2015). PDCA is also a useful tool in RCAs and when developing a new or improved design of a care delivery process. There are a number of Web-based, print, and program resources to help advanced nurses build expertise with the PDCA process and other QI methods (**BOXES 9-4** and **9-5**).

FOCUS-PDCA Quality Improvement Model

FOCUS is an acronym for *find, organize, clarify, understand,* and *select* (Zimnicki, 2015). FOCUS is frequently added as a forerunner to the PDCA cycle (**FIGURE 9-7**).

TABLE 9-5 PDSA/PDCA Process

STEPS	
Plan	Diagnose an opportunity. Consider a change idea. Plan the change. Determine metrics of success. Design data collection plan. Determine necessary sampling plan and numbers of subjects.
Do	Test the change. Conduct a small-scale study. Track the results, measures, challenges, and unintended consequence.
Study or Check	Review the methods. Analyze results. Identify findings and compare to predictions. Summarize and reflect.
Act	Take action based on what was learned in the study step. Depending on findings, planned change should be adopted, adapted, or abandoned.

Data from ASQ (2017b); Health Quality Ontario (2013).

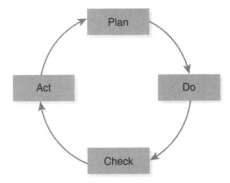

FIGURE 9-6 PDCA Cycle.
Data from ASQ Quality Press. © 2005 AmericanSociety for Quality

---

BOX 9-4 Quality Tools and Templates Available from ASQ

Tool Name

- Box and Whisker Plot
- Check Sheet
- Control Chart
- Design of Experiments Template
- FMEA Template
- Fishbone (Cause and Effect) Diagram

- Flowchart Template
- Gantt Chart
- Histogram
- Pareto Chart
- Scatter Diagram
- Stratification Diagram

Data from American Society for Quality. (2018). Learn about quality. Quality tools and templates. Retrieved January 28, 2018, from http://asq.org/learn-about-quality/tools-templates.html.

BOX 9-5 Quality Tools and Templates Available from IHI

Toolkit Content

- Cause and Effect Diagram
- Driver Diagram
- Failure Modes and Effects Analysis (FMEA) flowchart
- Histogram

- Pareto Chart
- PDSA Worksheet
- Project Planning Form
- Run Chart & Control Chart
- Scatter Diagram

Data from Institute for Healthcare Improvement. (2017). QI essentials tool kit. Retrieved January 28, 2018, from http://www.ihi.org/resources/Pages/Tools/Quality-Improvement-Essentials-Toolkit.aspx.

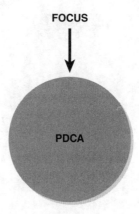

FIGURE 9-7 FOCUS-PDCA.

FOCUS facilitates the discovery process and problem identification required for PDCA to begin. The advanced nurse begins by finding a process requiring improvement. As mentioned, this process may be discovered using a variety of methodologies or it may be assigned to the advanced nurse as part of a department or institution initiative. Run charts can provide a useful depiction of the variability of the measure of interest (HQO, 2013). These charts can also be intriguing to staff and leadership and offer compelling support for why a particular measure is worthy of attention and effort.

Once a problem is found, the second step is to organize in order to improve the current state of the process. The nurse may elect to form an interprofessional committee, nursing committee, or may determine that the best organizational structure is to use an existing standing committee. Brainstorming with colleagues may offer unique insights.

It is imperative to establish a team that will be responsive, enthusiastic, and interested in knowledge building. Identifying appropriate team members is critical. The advanced nurse needs to make certain that key stakeholders are represented and that the individuals who know the way that the process *truly* works are included. This may also be a good opportunity to establish ownership of the project not only in terms of budgetary responsibility but also specific to authorship and presentation rights, should the activity result in a scholarly outcome. The leader should determine whether secretarial, technical, or fiscal supports are in place.

Clarification follows organization. This stage is concerned with accurately describing the process and identifying the details that may contribute to opportunities for improvement. Organizing activities may include searching the literature, examining available evidence, scrutinizing benchmarked data, flowcharting or diagramming current processes, or exploring the problem of interest using some type of descriptive data collection method including focus groups, interviews, or surveys, among others.

Organizing activities are important as they provide fodder for developing a clear understanding of the current processes and identifying the gaps and shortcomings. Chart audits and medical records reports may also provide useful information, depending upon the process requiring improvement. There are times when systems are needlessly complex and processes are onerous. Flowcharting or diagramming the process of interest in a step-by-step, detailed fashion is helpful.

Understanding or uncovering the sources of variation or the problems in the process is the fourth step. The team may discover that some of the problems cannot be solved. For example, if a group is working on improving patient wait times in a small but busy ED and a key problem area is a lack of physical space, there may not be a realistic way to correct this problem until a new waiting room is constructed. However, there may be other opportunities in the ED arrival process or bed assignment that could be addressed and that might contribute to reducing waiting room time.

The advanced nurse should think about variable measurement during this step. As previously noted, an important aspect of outcomes management and CQI is outcomes measurement. The team needs to consider the ways that variables and processes are measured and make certain that these measurements are useful and practical. Remember that data will need to be collected, compiled, and analyzed. It makes sense to establish a data collection plan early. If possible, take advantage of data collection processes that are already in play.

Once a process has been selected, dissected, and understood, PDCA activities begin. In general, PDCA should focus on particular aspects of the selected process. Complex processes should not be tackled all at once. Rather, the advanced nurse should start the process by selecting exactly what portion of the process will be examined. The selection criteria should include the feasibility of changing the selected process.

At this point, the advanced nurse and team plan the improvement. The working group needs to decide whether the identified changes will be made in a pilot program or initiated on a large scale. This decision depends upon the recommended change and the process.

For example, if the recommended change is dramatic and the consequences are not entirely understood, or if there is little in the literature or experientially that describes the potential impact of the change, a pilot study may be the wisest course. If the change is based upon research and is consistent with the recommendations of leading authorities, it may be acceptable to proceed on a larger scale. Remember that a data collection plan should be in place prior to implementing changes.

The next step is to *do* or implement the recommendation. Part of the challenge of "doing" is to make certain that the recommended changes are being done correctly and consistently. The advanced nurse should be auditing processes, talking with people involved in the implementation, and maintaining careful data collection that follows the developed data collection plan.

After implementing changes and collecting data, check for improvement, deterioration, or no change from the status quo. In the event of little or no positive change, the group needs to analyze how the intervention was implemented and whether the processes rather than the recommendation were deficient. Brainstorming and interviewing are effective strategies for collecting this information. Remember that there is a possibility that the change was not conducted as planned and that unaccounted intervening influences had a negative effect on the outcomes. Theory-driven evaluation strategies and considerations are necessary to avoid discarding appropriate changes to the system based upon faulty data (Chen, 2015).

As noted, the final step is *act*, but the team needs to keep in mind that PDCA is a circular model when used for QI. At this point, the advanced nurse and colleagues need to decide whether to adjust, abandon, or adopt the change. If data reveal that the change has positively affected the system, the group will need to devise strategies for establishing this change as fixed.

Final activities should include updating policies and procedures and informing key personnel of the changes. The team may also want to give thought to potential ways to continuously improve the process. Certainly it is important to monitor measures to ensure that process fixes are maintained rather than returning to the original baseline. It can be difficult to protect newly established or revised processes. Zimnicki (2015) offers an example of using FOCUS-PDCA to improve evidence-based preoperative stoma site markings. The FOCUS-PDCA model provided opportunities to identify barriers to consistent implementation of preoperative teaching and stoma site marking. The project was a successful endeavor but sustaining long-term change proved challenging. Zimnicki's efforts illustrate the importance of regular evaluation of outcomes measures to ensure that process improvements persist.

FOCUS-PDCA and PDCA are popular methods for QI endeavors. Advanced nurses will find these methods useful and user friendly as they guide planned change that is predicated upon careful analysis. Changing systems and processes takes time and FOCUS-PDCA is a careful, deliberate strategy. Certainly there are aspects of patient care that can be swiftly and effectively changed without engaging in PDCA; however, it is a very useful tool for correcting and improving processes based upon clear understanding that has arisen from careful, informed analysis.

The Six Sigma Revolution: A Measure of Quality Striving for Perfection

Six Sigma is a disciplined, data-driven approach and method for eliminating defects in any process (iSixSigma, 2017), including health care. It is an improvement process committed to excellence. Six Sigma originated in Motorola in the mid-1980s, and soon other industries, including General Electric, Allied Signal, Sony, Motorola, and Polaroid, became users as well (Chowdhury, 2001; Ha et al., 2016).

Six Sigma focuses on eliminating defects by reducing variability. Sigma is the Greek letter used to describe variability as standard deviation (**FIGURE 9-8**). The "six" standard deviation refers to the sixth standard deviation or a 99.9996% success rate (Chowdhury, 2001), or not more than 3.4 defects per million opportunities (Ha et al., 2016; iSixSigma, 2017). As the name implies, Six Sigma relies heavily on quantitative data analysis.

Six Sigma methodology is appealing to the health care industry because of its emphasis on variation or error reduction. Hospitals and health care systems continue to display variability in outcomes that contribute to patient dissatisfaction and inefficiencies in processes and outputs (Woodward, 2005). Six Sigma methodologies have

FIGURE 9-8 Greek Letter, Sigma.

been used to improve operating room turnover time (Adams, Warner, Hubbard, & Goulding, 2004) and operating room efficiencies (Bender et al., 2015), and improve quality and patient safety (Nimtz-Rusch & Thompson, 2008). Major and Huey (2016) used lean and Six Sigma methodology with significant success to reduce the incidence of intravenous infiltrates in hospitalized children. The U.S. Naval Academy has used Six Sigma to improve a mass immunizations process at the academy (Ha et al., 2016), and it has been used in combination with simulation and lean to improve the phlebotomy process (Huang & Klassen, 2016). A review of literature reveals the increasing popularity of Six Sigma methods in the United States and also internationally with demonstrated utility across a wide variety of health care processes in numerous settings.

Critics of Six Sigma may be concerned about the applicability of a QI process with its roots in manufacturing being reasonably applied to the health care industry. Six Sigma demands identification of specification limits that define acceptable performance. Health care systems are not always inclined to evaluate performance within tight, prescriptive constraints despite the fact that continuous improvement requires accurate measurements. During the early stages of Six Sigma's application to health care processes, Lazarus (2003) asserted that Six Sigma is adaptable to the development of best clinical practices and that the language of Six Sigma will benefit health care consumers. During the past two decades, Six Sigma has increased in its popularity as an important tool to improving various health care outcomes; and its utility will likely continue to increase as organizations put resources into establishing Six Sigma models for QI.

Improving an existing process using Six Sigma methodology follows a five-step analysis: (1) Define the opportunity, (2) measure to establish baseline performance; (3) analyze data and critical elements; (4) improve the new process; and (5) control the new process (DMAIC) (iSixSigma, 2017). DMAIC (pronounced "duh-may-ick") uses statistical analysis to find the most defective part of the process under scrutiny and applies rigorous control procedures to maintain improvement. A second key methodology in Six Sigma is DMADV (define, measure, analyze, design, and verify). DMADV is used to create new product or process designs (iSixSigma, 2017). DMAIC is the most popular Six Sigma methodology (ASQ, 2017c).

There are various Six Sigma definitions but when used in terms of quality, Six Sigma represents a process that is well controlled with tolerance limits driving toward six standard deviations from the mean to the nearest specification limit (ASQ, 2017c; iSixSigma, 2017). Differing Six Sigma definitions share some commonalities, including the use of teams assigned to clearly defined projects that directly affect the organization's bottom line; statistical thinking with some people, referred to as Black Belts, receiving extensive training in advanced statistics and project management; a prominent DMAIC approach; and a supportive management environment that values these efforts as an important business strategy (ASQ, 2017c).

Six Sigma creates new positions within the organization. These positions have names taken from the martial arts (**TABLE 9-6**). In addition to Belt designation, Six Sigma relies on champions that translate the company's vision, mission, goals, and objectives to create a deployment plan and to identify individual projects. These champions smooth the way for project work. Executives are needed to establish the Six Sigma program and keep it informed by the organization's culture and vision (ASQ, 2017d).

Change acceleration process identifies change barriers and works through them. Work-out is a process that brings approximately 10 to 12 key people together for 4

TABLE 9-6 Six Sigma Belts and Selected, Designated Responsibilities

Belt Color	Selected, Designated Responsibilities
Master Black Belt	Trains and coaches Black and Green Belts.
Black Belt	Project leader. Trains and coaches project teams.
Green Belt	Assists with data collection and analysis efforts. Leads Green Belt projects/teams.
Yellow Belt	Team participant.
White Belt	Aware of basic Six Sigma concepts. May work on local teams that support projects. May not be a Six Sigma project team member.

to 8 hours to concentrate on reaching the best decision for improvement or change (Adams et al., 2004). The basic working premise of Six Sigma is $Q \times A = E$ (Chowdhury, 2001). This formula denotes that the effectiveness of the results (E) is equal to the quality of the solution (Q) times the acceptance of the idea (A).

There is a substantial amount of training involved in Six Sigma, and it is not a trivial or insignificant commitment. As an example, Adams et al. (2004) describe the education commitment within their institution after having committed to using Six Sigma as 7 days for executive leadership training, 4 days for managers, 35 days for Green Belts, 7 days for change agents, and 21 days for team planning and training. When these days are distributed across a significant number of employees, the startup costs are high. In general, a quick Internet search for information specific to Six Sigma preparation, required resources, institutional supports, and other key words related to preparatory activities reveals the intensity of the Six Sigma initiation period.

Six Sigma is an increasingly popular methodology for QI. Health care institutions are looking for opportunities to reduce care process outcomes variances more than those provided in traditional QI models. The published results of Six Sigma are impressive and suggest that advanced nurses should at least be aware of and comfortable with the basic underlying premises of this method as it is likely that their exposure to Six Sigma methodologies may increase.

Lean Thinking

Lean is a process improvement strategy designed to eliminate unnecessary steps and redundancies that are not critical to quality for the user. Lean is often integrated with Six Sigma because they share the same goal of providing the customer with the best quality, cost, delivery, and nimbleness (ASQ, 2017c). Within the health care enterprise, this user, or customer, may be the nurse, physician, patient, or other key stakeholder who is the direct beneficiary of the particular service. Lean is meant to eliminate waste, identified as waste in inventory, overproduction, waiting, transportation, defects, excess motion or walking, and processing. Underutilizing employee skills is also considered wastage (ASQ, 2018).

This waste reduction emphasis differs from Six Sigma's emphasis on reducing variability but there is overlap and the two processes enhance each other when waste and variation coexist, a common finding when examining outcomes and the processes leading to such that require improvement. For example, Lean Six Sigma (LSS) may offer benefits to the purchasing departments of health care systems as they work to reduce waste while also lessening purchasing decision variations and errors. The tools and methodologies associated with LSS may have applicability to any number of health care processes (Barlow, 2008). Another difference between lean and Six Sigma is lean's reliance on tools that are not as statistically driven. One such example is lean's use of *kaizen*, an emphasis on continuous improvement that relies on small, incremental changes in work processes (Kaizen Institute, 2017).

Rapid Cycle Improvement Model

The rapid cycle improvement model (RCIM) builds on organizations' desires to accelerate the change process to make rapid improvements in outcomes. The model is also referred to as rapid cycle tests (RCTs) of change (Pape et al., 2005), rapid cycle change (RCC) methodology (Bisaillon, Kelloway, LeBlanc, Pageau, & Woloshyn, 2005), or rapid cycle improvements (Stover & Harpin, 2015). RCIM is based on the premise that traditional methods of QI are too slow, fail to engage people, and inadequately utilize current evidence (Bisaillon et al., 2005).

Even when advanced nurses use established QI methods like PDCA, these projects may take too long with end dates open or too far in the future. Lloyd Provost MS, Statistician, Associates for Process Improvement discussed troublesome end date challenges during his IHI Open School's video presentation, "How Long Should a PDSA Cycle Last?" (https://www.youtube.com/watch?time_continue=89&v=cWGs1Q-K6CM). Provost asserts that end dates should be set for PDSA cycles and these end dates should be shorter than what some teams might initially consider. PDSA/PDCA projects should be rapid tests of change and keeping true to this rapid approach is necessary for project success (IHI, 2017c).

RCIM builds on the position that if an organization wants to make rapid gains in quality, it must be able to answer three questions: (1) What does the organization want to accomplish? (2) How will change be recognized as an improvement and how will it be measured? (3) What changes can be made that will result in an improvement? (Martin, 2003).

Rapid change improvement (RCI) processes are often used in conjunction with DMAIC steps. The basic process is to follow the initial DMAIC steps and after analyzing the problem or gap, use RCIs to improve the system (Pape et al., 2005). RCIs may also be used in partnership with PDSA as a component of the "do" step. If results are positive, the improvements should be controlled and perpetuated. If results are not positive, or not positive enough, the action plan requires revision.

Stover and Harpin (2015) conducted a QI project to reduce ED wait times for patients needing psychiatric admission. Following a review and appraisal of available evidence, an established team guided evidence-based process changes to improve patient flow and reduce wait time. These advanced nurses used rapid cycle improvement methodology guided by the PDSA method. Seven PDSA cycles were conducted and data were evaluated to reveal that ED wait times were reduced (Stover &

Harpin, 2015). The entire project, including the seven PDCA cycles with RCIs, took place over a 12-month period. Information was not provided as to whether an end date was predetermined. It is also not clear if additional efficiencies could have reduced this yearlong timeframe; however, one important takeaway is that the project did not languish or continue as an ad infinitum approach to improvement efforts.

RCIM can be used in a variety of clinical venues. It has been used success-fully as a process for improving medication use systems by addressing nurses' distractions during medication administration (Pape et al., 2005). It has also been used to establish best practices in stroke care by incorporating small improve-ment changes, measuring results, and using the measured successes to facilitate further improvements in stroke care practices for both patients and care providers (Bisaillon et al., 2005). Terry, Disabata, and Krajicek (2015) used RCIM with PDCA to reduce the number of respiratory adverse events in pediatric patients undergoing surgery. Each cycle was described and a total of eight testing cycles were required. This project did improve identification of perioperative risk related to undiagnosed sleep disordered breathing.

IHI (2017d) offers tips for testing changes that should be considered when using RCTs. The suggestions include staying ahead of the tests based upon the possible findings that were identified in the study phase of PDSA efforts. Other recom-mendations include working with people who want to work on the project, picking changes that are simple and reasonable, scaling down the breadth of the tests when possible, and preparing to eliminate a change if it is not improving the measure of interest (IHI, 2017d).

Positive Deviance

PD describes uncommon, beneficial health behaviors that some people already prac-tice. Positive deviant behavior is atypical and confers benefits to people who practice it as compared to the rest of the community (Marsh, Schroeder, Dearden, Sternin, & Sternin, 2004) without any difference in available resources (Bertels & Sternin, 2003) and despite having characteristics that place them at high risk for unhealthy behaviors (Barbosa, Masho, Carlyle, & Mosavel, 2016). In the 1990s, the PD approach was first used to influence the nutritional status of children by Jerry and Monique Sternin in Vietnam during their efforts with Save the Children. The Sternins were the first to apply the PD approach, and subsequent efforts have built on their initiatives.

Since this time, PD has been used to affect changes via a variety of projects, including breastfeeding in rural Vietnam (Dearden et al., 2002); the eating strategies of low-income pregnant women (Fowles, Hendricks, & Walker, 2005); female genital cutting (UNICEF, 2008); persistent breastfeeding rather than formula feeding among low-income African American women (Barbosa et al., 2016); predictors of physical activity in adolescents (Spurr, Bally, & Trinder, 2016); and standardization of nursing operating procedures (Ausserhofer et al., 2016).

PD addresses problems that require behavioral or social change. The approach is consistent with Six Sigma because it provides a design that Six Sigma projects can amplify and replicate (Bertels & Sternin, 2003). For Six Sigma to be successful in reducing outcomes variability, Six Sigma projects must be replicable across entire organizations. Replication is challenging and yet is crucial to benefiting fully from Six Sigma project efforts. The PD approach offers a way for Six Sigma organizations to spread successes.

PD comprises six steps: define, determine, discover, design, discern, and disseminate (Bertels & Sternin, 2003). The focus of PD is on behavior replication. Rather than targeting the acquisition of knowledge related to why people behave in the ways that they do, PD demonstrates that it is possible to find successful solutions before all the underlying causes are addressed. Marsh et al. (2004) identify six steps to the PD approach with the community as an active partner. The approach includes the following:

1. Developing case definitions
2. Locating four to six people who have managed to achieve an unanticipated good outcome despite their high level of risk
3. Interviewing and observing these deviants to uncover the atypical behaviors or enabling factors that might explain the positive outcome
4. Analyzing the findings to confirm that the behaviors really are atypical and are available to the people who would benefit by adopting the behaviors
5. Designing activities to change behaviors and to encourage the community to adopt the new behaviors
6. Monitoring performance and evaluate outcomes

Marsh et al. (2004) suggest that there are three important processes that occur in response to the PD approach. The first is the positive reaction of community members when they learn that they are doing something right rather than hearing only negative feedback. The second process involves information seeking and gathering to identify the positive behaviors that may be spread and the factors that encourage this spread. The third process is the actual behavior change.

Dearden et al. (2002) provide an early example of the PD process as it relates to exclusive breastfeeding in a rural Vietnam village. The goal of the project was to improve breastfeeding practices. Examination of Vietnamese breastfeeding practices revealed that women who return to work were confronted with barriers that hindered exclusive breastfeeding. Data were collected and women were grouped into (1) those who were not exclusively breastfeeding and had returned to work; (2) women who were exclusively breastfeeding and had returned to work; (3) women who were not exclusively breastfeeding and had not yet returned to work; and (4) women who were exclusively breastfeeding and had not yet returned to work.

The women in the second group were identified as the positive deviants. These women were working and yet were able to maintain exclusive breastfeeding while other women in similar circumstances were not exclusively breastfeeding. The researchers explored the differences between these groups of women and determined the facilitators and barriers to exclusive breastfeeding. Based upon these findings, the researchers offered suggestions for programmatic changes that might increase the incidence of exclusive breastfeeding. The focus of the researchers' activities was to identify the experiences of the PDs in an effort to promote this deviant or abnormal behavior within the community of interest. Although this particular study was early in the trajectory of PD as an approach to improving health outcomes, it offers a clearly understood and uncluttered illustration of PD in action.

Sternin (2002) defines PD as "a departure, difference, or deviation from the norm resulting in a positive outcome" (p. 1). Sternin sees this deviance as proof that there are viable solutions to today's complex problems that can be utilized before addressing all the factors underlying the problem. In other words, the PD approach offers hope. Sternin offers this assertion within the context of childhood malnutrition and points out that these children need immediate help if they are to survive and thrive. These children do not have time to wait for problem analysis; rather, they need immediate solutions. PD offers these solutions. Sternin states:

> A critical component of the definition of "positive deviants" is that PD individuals have exactly the same resource base as their non-positive deviant neighbors. Hence, whatever they are doing, whatever resources they are using to achieve their successful outcomes, are by definition, accessible to their neighbors. By identifying the special beliefs and practices of the positive deviants and then making them accessible to the community, a *demonstrably successful* strategy is provided which can be acted upon *today.* (p. 2)

Sternin (2002) comments that if a project's objective is social or behavioral change and if there are some individuals exhibiting the behavior within the community, then PD is a useful tool. The advantage of PD is the sustainability that occurs because the resources required for change already exist within the community. In other words, external resources are not required. Positive deviants are successful with the resources that are available to them illustrating that the fundamental structure of PD is the belief that there is "wisdom and untapped resources" within the community of interest (Sternin, 2002, p. 6).

PD offers opportunities to improve outcomes and to sustain these changes within the health care system just as it offers opportunities within communities. Handwashing behaviors, best practice implementation, infection control practices, and nursing documentation are examples of health care concerns that fundamentally rely on behavior and social changes. If there are units within a hospital or nurses employed on a particular unit whose practices are associated with uncommon but positive outcomes, these individuals may be identified as positive deviants.

There are several examples illustrating the potential impact of PD on problem solving in health care. Robert Wood Johnson Foundation awarded a Pioneer Grant 2006–2008 for a project targeting methicillin-resistant *Staphylococcus aureus* (MRSA) infections in hospitals using the PD approach. As a consequence of this project, MRSA rates were lowered by 73% (Shaw, 2009). Cusano (2006) describes using the PD approach to improving medication use processes for patients at time of discharge and transfer. This medication reconciliation project included identification of positively deviant staff and practices related to those positively deviant patients who had no problems with their medical regimen after discharge. During the course of the study, the researchers identified that the uncommon but successful practices included following up discharge with a telephone call, using written instructions with specific information for complex regimens, providing instructions to caregivers, among other strategies. These practices were shared in small-group meetings with other professionals, and 6 months later, the PD team found that patients were 66% more likely to use their medications without troubles (Cusano, 2006).

Of course, one challenge following a successful endeavor is to figure out strategies for replicating the success across an entire organization. Difficulties duplicating successful results are the result of a lack in communication, transferability, processes and systems, and incentives (Bertels & Sternin, 2003). Six Sigma relies on the successful implementation and spread of changes that have been demonstrated as positive and useful via pilot studies or rapid change testing. If successes are not replicated, Six Sigma is ineffective as an improvement process. The PD approach may help to facilitate the spread of the improvements. Six Sigma pilots can be treated as positive deviants and then magnified. The potential connection between PD and Six Sigma may be useful to the advanced nurse employed by an organization who is using either or both of these approaches to QI. A basic understanding of the two methodologies and their interconnectedness may be helpful as nurse leaders begin to learn and implement both processes.

Bertels and Sternin (2003) caution that benchmarking and PD have similar objectives but that there are profound differences between the two concepts. They point out that the PD approach recognizes successful and accessible behaviors as critical while benchmarking targets efficiency and effectiveness. PD attends to the context of a process, and benchmarking applies the principles and attributes of an effective process as enacted by a different entity.

Finally, benchmarking focuses on opportunities external to the organization that may be borrowed and applied; PD looks for successful ideas from *within* the organization. Bertels and Sternin (2003) appreciate the benefits of benchmarking as a helpful process when organizations are seeking to redesign or duplicate results but note that benchmarking is more applicable to situations that require unconventional ideas; for example, thinking that is *outside the box*. PD works best when an organization is looking for results that can be nurtured and replicated.

In addition to using the PD approach to improving clinical outcomes, PD may also be useful to improve norms in the workplace, including those existing within health care organizations. The Center for Positive Organizations in the University of Michigan's Ross School of Business works to promote the positive workplace and positive leadership. PD focuses on replicating positive behaviors, similar to the goal of those in workplace situations who aspire to encourage honorable and excellent organizational behaviors, also referred to as positive organizational scholarship (POS). The Center for Positive Organizations (2018) offers several examples of research studies that have utilized a PD approach.

Nurses in advanced roles may find the PD-position organizational scholarship connection useful as they attempt to positively influence problems in nursing work environments including incivility or poor end-of-shift reports. PD may provide a method for exploring the positive deviants who nurture young, inexperienced staff members or who provide excellent, timely, and succinct end-of-shift reports. PD may be a wiser and more effective approach than telling staff what it is that they are doing that is wrong and inappropriate. The PD approach offers an alternative means of influencing behavioral and social outcomes within health care organizations and in clinical practice.

Failure Mode and Effects Analysis

FMEA is a proactive process focusing on *predicting* the negative outcomes of human, system, and machine failures (Senders, 2004). FMEA was created as an industrial tool and was developed by reliability engineers to evaluate complex processes in a systematic fashion, to identify the elements that may cause harm, and to prioritize remedial measures (Apkon, Leonard, Probst, DeLizio, & Vitale, 2004). It is a tool to guide systematic analysis of a process in which harm may occur (IHI, 2017e).

FMEA is based on the idea that the amount of risk associated with a process, system, machine malfunction, or human behavior relates not only to the probability of a failure occurrence but also to the degree of severity of the failure and the ease with which failure might be noticed and addressed before causing harm. FMEA uses a variety of information sources to determine failure rates and then predicts the behavior of a system in the event of failure (Apkon et al., 2004). Teams use FMEA to examine processes for potential failures and to prevent these failures by proactively correcting the processes rather than waiting for adverse events to occur and then reacting.

The FMEA is a challenging exercise that AHRQ (n.d.) evaluates as a difficult process that tends to take time. The process is useful for planning improvements to existing concerns or using preexisting processes, products, or services in new ways; forecasting errors; preventing mistakes; periodically evaluating existing concerns; or when examining failures (AHRQ, n.d.). Advanced nurses may be familiar FMEA because of TJC's requirement of hospitals to select one high-risk process and conduct a proactive risk assessment at least every 18 months (TJC, 2016b).

FMEA is important to outcomes because it offers a proactive strategy to potentially reduce harm. Adverse events should be consistently considered as opportunities to improve; although, ideally, health care organizations protect patients from harm rather than contribute to or cause harm. TJC views quality and safety as indivisible and identifies safety as a central aim of quality (TJC, 2016b). Quality management systems are charged with ensuring reliable processes, decreasing variability and waste, achieving better outcomes, and using evidence to safeguard satisfactory service delivery (TJC, 2016b). FMEA contributes to these responsibilities by facilitating risk assessment and identifying opportunities to improve outcomes.

Advanced nurses should take advantage of IHI resources available in its QI Essentials Toolkit specific to FMEA (IHI, 2017e). IHI provides instructions and resources, including an interactive FMEA Tool on its website. For those interested in using a hard-copy-based tool, IHI provides a nine-column table to guide the FMEA process. Step-by-step instructions are clearly developed, and scoring is described. A risk profile number (RPN) description is provided and tips are suggested for working toward RPN reduction based on proposed changes to the system (IHI, 2017e). An exemplar of a FMEA related to a medication dispensing process is included in the QI Toolkit.

Root Cause Analysis

RCA is frequently used by health professionals, including advanced nurses, to figure out how and why adverse events have occurred. It is a *retrospective* analysis as compared to the FMEA prospective considerations. IHI (2017f) has renamed the RCA process to Root Cause Analyses and Actions (RCA[2]) to make clear that RCA is conducted to understand how medical errors, adverse events, and near misses have occurred with the ultimate goal of taking action to prevent future harm. Advanced nurses often have a vantage point in the practice setting that contributes to keen insights on system vulnerabilities. Working with nursing colleagues and other interprofessional team members to clearly delineate processes and structures that contributed to harm, advanced nurses have opportunities to improve quality for those dependent on the health care system and its representatives for safe, effective, evidence-based care.

The RCA[2] process was designed under the leadership of the National Patient Safety Foundation (NPSF) in 2015. The second version of this best practice document is available on the IHI website (IHI, 2017g). The tool is richly detailed and a terrific resource for advanced nurses, regardless of RCA skill level. Content includes information about selecting events appropriate for RCA[2] review, event classifications, RCA[2] timing and team membership, interviewing strategies, and the event review process. Appendices offer terrific opportunities for guidance and skill acquisition.

Practical information is highlighted via the use of textbox summaries. For example, one such narrative responds to the question, "Why is 'human error' not an acceptable root cause?" The discussion emphasizes that human error may be involved in adverse events because it is inevitable; however, the point of the RCA is to understand system factors that allow such errors to occur and then identify solutions that will remove the error possibility or mitigate its effects (IHI, 2017g).

FMEA and RCA processes do improve health care outcomes and are useful for improving patient safety systems. Senders (2004) labels FMEA and RCA acronyms as "mantras of modern risk management" (p. 249). It is obvious that simply because a potential error is identified and associated with quantified risk does not guarantee a cause-effect relationship between one specific error and one specific injury. However, Senders (2004) points out that a benefit of using FMEA and RCA methodologies is their potential protective influence against lawsuits given that diligent use of these methodologies demonstrates a genuine organizational commitment to preventing avoidable patient injuries.

Advanced nurses need familiarity with FMEA and RCA processes and, in some instances, need a more advanced understanding to participate in these activities as a fully engaged member of a multidisciplinary committee. Staff may be more familiar with RCAs, particularly those practicing in acute care settings, because of the linkage between RCAs and sentinel event reporting requirements through TJC. TJC (2017c) defines a sentinel event as a patient safety event that reaches the patient and results in death, permanent harm, or severe temporary harm and intervention required to sustain life. Organizations are required to report sentinel events to TJC.

TJC requires an analysis of the root causes of sentinel events and an action plan. However, this is a retrospective review that may improve outcomes for future patients but does not work to prevent the event from occurring in the first place. FMEA may assist by providing a prospective analysis of risk thereby enhancing improved outcomes management and measurement. It is very likely that advanced nurses of all types will have opportunities to participate on teams conducting FMEA and RCA procedures as health care professionals continue to attend to improving quality and ensuring safe outcomes for patients.

Flowcharts and Diagrams: Visual Tools to Guide Outcomes Improvements

The use of flowcharts and diagrams as pictorial representations of a process is a common practice in QI initiatives. To improve outcomes, advanced nurses must understand the processes leading to the outcome. Many people grasp material best when information is presented using a variety of modalities. Graphic representations of processes and group discussions that "fill in" gaps and ensure accuracy in the diagrammed steps are very important to multidisciplinary QI efforts. IHI's (2017e) QI Toolkit provides helpful process tools including flowcharts, cause-effect or fishbone diagrams (also known as Ishikawa diagrams), histograms, and Pareto diagrams as well as instructional videos. ASQ (2017e) offers a number of process analysis tools on its website, including a flowchart template in Microsoft Excel.

In general, providing that the process under scrutiny is not too complicated, flowcharts can be user friendly and efficient. They may also serve as a blueprint for group activities. There are common symbols used in flowcharts. Microsoft Word has a flowchart option in its AutoShapes feature. Each shape is tagged with an identifier

Symbol	Meaning
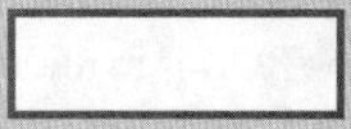	Process
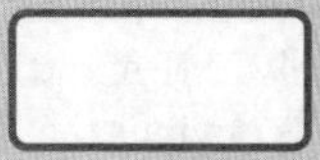	Alternate process
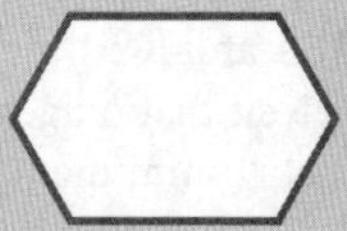	Preparation
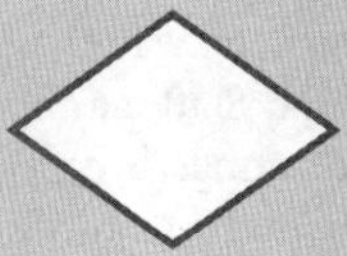	Decision
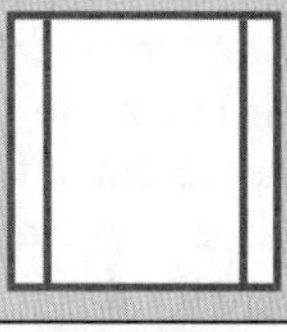	Predefined process

FIGURE 9-9 Select Microsoft™ Office Professional Plus 2013 Shapes/Flowchart.

making it easy for the novice flowchart creator to depict simple processes (**FIGURE 9-9**). There are also flowchart software programs available for purchase.

Cause-effect or Ishikawa diagrams are useful to explore sources of variability within a process (**FIGURE 9-10**). This diagram appears as a fishbone skeleton. The name of the problem of interest is on the right side of the diagram at the end of the main "backbone" of the fish. The possible causes of the problem are pictorially represented as bones off the backbone. Ishikawa diagram templates are available through Microsoft's website as a PowerPoint download. ASQ (2017f) has a number of templates (see Box 9-4) for use, most in Excel, and training is also available. AHRQ provides a *Practice Facilitation Handbook* (Knox & Brach, 2013a) to support the training of new practice facilitators who will be working to promote meaningful primary care improvement practices. The handbook is composed of 21 training modules and each module contains a trainer's guide. Advanced nurses may elect to complete some or all of these modules given their relevance to improving care processes and outcomes across a variety of health care settings. The appendices are quite useful and Module 5 Appendix provides a guide on workflow mapping formatted in PowerPoint (Knox & Brach, 2013b).

Pareto diagrams depict the variables that contribute to a particular outcome or overall effect. Variables are arranged in the order of their contribution to the outcome

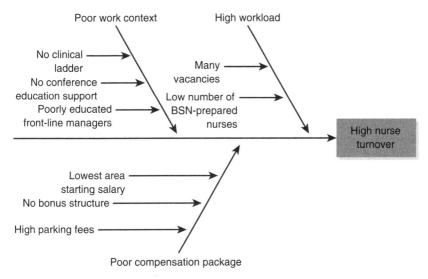

FIGURE 9-10 Cause-Effect or Fishbone Diagram.

of interest as a histogram or bar graph (IHI, 2017h). Identifying the influences responsible for the greatest effects assists team members with making decisions as to which variables should be addressed in terms of costs and benefits. In other words, team members can use the chart to determine the factors that require the most attention. The contributions of the variables should be determined in a rigorous, objective fashion rather than through opinion gathering.

Advanced nurses may find it useful to incorporate diagramming and flowcharting activities into group discussions, staff meetings, and multidisciplinary committee work. Visual aids are useful in establishing a common perspective and facilitate communication. There are times when problems become self-evident once details are diagrammed.

▶ Standardizing the Language of Nursing

As national progress is made in advancing electronic health records (EHRs), the need for nursing language standardization becomes more acute. Advanced nurses likely recognize that sharing data requires a common nursing language such as the nomenclature published by NANDA International, the Nursing Interventions Classification (NIC), and the Nursing Outcomes Classification (NOC). Collectively, NANDA, NIC, and NOC may be referred to as NNN, the standardized language of nursing.

An EHR facilitates data aggregation that encourages knowledge development, including a better understanding of outcomes and quality (Lunney, 2006). To examine the quality of nursing care and its associated costs, outcomes and interventions must be connected in the clinical record to the relevant nursing diagnoses (Moorhead & Johnson, 2004). To date, NNN is not well captured in the EHR specific to nursing practice and patient outcomes. Flanagan and Weir-Hughes (2016) express concern that EHR development has excluded NNN and, as a result, nursing's voice is lost.

EHR progression consists of three stages (CMS, 2017b). The first stage set the foundation by establishing requirements for the electronic recording of clinical data as well as providing patients with electronic access to their health information. This first stage has concluded. Stage 2 focuses on advancing clinical processes and ensuring that the meaningful use of EHRs supports the target and priorities of the National Quality Strategy. Stage 3 began in 2017 and focuses on improving health outcomes (CMS, 2017b). Flanagan and Weir-Hughes (2016) point out that hospitals in Europe and the United Kingdom have adopted American EHR provider's solution and, as a result, the system is driven by medicine. Nursing's voice will be extinguished if NNN is unaddressed in EHR systems and the rich data supporting nursing's contributions to improved patient outcomes will be unobtainable.

With this backdrop in mind, advanced nurses are cautioned to attend to NNN and contribute to EHR visibility efforts. A necessary first step is for advanced nurses to develop their understanding of NNN. Using the standardized languages of NANDA, NIC, and NOC differs from using the familiar and customary *nursing process*. NNN compel data *interpretation* rather than data collection. NNN provides outcome data and nursing intervention using a standardized format rather than the narrative forms with which many nurses are familiar. Narrative documentation can be difficult to interpret owing to inconsistencies, inadequacies, and different style forms that make drawing comparisons difficult. NNN in an EHR supports consistency because the names used for patient outcomes and nursing interventions are available to all nurses (Lunney, 2006).

Lunney (2006) suggests that both novice nurses and advanced beginners are capable of proficiently learning and using NNN. More experienced nurses, including advanced nurses, may need encouragement to document and think differently than the status quo. As the EHR is further integrated into the health care system, nurses will become more accountable for their diagnoses, outcomes, and interventions and the impact these processes will have on cost and quality. Educators will need to make certain that nursing curriculums include NNN so that nurses learn how to collect data, rule in or rule out diagnoses, and perform complex nursing interventions (Lunney, 2006). Staff development experts and those in administration will also need to be certain that nursing professionals are well versed in NNN.

A good source of information is the website of the University of Iowa College of Nursing's Center for Nursing Classification and Clinical Effectiveness (CNC) (2017). The center's home page offers information about NIC and NOC and has resources for purchase, translations, and reports available for review. An extensive list of hyperlinks provides starting points for knowledge acquisition (University of Iowa College of Nursing, 2017).

▶ Conclusion

Advanced nurses practicing in direct and indirect care roles have significant responsibility for outcomes measurement and management. Patient safety, catapulted to the forefront of public attention with the published report *To Err Is Human* (IOM, 1999), is a critical quality indicator in health care that has a broad and deep reach across all aspects of the national health care system—and rightly so.

Advanced nurses must recognize the partnership between outcomes, QI processes, and EBP. Outcomes measures provide indicators of quality that may be improved through the use of systematically applied evidence. In addition to using outcomes measures to demonstrate QIs within systems and processes, nurses are challenged to demonstrate their impact on patients/families, nurses, and organizations by using outcomes measures that are sensitive to their unique contributions. More attention must be paid to integrating the language of nursing into the EHR.

Selecting measurable and meaningful outcomes is not an easy task. It can be challenging to discern the "best" outcome measure out of the many potential outcomes that could exist related to a specific aspect of health care. Garnering input from interprofessional colleagues via working teams can be very helpful. Advanced nurses should use established resources that are available to them from the exceptional foundations, agencies, and organizations that have made outcomes improvement their reveille call. Tools from these experts provide valid and reliable measures of quality. Outcomes management and QI can be overwhelming to new advanced nurses or to those unfamiliar with this burgeoning area of inquiry; however, starting with unit projects or small-scale department activities can be a good way to develop a repertoire of QI process tools.

References

Adams, R., Warner, P., Hubbard, B., & Goulding, T. (2004). Decreasing turnaround time between general surgery cases: A Six Sigma initiative. *Journal of Nursing Administration, 34*(3), 140–148.

Agency for Healthcare Research and Quality. (n.d.). Failure mode and effects analysis. Retrieved January 28, 2018, from https://healthit.ahrq.gov/health-it-tools-and-resources/evaluation-resources /workflow-assessment-health-it-toolkit/all-workflow-tools/fmea-analysis.

Agency for Healthcare Research and Quality. (2000). Outcomes research. Fact sheet (AHRQ Publication No. 00-P011). Retrieved January 12, 2009, from http://www.ahrq.gov/clinic/outfact.htm.

Agency for Healthcare Research and Quality. (2016, October). AHRQ's role in the patient-centered outcomes research (PCOR) cycle. Retrieved December 27, 2017, from https://www.ahrq.gov /pcor/dissemination-of-pcor/ahrq-role-in-pcor-cycle.html.

Agency for Healthcare Research and Quality. (2017). Communication and optimal resolution (CANDOR) toolkit. Retrieved December 27, 2017, from www.ahrq.gov/professionals/quality -patient-safety/patient-safety-resources/resources/candor/introduction.html.

Aiken, L. H., Clarke, S. P., Sloane, D. M., Sochalski, J., & Silber, J. H. (2002). Hospital nurse staffing and patient mortality, nurse burnout, and job dissatisfaction. *Journal of the American Medical Association, 288*, 1987–1993.

Aiken, L. H., Simiotti, J., Sloane, D. M., Smith, H. L., Flynn, L., & Neff, D. (2011). The effects of nurse staffing and nurse education on patient deaths in hospitals with different nurse work environments. *Medical Care, 49*, 1047–1053.

American Association of Colleges of Nursing. (2004, October). Position statement on the practice doctorate in nursing. Retrieved January 7, 2009, from http://www.aacn.nche.edu/DNP/pdf /DNP.pdf.

American Association of Nurse Practitioners. (2013). Discussion paper. Doctor of nursing practice. Retrieved December 20, 2017, from https://www.aanp.org/images/documents/publications /doctorofnursingpractice.pdf.

American Association of Nurse Practitioners. (2017). Press releases and announcements. American Association of Nurse Practitioners responds to American Medical Association amendment to Resolution 214. Retrieved December 19, 2017, from https://www.aanp.org/press-room /press-releases/173-press-room/2017-press-releases/2156-aanp-responds-to-ama-amendment -to-resolution-214.

American College of Nurse-Midwives. (2012). Midwifery education and the doctor of nursing practice (DNP). Retrieved December 20, 2017, from http://www.midwife.org/ACNM/files /ACNMLibraryData/UPLOADFILENAME/000000000079/Midwifery%20Ed%20and%20DNP%20 Position%20Statement%20June%202012.pdf.

American Medical Association. (2017). American Medical Association. House of Delegates (I-17). Report of Reference Committee B. Retrieved December 19, 2017, from https://www.ama-assn .org/sites/default/files/media-browser/public/hod/i17-refcommb-rpt.pdf.

American Nurses Association. (1995). *The nursing care report card for acute care.* Washington, DC: Author.

American Nurses Association. (1999). Nursing-sensitive quality indicators for acute care settings and ANA's safety and quality initiative. Retrieved January 12, 2009, from http://www.nursingworld .org/MainMenuCategories/ThePracticeofProfessional Nursing/PatientSafetyQuality/NDNQI /Research/QIforAcuteCareSettings.aspx.

American Organization of Nurse Executives. (2007). Consideration of the doctorate of nursing practice. Retrieved December 20, 2017, from http://www.aone.org/resources/doctorate-nursing -practice.pdf.

American Society for Quality. (2017a). About ASQ. Retrieved December 27, 2017, from https://asq .org/about-asq.

American Society for Quality (2017b). Plan-do-check-act cycle. Retrieved January 28, 2018, from http://www.asq.org/learn-about-quality/project-planning-tools/overview/pdca-cycle.html.

American Society for Quality. (2017c). What is Six Sigma? Retrieved December 30, 2017, from http:// asq.org/learn-about-quality/six-sigma/overview/overview.html.

American Society for Quality. (2017d). Six Sigma belts, executives and champions, what does it all mean? Retrieved December 30, 2017, from http://asq.org/learn-about-quality/six-sigma/overview /belts-executives-champions.html.

American Society for Quality. (2017e). Process analysis tools. Retrieved December 31, 2017, from http://asq.org/learn-about-quality/process-analysis-tools/overview/overview.html.

American Society for Quality. (2017f). Quality tools & templates. Retrieved December 31, 2017, from http://asq.org/learn-about-quality/tools-templates.html.

American Society for Quality. (2018). What is LEAN? Retrieved January 28, 2018, from http://asq .org/learn-about-quality/lean/overview/overview.html.

American Society of Anesthesiologists. (2017). Nurse anesthetist care not equal to physician anesthesiologist -led care, comprehensive evidence-based review finds, American Society of Anesthesiologists® calls for further examination. Retrieved from http://www.asahq.org/about-asa/newsroom /news-releases/2014/08/nurse-anesthetist-care-not-equal-to-physician-anesthesiologist-led-care.

American Urological Association. (2017). AMA House of Delegates interim meeting update: November 14, 2017. Retrieved December 19, 2017, from https://community.auanet.org/blogs /policy-brief/2017/11/14/ama-house-of-delegates-interim-meeting-update-november-14-2017.

Apkon, M., Leonard, J., Probst, L., DeLizio, L., & Vitale, R. (2004). Design of a safer approach to intravenous drug infusions: Failure model effects analysis. *Quality and Safety in Health Care, 13,* 265–271.

Ausserhofer, D., Rakic, S., Novo, A., Dropic, E., Fisekovic, E., Sredic, A., & Van Malderen, G. (2016). Improving the safety and quality of nursing care through standardized operating procedures in Bosnia and Herzegovina. *International Nursing Review, 63,* 208–217. doi:10.1111/inr.12237

Barbosa, C. E., Masho, S. W., Carlyle, K. E., & Mosavel, M. (2016). Factors distinguishing positive deviance among low-income African American women: A qualitative study on infant feeding. *Journal of Human Lactation, 33,* 368–378. doi:10.1177/089033441667

Barlow, R. D. (2008). Erasing the stigma of Six Sigma and LEAN principles. *Healthcare Purchasing News.* Retrieved January 28, 2018, from https://www.hpnonline.com/inside/2008-08/0808-PS -sixsigma.html.

Bender, J. S., Nicolescu, T. O., Hollingsworth, S. B., Murer, K., Wallace, K. R., & Ertl, W. J. (2015). Improving operating room efficiency via an interprofessional approach. *The American Journal of Surgery, 209,* 447–450. doi:http://dx.doi.org/10.1016/j.amjsurg.2014.12.007

Bertels, T., & Sternin, J. (2003). Replicating results and managing knowledge. In T. Bertels (Ed.), *Rath & Strong's Six Sigma leadership handbook* (pp. 450–457). Hoboken, NJ: John Wiley & Sons.

Bisaillon, S., Kelloway, L., LeBlanc, K., Pageau, N., & Woloshyn, N. (2005). Best practices in stroke care. *Canadian Nurse, 101*(8), 25–29.

Burston, S., Chaboyer, W., & Gillespie, B. (2013). Nurse-sensitive indicators suitable to reflect nursing care quality: A review and discussion of issues. *Journal of Clinical Nursing, 23,* 1785–1795. doi:10.1111/jocn.12337

Center for Positive Organizations. (2018). Search results for positive deviance. Retrieved January 28, 2018, from http://positiveorgs.bus.umich.edu/?s=positive+deviance.

Centers for Medicare & Medicaid Services. (2008). Medicare takes new steps to help make your hospital stay safer. Retrieved January 28, 2018, from https://www.cms.gov/Newsroom/MediaReleaseDatabase

/Fact-sheets/2008-Fact-sheets-items/2008-08045.html?DLPage=1&DLFilter=hospital%20 care&DLSort=0&DLSortDir=descending.

Centers for Medicare & Medicaid Services. (2015). Hospital-acquired conditions. Retrieved January 28, 2018, from https://www.cms.gov/medicare/medicare-fee-for-service-payment/hospitalacqcond /hospital-acquired_conditions.html.

Centers for Medicare & Medicaid Services. (2017a). ICD-10-CM/PCS MS-DRGv33 definitions manual. Appendix I. Hospital acquired conditions (HACS) list. Hospital acquired conditions. Retrieved December 28, 2017, from https://www.cms.gov/ICD10Manual/version33-fullcode-cms/fullcode_cms/P1059.html.

Centers for Medicare & Medicaid Services. (2017b). Electronic health records (EHR) incentive programs. Retrieved December 31, 2017, from https://www.cms.gov/Regulations-and-Guidance /Legislation/EHRIncentivePrograms/index.html?redirect=/EHRIncentivePrograms/.

Chen. H. (2015). *Practical program evaluation. Theory-driven evaluation and the integrated evaluation perspective* (2nd ed.). Newbury Park, CA: Sage Publishing.

Chowdhury, S. (2001). *The power of Six Sigma*. Chicago, IL: Dearborn Trade.

Cusano, A. J. (2006). Use of the positive deviance approach to improve reconciliation of medications and patients medication management after hospital discharge: The experience of Waterbury Hospital (Connecticut). Retrieved January 7, 2009, from http://www.positivedeviance.org /projects/waterbury/waterbury_narrative_final.pdf.

Dearden, K., Quan, L. N., Do, M., Marsh, D. R., Pachón, H., Schroeder, D. G., & Lang, T. T. (2002). Work outside the home is the primary barrier to exclusive breastfeeding in rural Viet Nam: Insights from mothers who exclusively breastfed and worked. *Food and Nutrition Bulletin, 23*(4), 99–106.

Elliott, N., Begley, C., Kleinpell, R., & Higgins, A. (2014). The development of leadership outcome-indicators evaluating the contribution of clinical specialists and advanced practitioners to health care; A secondary analysis. *Journal of Advanced Nursing, 70,* 1078–1093. doi:10.1111/jan.12262

Flanagan, J., & Weir-Hughes, D. (2016). NANDA-I, NIC and NOC, the EHR, and meaningful use. *International Journal of Nursing Knowledge, 27,* 183.

Fowles, E. R., Hendricks, J. A., & Walker, L. O. (2005). Identifying healthy eating strategies in low-income pregnant women: Applying a positive deviance model. *Health Care for Women International, 26*(9), 807–820.

Given, B., & Sherwood, P. (2005). Nursing-sensitive patient outcomes: A white paper. *Oncology Nursing Forum, 32*(4), 773–784.

Ha, C., Mccoy, D. A., Taylor, C. B., Kirk, K. D., Fry, R. S., & Modi, J. R. (2016). Using Lean Six Sigma methodology to improve a mass immunizations process at the United States Naval Academy. *Military Medicine, 181,* 582–588. doi:10.7205/MILMED-D-15-00247

Health Quality Ontario. (2013). Quality improvement primers. Measurement for quality improvement. Retrieved December 28, 2017, from http://www.hqontario.ca/Portals/0/documents/qi/qi -measurement-primer-en.pdf.

Huang, Y., & Klassen, K. (2016). Using Six Sigma, lean, and simulation to improve the phlebotomy process. *Quality Management Journal, 23,* 6–21. doi: https://doi.org/10.1080/10686967.2016.11918468

Institute for Healthcare Improvement. (n.d.). Overview. Protecting 5 million lives from harm. Retrieved January 27, 2018, from http://www.ihi.org/Engage/Initiatives/Completed/5MillionLivesCampaign /Pages/default.aspx.

Institute for Healthcare Improvement. (2012). How-to-guide. Prevent central line-associated bloodstream infections. Retrieved January 27, 2018, from http://www.ihi.org/resources/Pages /Tools/HowtoGuidePreventCentralLineAssociatedBloodstreamInfection.aspx.

Institute for Healthcare Improvement. (2017a). Patient safety. Retrieved December 27, 2017, from http://www.ihi.org/Topics/PatientSafety/Pages/default.aspx.

Institute for Healthcare Improvement. (2017b). Resources. Retrieved December 27, 2017, from http:// www.ihi.org/resources/Pages/default.aspx.

Institute for Healthcare Improvement. (2017c). How long should a PDSA cycle last? Retrieved December 30, 2017, from http://www.ihi.org/education/IHIOpenSchool/resources/Pages /Activities/Provost-HowLongShouldAPDSACycleLast.aspx.

Institute for Healthcare Improvement. (2017d). Science of improvement. Tips for testing changes. Retrieved December 30, 2017, from http://www.ihi.org/resources/Pages/HowtoImprove /ScienceofImprovementTipsforTestingChanges.aspx.

Institute for Healthcare Improvement. (2017e). QI essentials toolkit: Failure modes and effects analysis (FMEA). Retrieved January 28, 2018, from http://www.ihi.org/resources/Pages/Tools /FailureModesandEffectsAnalysisTool.aspx.

Institute for Healthcare Improvement. (2017f). RCA2: Improving root cause analyses and actions to prevent harm. Retrieved December 31, 2017, from http://www.ihi.org/resources/Pages/Tools /RCA2-Improving-Root-Cause-Analyses-and-Actions-to-Prevent-Harm.aspx.

Institute for Healthcare Improvement. (2017g). National Patient Safety Foundation RCA^2 improving root cause analyses and actions to prevent harm (Version 2). January 2016. Retrieved December 31, 2017, from http://www.ihi.org/resources/_layouts/download.aspx?S ourceURL=%2fresources%2fKnowledge+Center+Assets%2fTools+-+RCA2ImprovingRootC auseAnalysesandActionstoPreventHarm_f65ed89f-eb0c-490f-b05a-a772a68fd6d9%2fRCA2 _ImprovingRootCauseAnalysesandActionstoPreventHarm.pdf.

Institute for Healthcare Improvement. (2017h). Pareto chart. Retrieved December 31, 2017, from http://www.ihi.org/resources/Pages/Tools/ParetoDiagram.aspx.

Institute for Healthcare Improvement. (2018). The IHI triple aim. Retrieved January 28, 2018, from http://www.ihi.org/Engage/Initiatives/TripleAim/Pages/default.aspx.

Institute of Medicine. (1999). *To err is human: Building a safer health system.* Washington, DC: National Academies Press.

Institute of Medicine. (2010). The future of nursing: Leading change, advancing health. Retrieved December 18, 2017, from http://books.nap.edu/openbook.php?record_id=12956&page=R1.

iSixSigma. (2017). Six Sigma—What is Six Sigma? Retrieved December 30, 2017, from http://www .isixsigma.com/sixsigma/six_sigma.asp.

Jones, T. (2016). Outcome measurement in nursing: Imperatives, ideals, history, and challenges. *OJIN: The Online Journal of Issues in Nursing, 21*(2), manuscript 1. doi:10.3912/OJIN.Vol21No02Man01

Kaizen Institute. (2017). KAIZEN™ guiding principles. Retrieved December 30, 2017, from http://asq .org/learn-about-quality/six-sigma/overview/belts-executives-champions.html.

Kirby, K. K. (2015). Hours per patient day: Not the problem, nor the solution. *Nursing Economics, 33*, 64–66.

Kleinpell, R., & Gawlinski, A. (2005). Assessing outcomes in advanced practice nursing practice: The use of quality indicators and evidence-based practice. *AACN Clinical Issues, 16*(1), 43–57.

Knox, L., & Brach, C. (2013a). *The practice facilitation handbook: Training modules for new facilitators and their trainers.* (Prepared by LA Net through a subcontract with the University of Minnesota under Contract No. HHSA29000710010 TO 3.). Rockville, MD: Agency for Healthcare Research and Quality. AHRQ Publication No. 13-0046-EF. Retrieved December 31, 2017, from https:// www.ahrq.gov/sites/default/files/publications/files/practicefacilitationhandbook.pdf.

Knox, L., & Brach, C. (2013b). *The practice facilitation handbook: Training modules for new facilitators and their trainers. Appendix.* (Prepared by LA Net through a subcontract with the University of Minnesota under Contract No. HHSA29000710010 TO 3.). Rockville, MD: Agency for Healthcare Research and Quality. AHRQ Publication No. 13-0046-EF. Retrieved December 31, 2017, from https://www.ahrq.gov/sites/default/files/publications/files/pfchandbookappendices.pdf.

Lazarus, I. (2003). Six Sigma. Raising the bar. Managed Healthcare Executive. Retrieved January 28, 2018, from http://www.managedhealthcareexecutive.com/mhe/article/articleDetail.jsp?id=43331.

Lean Enterprise Institute. (2012). Waste walk. Retrieved January 27, 2018, from http://oe.ucdavis .edu/Lean/Lean%20docs/Waste%20Walk_FINAL.docx.

Leapfrog Group. (n.d.). Home page. About the Leapfrog Group. Retrieved December 27, 2017, from http://www.leapfroggroup.org/.

Lunney, M. (2006). Helping nurses use NANDA, NOC, and NIC: Novice to expert. *Journal of Nursing Administration, 36*(3), 118–125.

Major, T. W., & Huey, T. K. (2016). Decreasing IV infiltrates in the pediatric patient—system-based improvement project. *Pediatric Nursing, 42*, 14+. Retrieved December 30, 2017, from http://link .galegroup.com/apps/doc/A445116641/AONE?u=drexel_main&sid=AONE&xid=13995191.

Marsh, D. R., Schroeder, D. G., Dearden, K. A., Sternin, J., & Sternin, M. (2004). The power of positive deviance. *British Medical Journal, 329*, 1177–1179.

Martin, M. L. (2003). Rapid-cycle improvement in pediatric health care: A solution for patients with similar or same last names. *Journal for Specialists in Pediatric Nursing, 8*(4), 148–154.

Montalvo, I. (2007). The National Database of Nursing Quality Indicators™ (NDNQI®). *OJIN: The Online Journal of Issues in Nursing, 12*(3), manuscript 2. Retrieved December 26, 2017, from

http://www.nursingworld.org/MainMenuCategories/ANAMarketplace/ANAPeriodicals/OJIN
/TableofContents/Volume122007/No3Sept07/NursingQualityIndicators.html. doi:10.3912/OJIN.
Vol12No03Man02

Moore, K., Lynn, M., McMillen, B., & Evans, S. (1999). Implementation of the ANA Report Card.
Journal of Nursing Administration, 29(6), 46–54.

Moorhead, S., & Johnson, M. (2004). Diagnostic-specific outcomes and nursing effectiveness research.
International Journal of Nursing Terminologies and Classifications, 15(2), 49–57.

National Association of Clinical Nurse Specialists. (2017). Position statement on the doctor of nursing
practice. Retrieved December 20, 2017, from http://nacns.org/advocacy-policy/position-statements
/position-statement-on-the-doctor-of-nursing-practice/.

National Committee for Quality Assurance. (n.d.). HEDIS® and Quality Compass®. Retrieved December
27, 2017, from http://www.ncqa.org/hedis-quality-measurement/what-is-hedis.

National Committee for Quality Assurance. (2016). 2016 State of health care quality table of
contents. Retrieved December 27, 2017, from http://www.ncqa.org/report-cards/health-plans
/state-of-health-care-quality/2016-table-of-contents.

National Council of State Boards of Nursing. (2017a). CNS independent practice map. Retrieved
December 18, 2017, from https://www.ncsbn.org/5406.htm.

National Council of State Boards of Nursing. (2017b). Independent prescribing-CNS. Retrieved
December 18, 2017, from https://www.ncsbn.org/5410.htm.

National League for Nursing. (2018). Interprofessional education (IPE). Retrieved January 28,
2018, from http://www.nln.org/professional-development-programs/teaching-resources
/interprofessional-education-(ipe).

National Practitioner Data Bank. (n.d.[a]). About us. Retrieved December 27, 2017, from https://
www.npdb.hrsa.gov/topNavigation/aboutUs.jsp.

National Practitioner Data Bank. (n.d.[b]). NPDB history. Retrieved December 27, 2017, from https://
www.npdb.hrsa.gov/topNavigation/timeline.jsp.

National Provider Identifier Registry. (2017). NPI lookup from the NPI Registry—National Provider
Identifier Database (NPIdb). Retrieved December 27, 2017, from https://npidb.org/.

National Quality Forum. (2018a). About us. Retrieved June 5, 2018, from https://asq.org/about-asq.

National Quality Forum. (2018b). NQF's work in quality measurement. Retrieved June 5, 2018, from
http://www.qualityforum.org/about_nqf/work_in_quality_measurement/.

Nester, J. (2016). The importance of interprofessional practice and education in the era of accountable
care. *North Carolina Medical Journal, 77*, 128–132. doi:10.18043/ncm.77.2.128

Nimtz-Rusch, K., & Thompson, J. (2008). Nursing and Six Sigma: A perfect match for safety and
quality improvement. *CHART, 105*(3), 10–13.

Owens, L. D., & Koch, R. W. (2015) Understanding quality patient care and the role of the practicing
nurse. *Nursing Clinics North America, 50*, 33–43. doi:10.1016/j.cnur.2014.10.003

Pape, T. M., Guerra, D. M., Muzquiz, M., Bryant, J. B., Ingram, M., Schranner, B., et al. (2005).
Innovative approaches to reducing nurses' distractions during medication administration. *Journal
of Continuing Education in Nursing, 36*(3), 108–116.

Pennsylvania General Assembly. (2015). House Bill No. 1238. Session of 2015. Printer's No. 1633.
Retrieved May 18, 2018, from http://www.legis.state.pa.us/cfdocs/legis/PN/Public/btCheck
.cfm?txtType=PDF&sessYr=2015&sessInd=0&billBody=H&billTyp=B&billNbr=1238&pn=1633

Peterson, J., Adlard, K., Hayakawa, J., McClean, E., & Feidner, S. C. (2015). Clinical nurse specialist
collaboration to recognize, prevent, and treat pediatric pressure ulcers. *Clinical Nurse Specialist,
29*, 276–282. doi:10.1097/NUR.0000000000000135

Press Ganey. (n.d.). Magnet nursing data. Retrieved December 26, 2017, from https://helpandtraining
.pressganey.com/resources/magnet-nursing-data.

Press Ganey. (2015). Press Ganey acquires National Database of Nursing Quality Indicators
(NDNQI®). Retrieved December 20, 2017, from http://www.pressganey.com/resources/reports
/press-ganey-acquires-national-database-of-nursing-quality-indicators-(ndnqi-).

Press Ganey. (2017). Resources and research. Retrieved December 26, 2017, from http://www
.pressganey.com/resources#?t=Select%20all/none?t=Clinical%20Quality?t=Nursing%20
Quality:%20NDNQI?t=Core%20Quality%20Measures?t=Patient-Reported%20Outcomes%20
(PROMS)?t=Engagement?t=Caregiver%20Burnout?t=General?t=Patient%20Experience?t=CAHPS%20
Programs?t=Transparency?t=Nursing?t=Safety?m=Articles?m=Blog?m=Video?m=Webinar?m

=Report?s=ACO/Cross-Continuum?s=Acute?s=Dialysis/ICH?s=ED?s=General?s=Hospitals?s=ICU?s=NDNQI?s=Nursing?s=Pediatrics?s=Rehabilitation?s=Safety?s=Transparency.

Santiago, A. C. (2017). States that allow CRNAs to practice without physician supervision. State laws dictate CRNA work. Retrieved December 19, 2017, from https://www.verywell.com/which-states-allow-crnas-to-practice-independently-1736102.

Senders, J. W. (2004). FMEA and RCA: The mantras of modern risk management. *BMJ Quality and Safety in Healthcare, 13,* 265–271. Retrieved January 28, 2018, from http://qhc.bmjjournals.com/cgi/content/full/13/4/249. doi:10.1136/qshc.2003.007443

Shaw, G. (2009). Robert Wood Johnson Foundation. Program results report. Mastering MRSA: Pilot project lowers rates 73 percent. Retrieved December 30, 2017, from https://www.rwjf.org/content/dam/farm/reports/program_results_reports/2009/rwjf48863.

Spurr, S., Bally, J., & Trinder, K. (2016). Predictors of physical activity in positive deviant adolescents. *Journal of Pediatric Nursing, 31,* 311–318. doi:10.1016/j.pedn.2015.11.006

Sternin, J. (2002, Spring). Positive deviance: A new paradigm for addressing today's problems today. *The Journal of Corporate Citizenship,* 57+. Retrieved December 30, 2017, from http://link.galegroup.com.ezproxy2.library.drexel.edu/apps/doc/A84669002/AONE?u=drexel_main&sid=AONE&xid=2b1487c0.

Stover, P. R., & Harpin, S. (2015). Decreasing psychiatric admission wait time in the emergency department by facilitating psychiatric discharges. *Journal of Psychosocial Nursing and Mental Health Services, 53*(12), 20–27. doi:10.3928/02793695-20151020-02

Szablewski, S., Zuzelo, P., Thomas, L., & Morales, M. (2009). Describing saline-lock usage patterns on a telemetry unit: A retrospective study. *Clinical Nurse Specialist, 23,* 296-304.

Terry, K. L., Disabata, J., & Krajicek, M. (2015). Snoring, trouble breathing, un-refreshed (STBUR) screening questionnaire to reduce perioperative respiratory adverse events in pediatric surgical patients: A quality improvement project. *American Association of Nurse Anesthetists Journal, 83,* 256–262.

The Interprofessional Education Collaborative. (2017). Home. Retrieved January 28, 2018, from https://www.ipecollaborative.org/.

The Joint Commission. (2016a). Facts about Quality Check® and Quality Reports®. Retrieved December 27, 2017, from https://www.jointcommission.org/facts_about_quality_check_and_quality_reports/.

The Joint Commission. (2016b). Patient safety systems. Retrieved December 31, 2017, from https://www.jointcommission.org/assets/1/18/PSC_for_Web.pdf.

The Joint Commission. (2017a). Pioneers in Quality™. About the program. Retrieved December 27, 2017, from https://www.jointcommission.org/topics/pioneers_in_quality.aspx.

The Joint Commission. (2017b). Facts about Pioneers in Quality™. Retrieved December 27, 2017, from https://www.jointcommission.org/facts_about_pioneers_in_quality/

The Joint Commission. (2017c, June 29). Sentinel event policy and procedures. Retrieved December 31, 2017, from https://www.jointcommission.org/sentinel_event_policy_and_procedures/.

The Josiah Macy Jr. Foundation. (2015). About the foundation. Retrieved January 28, 2018, from http://macyfoundation.org/.

UNICEF. (2008, April 24). Female genital mutilation abandonment program. Evaluation summary report. Retrieved December 30, 2017, from https://www.unicef.org/evaldatabase/files/EGY_FGM_AP_report.pdf.

University of Iowa College of Nursing. (2017). Center for nursing classification and clinical effectiveness. Retrieved December 31, 2017, from https://nursing.uiowa.edu/center-for-nursing-classification-and-clinical-effectiveness.

Williams, H., & Fallone, S. (2008). CQI in the acute care setting: An opportunity to influence acute care practice. *Nephrology Nursing Journal, 35*(5), 515–517.

Woodward, T. (2005). Addressing variation in hospital quality: Is Six Sigma the answer? *Journal of Healthcare Management, 50*(4), 226.

Zimnicki, K. M. (2015). Preoperative teaching and stoma marking in an inpatient population. A quality improvement process using a FOCUS-plan-do-check-act model. *Journal of Wound Ostomy Continence Nursing, 42,* 165–169.

Zuzelo, P. (2006). Evidence-based nursing and qualitative research: A partnership imperative for real-world practice. In P. Munhall (Ed.), *Nursing research: A qualitative perspective* (4th ed.). Sudbury, MA: Jones and Bartlett.

CHAPTER 10

Recognizing and Responding to Risk, Harm, and Liability

Patti Rager Zuzelo, EdD, RN, ACNS-BC, ANP-BC, CRNP, FAAN and
Joanne Farley Serembus, EdD, MSN, RN, CCRN (Alumnus), CNE

PART ONE

Harm Recognition and Reduction

Patti Rager Zuzelo, EdD, MSN, RN, ACNS-BC, ANP-BC, FAAN

Nurses' work is complex and largely relates to advocating for patients by prioritizing their needs and recognizing risks, preventing harm, and ensuring safety during delivery of high-quality, patient-centered care that achieves excellent outcomes. These efforts are demanding and stressful, particularly when provided within a practice context that is often underresourced, unpredictable, and sometimes chaotically organized despite best team efforts. However, nursing is certainly a rewarding profession that the public highly regards and trusts. Given this trust, nurses and advanced nurses practicing in various roles that have direct and indirect responsibilities for patient care feel tremendously responsible for making certain that patients do not experience harm.

Prioritization of harm avoidance and risk reduction is consistent with Provision 3 of the Code of Ethics for Nurses (American Nurses Association [ANA], 2015) that declares, "The nurse promotes, advocates for, and protects the rights, health, and safety of the patient" (p. 9). This particular provision specifically addresses the rights of privacy, confidentiality, protection of human participants in research, performance standards and review mechanisms, responsibilities in promoting a culture of safety, protection of patient health and safety by action on questionable practice as well as impaired practice (Fowler, 2015).

Advanced nurses respond to the expectations of Provision 3 through constant surveillance and risk management strategies that include risk assessment, threat recognition, response prioritization, and protective interventions across an array of potential harm opportunities (Groves, Finfgeld-Connett, & Wakefield, 2014). Experienced nurses appreciate that some degree of risk is innate to health care encounters, whether it is a mild risk of being exposed to some sort of viral or bacterial infection while waiting in the reception area, moderate risk of postoperative complications or fluid/electrolyte imbalances secondary to preparation for procedures, or major risk affiliated with concerning comorbidities that increase the likelihood of cardiovascular or pulmonary complications. Each encounter entails risk of harm. Experienced advanced nurses have knowledge of the risks of health care that are often poorly appreciated by those seeking care. Nurses use this knowledge to protect patients and advocate for them throughout episodes of care delivery, including hospitalization.

Patients and their families want to feel safe during health care interactions. *Feeling* safe is important and certainly nurses work hard to reassure patients that care will be correctly delivered; however, feeling safe and secure is not the equivalent to actually *being* safe (Mollon, 2014). Recognizing some risk is likely easy enough for many laypeople, depending on the circumstances of the potentially harmful event or process; however, the sorts of risk that advanced nurses spot are based on expertise, experience, and clinical intuition. Mollon (2014) conducted a concept analysis of feeling safe using an established eight-step process and explicated a safe feeling as "an emotional state where perceptions of care contribute to a sense of security and freedom from harm during an inpatient hospitalization" (p. 1729).

Findings revealed 40 characteristics associated with feeling safe and these traits clustered into four major themes: trust, cared for, presence, and knowledge (Mollon, 2014). Advanced nurses should reflect on these themes and consider how they might work with interprofessional and nurse colleagues to maximize the opportunities for patients to experience safe feelings by responding to concerns using unique and shared interventions. *Trust* was revealed as important to feeling safe and was appreciated as a principle value in the nurse-patient relationship. Keeping commitments to patients, including simple promises such as when the nurse will return to the room, can support trust development. Nurse authenticity and expertise were recognized as important to the *cared for* and *knowledge* clusters while *presence* represented having nurses and family members present during the hospitalization event in ways that were important to the patient (Mollon, 2014). Bedside availability of family and friends is well-supported by research as an important component of patient-centered care when desired by the patient and appropriate to the care delivery at the time.

One strategy for keeping patients safe is to consider risk as best avoided in all cases, particularly if lawsuit or disciplinary actions are practice drivers. Since nurses are often viewed as responsible when risk begets harm, they may be particularly risk averse. Keeping patients free from harm is a requisite responsibility of professional nurses; however, Clarke and Mantle (2016) note that risk avoidance can contribute to "silent harm" (p. 3). They explore this concern specific to person-centered dementia care, when afflicted persons find important aspects of their personhood removed as a strategy for keeping them safe. In this scenario, the individual living with dementia may find cooking, driving, or outside strolling no longer permitted in what had been a customary and enjoyable daily routine. Clarke and Mantle (2016) recommend that nurses reflect on people's vulnerabilities as one influence existing within the context of the person's life and manage these risks accordingly rather than seeing the risks as disabling barriers that exist within the individual. Avoiding silent harm in the interest of eliminating risk has its own harmful effects on patient outcomes.

The previous chapters leading up to this discussion about risk, safety, and harm have often addressed potentials for risk albeit, at times, in limited or subtle fashion; specifically, most chapters have recognized sources of risk and harm in meaningful, practical ways and generally in ways that need to be strategically addressed or avoided. Throughout these earlier discussions, the words *harm, adverse events* (AEs), and *injuries* are used interchangeably or in a fashion that suggests partnership. In actual fact, these terms share commonalities, but they are distinct and unique. Harm is defined as an outcome that has had a negative impact on health or quality of life. Adverse events do result in *unintended* harm to the patient directly related to the proffered care or services rather than occurring secondarily to an underlying medical condition (Parry, Cline, & Goldmann, 2012), but harm may be broader than recognized negative outcomes. There is increasing recognition of the need to measure and track national harm trends so that health care leadership and stakeholders can accurately determine improvement in harm rates caused by any type of circumstance or event—not only AEs (Parry et al., 2012).

The harm field of study is complex and relatively new. The concept of harm is not fully explicated, and it is not yet known whether harm is always detectable; perhaps patients could be harmed in ways or through processes that are not yet understood (Jackson & Wilson, 2016). Another unsettled question is whether harms that are not preventable or not caused by modifiable events or processes should be considered as harms (Jackson & Wilson, 2016).

Error is unique from harm and is often not associated with injury to the patient (Institute for Healthcare Improvement [IHI], 2009). This is one reason why a culture of safety is best served by focusing on harmful events rather than on errors. The driving point is to focus on improving outcomes, reducing or avoiding harm, rather than blaming or attributing errors to individuals—particularly given that most errors have no association to harm (IHI, 2009).

These thought-provoking questions are important in practical ways. Advanced nurses should keep abreast of evolving harm measurement standards and opportunities. Advanced nurses practicing in a variety of roles are often responsible for reporting, addressing, and tracking AEs. For the most part, nurses mostly examine harm in the context of root-cause analyses after an AE has occurred. Nurses at the sharp point of care monitor for harm potential by comparing what is occurring in the care context to a recognized normal that is informed by their expertise, education, and practice experiences. Nurses are simultaneously careful to avoid attributing what they observe as potentially harmful to a preconceived or preestablished diagnosis rather than considering the possibility of a unique condition that may be related to a harmful experience or AE (Groves et al., 2014). One example of this ongoing clinical harm surveillance is when a patient becomes sweaty, clammy, and dyspneic during a hospital stay. Rather than automatically assuming that this symptom experience is related to the patient's diabetes or asthma, the nurse contemplates all possibilities and discusses the need for an immediate electrocardiogram (ECG) with the provider.

▶ Measuring Harm

Several tools are available for measuring harm. Keep in mind that harm, by definition, is an outcome whereas an AE is an occurrence that has resulted in unintended harm (Parry et al., 2012). Some harm measurements focus on particular types of harm while others address all-cause harm; the most common all-cause harm measurement is the Global Trigger Tool (GTT) (IHI, 2009). Another tool is the Harvard Medical Practice Study (HMPS), best recognized for methods that were developed to identify AEs and estimate their occurrence. HMPS developers were initially interested in establishing whether the tort system at the time was effective in compensating those who were injured as a result of their hospital care experience and in assessing the economic impact of such injuries. HPMS established that AEs commonly occurred in hospital care and this finding took a preeminent position over evaluation of the tort system and its costs (Brennan et al., 2004).

A major conclusion of the HPMS study was there is a significant amount of injury sustained by patients from medical care provision and much of this injury is the result of substandard care (Brennan et al., 2004). Baker (2004) pointed out that the HMPS study established the standard by which AEs are measured and it provided the groundwork for patient safety policy discussions in the United States and in other countries. The HMPS study contributed important evidence to policy debates that followed the Institute of Medicine report, *To Err Is Human* (Kohn, Corrigan, & Donaldson, 2000). Advanced nurses would be well served to have a general appreciation for the HMPS study and its influence on quantifying the impact of the harm associated with AEs on patients.

The Medicare Patient Safety Monitoring System (MPSMS) provides another measure of harm. This national surveillance program was designed to identify occurrence rates of selected AEs within the Medicare recipient population (Hunt et al., n.d.). This system pulls AEs from randomly selected Medicare discharges and administrative data to provide national rates of AEs. The system focuses on patient harm rather than error; the well-being and perspective of the patient is the primary consideration (Hunt et al., n.d.). The particular AEs that are of interest to MPSMS are selected from prioritized patient safety topics compiled by the Agency for Healthcare Research and Quality (AHRQ). MPSMS was initiated in the year 2000 and it continues as a chart review–based surveillance system to provide rates for 21 selected measures of advanced events, including some hospital-acquired conditions (**TABLE 10-1**). In 2014, the MPSMS national sample drew from over 1,100 hospitals and included about 20,000 medical records (Brady, 2016).

AHRQ is working to replace MPSMS with a new system, the Quality and Safety Review System (QSRS) (Eldridge, 2016). MPSMS is recognized as old and impractical for use beyond Centers for Medicare & Medicaid Services' Clinical Data Abstraction Center. The system does not cover some important hospital-associated conditions including other adverse drug events such as opioid and allergy-related incidents, venous thromboembolic events in nonsurgical patients, surgical site infections, and some obstetric and neonatal events (Eldridge, 2016).

The QSRS system is designed to use clinical information from medical records and will also use other reliable, structured data. The new system will generate AE rates, trend performance over time, and will also serve as a local hospital and health system tool to identify and measure AEs (AHRQ, 2017). Among other features, the QSRS will also capture an "all-cause harm" measurement that can be used to better

TABLE 10-1 MPSMS Measures

Adverse Drug Events

Drug Name	Digoxin Hypoglycemic agents Intravenous heparin Low-molecular-weight heparin Warfarin

Hospital-Acquired Infections

Infection Type	*Clostridium difficile* infection Catheter-associated urinary tract infections Central venous catheter–associated bloodstream infections Methicillin-resistant *Staphylococcus aureus* (MRSA) infection in a sterile site Vancomycin-resistant enterococci (VRE) in a sterile site Ventilator-associated pneumonia

Surgical/Procedure-Related Events

Surgery/Procedure Type	Postoperative cardiac event (in cardiac and noncardiac surgery patients) Postoperative venous thromboembolic patient Postoperative pneumonia Adverse events after hip replacement Adverse events after knee replacement Adverse events after femoral artery puncture for angiography Nephropathy associated with contrast dye Mechanical adverse effects associated with central venous catheter placement

Patient Care/General Events

Event Type	Falls Pressure ulcers

Data from AHRQ. (2014). Retrieved January 4, 2018, from https://www.ahrq.gov/professionals/quality-patient-safety/pfp/methods.html

target and measure quality improvement efforts. Taxonomy will be standardized and consistent with definitions and algorithms used by the AHRQ Common Formats for Event Reporting, so that events can be compared and terms can be refined to share a consistent meaning across agencies and institutions (AHRQ, 2017).

The IHI's (2009) GTT identifies AEs (harm) and measures the rate of these harmful events over time. Its methodology is a retrospective review of randomly selected inpatient hospital records that looks for triggers to identify possible AEs. An important caveat is that the GTT does not intend to identify every single AE within an individual record. Its particular benefit is that AEs over time can be tracked to determine whether AEs are reduced over time in response to improvement efforts (IHI, 2009).

The GTT has been used in hundreds of hospitals around the world. IHI provides a white paper, now in its second edition, that advanced nurses can use to better understand the background of the measurement tool, including the severity ratings and trigger selections. The white paper is a comprehensive resource that provides a "nuts and bolts" review of the tool and the instructions necessary for correct use.

IHI's GTT is a highly recognized tool for measuring harm trends; however, it is a manual method that requires expert reviewers and it can be challenging to secure the reviewers given the varied and challenging responsibilities facing most providers (Martin et al., 2016). The best accepted method to determine harm is the full manual chart review; however, this technique requires highly skilled health professionals to review medical records and identify harm that has occurred to patients as a result of care (Martin et al., 2016). A manual review comes with concerns about availability of trained and skilled professionals as well as the costs associated with such intense review.

Another harm tracking option is voluntary incident reporting; however, voluntary reporting requires a strong safety culture and generally does not yield the number of AEs that have likely occurred (Mortaro et al., 2017). Typical event reporting systems identify approximately 10% to 20% of AEs (Edwards, 2017; IHI, 2018) and of these reported events, 90% to 95% cause no harm to patients. As a result, there was an identified need for a more effective measure to identify incidents that are harmful to patients so that changes could be selected and tested, and harm could be reduced. This need motivated IHI to develop the first Trigger Tool. With time came changes, and the IHI Trigger Tool is the result of multiple combinations of tools into a single tool that measures harm at the hospital system level (IHI, 2018). The IHI GTT provides three measures: (1) AEs per 1,000 patient days; (2) AEs per 100 admissions, and (3) percent of admissions with an AE (IHI, 2018).

If an advanced nurse practices at a hospital that uses the GTT or is considering its use, understanding possible limitations is important. Mortaro et al. (2017) implemented the Italian version of the GTT and evaluated efforts to improve interrater reliability over time. Mortaro et al. (2017) noted that there is substantial variation in measured harm rates as reported by different review teams and that only moderate agreement has been found. Mortaro et al. (2017) explored whether continuous training and crafting specific review guidelines would improve the interrater reliability. Study findings confirmed that combining training with a more structured review process did enhance reliability. Advanced nurses may need to advocate for a more structured, training-intensive approach when implementing IHI's GTT.

Walsh et al. (2017) address reliability issues in harm measurement by using a generalizability theory framework to estimate the impact of the number, experience, and provider type of raters on reliability. Walsh et al.'s (2017) examination of reliability was not specific to the GTT but rather lends support to the available evidence describing the high variability of clinician AE severity ratings. Physicians, nurses, and pharmacists served as the raters. Findings revealed that pharmacists were more precise in their ratings than physicians and nurses. High experience raters were more precise than medium or low experience raters; however, if the number of raters was increased, two medium or low experienced raters would be more precise than a single experienced rater. When the number of raters was increased from one to two raters, the ratings' reliability increased (Walsh et al., 2017). This study was not specific to the GTT but it serves as a interesting reminder to advanced nurses that the "who" underlying reviews and the number of them may make a difference in reliability. Additionally, training and structured review sessions to share perspectives are likely worth the time and effort.

Harm measures are critically important to quality improvement efforts, including those efforts in which advanced nurses lead and participate. Zero preventable harm is the long-term goal and there has been some progress, albeit very slow in coming. Some suspect that it is an unrealistic goal that is not achievable (Edwards, 2017). Perhaps in response to this lack of meaningful progress on the provider and system input side, there is an increasing push to involve patients in harm reduction and safety strategies. Patients are increasingly being asked to monitor health care providers' (HCPs) consistent follow-through with infection prevention procedures such as handwashing (Pittet et al., 2011). Many safety projects emphasize patients' responsibilities regarding safe medication use practices and emphasize the patient's role in making certain that medications provided by health care professionals or other caregivers are correct.

Research findings suggest that patients may not be comfortable with self-advocacy, particularly when it involves confronting physicians (Davis, Briggs, Arora, Moss, & Schwappach, 2014). Patients are generally more comfortable challenging nurses than physicians, perhaps, in part, because nurses may also be more receptive to this kind of feedback. A cross-sectional factorial survey study was designed to explore HCPs' attitudes toward patients' participation in efforts to prevent possible medication errors and remind providers of missed handwashing efforts. Data were collected from physicians and nurses working in four different inner-city hospitals in London. The participants responded to vignettes developed around the two scenarios. HCPs (N = 216) responded favorably to the patient interventions, although less positively toward the hand hygiene error than the medication error vignette. HCP responses were influenced by the communication style of the patients; confrontational communication was less supported by HCPs (Davis et al., 2014).

Davis et al. (2014) suggest that patients appear reluctant to participate in behaviors that they perceive as undercutting the clinical skills and expertise of HCPs. Advanced nurses need to consider patient and family-focused harm reduction programs as potential opportunities to support a more inclusive approach to safety and harm prevention efforts, particularly needed since patients tend to have only a passive and marginal role in health care systems' safety agendas. Patients need to feel supported in order to feel comfortable with asking questions and advocating for quality care. Advanced nurses have responsibility for guiding patients toward self-advocacy so that they can contribute to harm-free care.

Acknowledging Harm and Disclosing Errors to Patients

When patients experience harm as a result of preventable AEs, they experience distress, particularly when providers and agents of the institution are less than forthcoming about the cause(s) of the event (Harrison et al., 2015). A systematic review of patients' experiences of AEs in health care was conducted using the Preferred Reporting Items for Systematic Reviews and Meta-Analyses (PRISMA) statement. Extracted studies were assessed using the Quality Assessment Tool for Studies with Diverse Designs. Studies (N = 33) that satisfied the eligibility requirements were selected for review (Harrison et al., 2015). Most studies were not informed by a theory or conceptual model. Other limitations included the lack of power analyses or sample size justifications and lack of rationale for chosen data collection tools.

Findings revealed that patients view AEs differently than health professionals who often interpreted the patients' perceived AEs as misunderstandings rather than mistakes (Harrison et al., 2015). Most AEs experienced as such by patients were not included in the medical record, ostensibly because the provider did not share the belief that an AE had occurred. At times, patients described their event experience rather than discussing whether the harm was preventable (Harrison et al., 2015). Studies also addressed perceived harm resulting from AEs, including physical, financial, and/ or psychological. The studies reported on varying types of AEs.

Harrison et al. (2015) found that medication errors and communication problems are high-frequency occurrences across a range of health care settings. Patients are aware when events go wrong and their knowledge of events could be useful to prevent further harm events; however, their input is rarely solicited and is often not included in medical records. The researchers point out that there is a need to further investigate patients' experiences with AE. They recommend that experiential data should be routinely collected to inform a comprehensive understanding.

Advanced nurses should consider error disclosure as a component of an organizational culture that values safety and transparency. Although patients want to be informed of errors, regardless of whether harm or risk is involved, few are provided with this information, in part because providers are not trained to disclose errors to patients (Etchegaray, Gallagher, Bell, Sage, & Thomas, 2017). IHI offers a number of tools, including case studies, selected bibliography, strategies for involving patients in root-cause and system failure analyses, and other resources related to error disclosure (**TABLE 10-2**).

TABLE 10-2   Select IHI Resources for Building Error Disclosure Expertise

Title	Type of Resource	Website Address (Retrieved January 8, 2018)
The Wrong Shot: Error Disclosure (AHRQ)	Case Study	http://www.ihi.org/education /IHIOpenSchool/resources/Pages /Activities/AHRQCaseStudyWrong ShotErrorDisclosure.aspx
Respectful Management of Serious Clinical Adverse Events	White Paper plus three tools to guide practice	http://www.ihi.org/resources/Pages /IHIWhitePapers/RespectfulMan- agementSeriousClinicalAEsWhite- Paper.aspx
When Things Go Wrong: Responding to Adverse Events	Consensus Statement of the Harvard Hospitals	http://www.ihi.org/resources /Pages/Publications/When ThingsGoWrongRespondingto AdverseEvents.aspx
Including Patients in Root Cause and System Failure Analysis: Legal and Psychological Implications	Publication	http://www.ihi.org/resources/Pages /Publications/IncludingPatients RootCauseSystemFailureAnalysis .aspx

The Impact of Adverse Events on Providers

Adverse events are *unintentionally* harmful to patients. Harm may be experienced as temporary or permanent, including fatal. Some AEs are the result of errors caused by acts of commission (doing something wrong) or omission (failing to do the right thing). Preventable AEs are the result of either an error or a failure to enact a prevention strategy. Ameliorable AEs are likely not preventable, but the patient could have experienced less resultant harm if the care response had been different (PSNet, 2017). An example of an ameliorable AE is when a patient with no known drug allergies receives a necessary intravenous antibiotic for the first time and experiences anaphylaxis but the provider response to this shock event was slow and disorganized leading to transfer to an intensive care unit and postanaphylaxis complications. In this situation, the anaphylaxis could not have been predicted; however, the care response to this unanticipated event should have been rapid and organized to avoid or minimize temporary or permanent patient harm.

AEs and errors impact patients and HCPs, particularly those directly connected to the incident. Experienced advanced nurses likely recognize that many errors are unreported by the responsible provider, typically those that do not cause obvious patient harm, and near-miss events are also underreported. In part, this underreporting is likely due to a fear of possible consequences, including reputation damage, fear of professional reprisals, lawsuit risks, and other worries. A significant number of errors are associated with medication use systems, including medication prescription and administration. Wolf, Serembus, Smetzer, Cohen, and Cohen (2000) explored the responses and concerns of HCPs to medication errors almost 20 years ago, and it is somewhat discouraging that their findings have continued relevance to the current practice environment.

Wolf et al. (2000) observed that "providers make mistakes that have human consequences" (p. 278) and that suffering related to these errors is not confined to patients and families but also to the involved provider(s). Wolf et al. (2000) conducted a descriptive, correlational study to explore the responses and concerns of HCPs to making medication mistakes and to determine the relationship of these factors with estimated patient harm. Most study subjects (N = 402), medical doctors, professional nurses, and pharmacists recalled that they feared that patients experienced more harm post error than they actually had experienced. They felt guilty, worried, and nervous in response to medication errors, and they were also fearful for the patient. Providers were haunted by the errors that led to fatality or permanent harm.

A secondary analysis of the Wolf et al. (2000) study data focused on the providers (N = 11) involved in fatal medication errors (Serembus, Wolf, & Youngblood, 2001). The average number of years elapsed since the fatal error had occurred was 22.7. After the error, subjects acknowledged reactions that in order of highest to lowest frequency included: wanting to make amends, immobilized, nervous, fearful, unable to sleep, denial, cried, lost confidence, and other reactions. Their predominant fears centered around concerns for the patient followed by fears of license suspension, judgment of incompetence by coworkers, fear of license loss, and other noteworthy dreads and uncertainties (Serembus et al., 2001).

These exemplars offer support for the premise that HCPs suffer when errors occur, and their suffering is prolonged, intense, and detrimental to their state of well-being when the inflicted harm of the AE is life altering or life ending for the patient. *Just Culture* was popularized around the year 2000 when patient safety experts began to emphasize the importance of a nonblame, nonpunitive approach to error response (ANA, 2010a). Although incremental progress is evident within and across health care delivery systems toward providers who are involved in AEs, including medication errors that cause harm, there is evidence that work must continue to support affected providers.

Winning et al. (2018) explored the emotional impact of errors or AEs on HCPs practicing in a neonatal intensive care unit and the potentially moderating effect of coworker support. The cross-sectional online survey was completed by HCPs (N = 463) that assessed respondents' experiences with AE or error and their anxiety, depression, professional quality of life, and coworker support (Winning et al., 2018). The neonatal intensive care unit serves a particularly vulnerable population and, as a result, there is little margin for error and low patient tolerance for mistakes.

Data were collected via the hospital anxiety and depression scale (HADS), professional quality of life questionnaire (ProQOL), and the survey of perceived coworker support (SPCS). Each measure had established reliability (Winning et al., 2018). A majority of respondents were registered nurses (RNs) (n = 311) followed by nurse practitioners (NPs) (n = 40). Findings revealed that providers who observed or were involved in an error or AE self-reported significantly more anxiety, depression, burnout, and secondary traumatic stress than those who did not directly or indirectly experience a mistake or AE. Winning et al. (2018) found through post hoc analyses that when coworker support was low, errors or AEs were associated with higher levels of anxiety or depression than when this support was high. Colleagues' support was not found to influence compassion satisfaction, burnout, or secondary traumatic stress.

Winning et al. (2018) acknowledged that the study findings were limited by several possible concerns including the use of self-report that may have been influenced by social desirability bias and a majority of white, female nurses as respondents. Nonetheless, the study supports that AEs and errors continue to have a persistent negative effect on HCPs, including anxiety and depression, and suggests that coworker support is critical.

Recognizing and Responding to the Legal Ramifications of Real and Perceived Harm and Error

Advanced nurses recognize that there is liability risk secondary to AEs and errors, actual or perceived, which have occurred during a care event that has yielded less than desirable outcomes so far as the patient is concerned. Malpractice and negligence claims are real and frequent events when AEs occur that have led to unintended harms. Patient perceptions of poor quality of care, particularly when coupled with the belief that HCPs have been dishonest or not forthcoming, can certainly lead to lawsuits.

Just cultures, quality measurement and improvement activities, and other efforts to ensure safe, excellent care assist in mitigating legal risks. Adelman and Allen (2014) offer additional suggestions that are unique to assisted living communities but by extension have relevance to other types of health care settings. One caution is for HCPs and administrators to avoid inconsistencies between admission assessments and the provided level of care that the resident is assigned to receive. Adelman and Allen (2014) advise that there should not be inconsistencies between the resident's condition, any changes in this condition, and ongoing assessment findings within the context of the provided care arrangements. Discussions with team members should be documented and all paperwork or electronic record keeping should be complete and accurate. Advanced nurses may need to consider these same sorts of recommendations specific to hospitalized patients. When care demands change and nursing care needs increase, it is imperative that records reflect an appropriate response from HCPs to place the patient in a situation that is able to meet the increasingly complex care needs that have been assessed by care professionals.

Adelman and Allen (2014) note that liability risks increase when residents remain in assisted living facilities that cannot provide appropriate care. This same risk is incurred when hospitalized patients remain in units that are not staffed or resourced to meet the acute or rapidly changing needs of the patient exhibiting condition deterioration. Staffing adequacy and ratios need to be regularly monitored and adjusted as patient needs change.

One interesting recommendation is to review marketing materials, Internet advertisements, admission agreements, and resident handbooks to ensure consistency of terms and to make certain that promises meet level of services and opportunities that are available (Adelman & Allen, 2014). This suggestion is readily applied to assisted living facilities given their wide variability in terms of amenities and care provision options but may be less obviously connected to hospitals. However, many hospitals advertise services and amenities in marketing materials, Web-based advertisements, and radio announcements that suggest a particular level of guaranteed quality of care.

These risk-reducing strategies may be useful for advanced nurses to keep in mind as they work with colleagues to draft unit-based descriptions of nursing routines, family options, discharge planning commitments, and other commitments that patients come to expect. They also point out how important it is for policies, procedures, and institutional standards of care to match deliverables. Of course, legal risks and litigation efforts will continue in health care and advanced nurses need to know how to appropriately and wisely respond. The next section of the chapter addresses these needs and offers information to advanced nurses interested in developing business opportunities as legal nurse consultants and also those nurses in need of a good, basic understanding of the legal process when plaintiffs submit complaints about care.

PART TWO

Responding to Legal Charges: Malpractice, Negligence, and Claims of Harm

Joanne Farley Serembus, EdD, RN, CCRN (Alumnus), CNE

Advanced role nurses are at the forefront of care and, therefore, need to protect themselves and coworkers against the risk of being sued for malpractice. Nurses account for 2% of all medical malpractice payments, according to the National Practitioner Data Bank, operated by the U.S. Department of Health and Human Services (USDHHS, n.d.). While once a rarity, over the last 10 years, malpractice suits against nurses have been on the rise. Nurses may find themselves named in a suit against the facility for which they work and could potentially be named as individual defendants. The latter is quickly becoming a trend (Relias, 2016). Nurses in all roles need to be aware of the risks involved and how to prevent them.

▶ Negligence and Malpractice

Negligence is defined as doing something or failing to do something that a prudent, careful, and reasonable nurse would do or not do in the same or similar situation. Negligence also generally refers to acts or failures to act that are unintentional rather than intentional (Mathes & Reifsnyder, 2014). Professional malpractice is a form of negligence and refers to negligence committed in carrying out professional duties (Jacoby & Scruth, 2017). *Malpractice* is negligence, misconduct, or breach of duty by a professional person that results in injury or damage to a patient. In most cases, it includes failure to meet a standard of care or failure to deliver care that a reasonably prudent nurse would deliver in a similar situation (Reising, 2007). To prove a claim for malpractice, the following elements must be met: (1) the existence of a legal duty on the part of the nurse, (2) breach of that duty, (3) causal relationship between the breach of duty and injury to patient, and (4) the existence of damages flowing from the injury (Bal, 2009). The burden for proving malpractice lies with the plaintiff.

Common Types of Malpractice

Some of the most common types of medical malpractice claims against nurses include (1) failure to follow standards of care, (2) failure to communicate properly, (3) failure to document thoroughly, (4) failure to assess and monitor a patient, (5) failure to use equipment in a responsible manner, and (6) failure to delegate properly (Croke, 2003; Reising, 2007) (**TABLE 10-3**).

Standards of care are established to protect patients from substandard nursing practice. Standards of care provide criteria for determining whether a nurse has breached a duty in the care owed to the patient. These include an agency's policies and procedures, agency protocols, the state boards of nursing (BONs) and professional

TABLE 10-3 Nursing Malpractice Vignettes	
Medication Error	Mr. A is ordered to receive his clonidine (Catapres) tablet 0.1 mg by mouth for hypertension. The nurse mistakenly administers 3 tablets (0.3 mg total) and the patient's blood pressure drops leading to cardiac arrest. Due to the combination with other medications and patient comorbidities, he dies.
Failure to Use Equipment Correctly	Mr. T is receiving continuous tube feedings via a small-bore silicone feeding tube. The nurse measures the distance from the tip of the tube to the patient's nose and notes that the measurement is several centimeters greater than documented on the previous shift. She takes the guide wire and reinserts it to place the tube further into the gastrointestinal tract. Several hours later, the patient becomes extremely short of breath, arrests, and dies. Subsequent postmortem examination reveals that the feeding tube guide wire punctured the esophagus and bronchus with the enteral feeding infusing into the patient's left lung.

TABLE 10-3 Nursing Malpractice Vignettes	*(continued)*
Failure to Notify Physician	Ms. F is admitted with acute abdominal pain and is treated for diverticulosis. She is ordered to receive intravenous fluids and be NPO by the physician. The patient complains of nausea and increasing abdominal distention over 3 days. The patient complains on day 4 of vomiting several times during the night; however, the patient did not save the emesis for the nurse to assess and did not notify the nurse at the time of the events. Later that day, the patient is so distended she is unable to lay in bed and must sit up in a chair. Her abdomen is noted to be hard, distended, and with absent bowel sounds. The physician is not notified. Later that day, the patient has projectile vomiting leading to aspiration and dies 24 hours later.
Lack of Timely Monitoring of Patient	Mrs. L is a patient with type II diabetes admitted to the hospital for an unrelated diagnosis. She recently experienced a hypoglycemia event requiring treatment with glucagon IM several times. The physician has ordered fingerstick blood glucose monitoring every 2 hours. The nursing documentation records a blood glucose at 2 AM = 90 mg/dL and blood glucose at 4 AM = 70 mg/dL. The nurse did not measure the 6 AM blood glucose. The patient is found unconscious at 9 AM with a fingerstick blood glucose of 35 mg/dL. She experiences a seizure and is transferred to the intensive care unit after being administered glucagon intravenously. The patient never recovers and dies 2 days later.
Failure to Document	Mrs. S is 2 days post hysterectomy. While placing the thromboembolic stockings on the patient, the nurse notes the right calf to be swollen and reddened. She notifies the physician who instructs her to proceed with the patient orders as written. The patient is ambulated three times that day and at 8 PM complains of chest pain and shortness of breath. The patient is diagnosed with a pulmonary embolus and transferred to intensive care. The physician denies receiving the call earlier in the day regarding the change in the patient's status. The nurse did not document the phone call to the physician and resultant orders to continue care as previously ordered. The nurse is named in a lawsuit brought by the patient several months later.
Failure to Delegate Properly	A registered nurse (RN) delegates the administration of an intermittent intravenous antibiotic dose via a subclavian central line access to the licensed practical nurse (LPN) with whom she is working. The RN is busy caring for another critically ill patient when the LPN tells her that the medication is not properly infusing. The RN asks the LPN to flush the intravenous access, anticipating that this intervention would facilitate the infusion. The LPN returns to the RN after 10 minutes stating that she pushed 10 mL of normal saline and had to push very hard. Since doing so, the patient "turned blue" and is "short of breath." The patient later codes and is noted to have a pulmonary embolism and dies. The RN failed to delegate the right task (intravenous push of fluid), to the right person (LPN), in the right circumstances (critically ill patient receiving intravenous infusions). This error in judgment was compounded by not providing adequate supervision.

nursing associations, and guidelines from federal organizations such as the Joint Commission (TJC) and the Centers for Disease Control and Prevention (CDC).

Communication issues arise when a nurse fails to communicate changes in a patient's status in a timely manner or fails to relay all patient information about the patient to the physician. Nurses can also flounder when they do not provide a full report to the oncoming nurse or nurse covering for them during a break. Additionally, nurses are relied upon to provide ample instruction upon patient discharge. Sometimes, these conversations are not documented, making it difficult to prove that they took place. On occasion, failure to communicate can cause or contribute to failure to act on a patient condition leading to a patient's demise.

Clear, accurate, and accessible documentation is an essential element of safe, high quality, evidence-based nursing practice. The purpose of documentation is to communicate patient information among HCPs. Lack of proper documentation of events in the care of patients or their response to treatment can set a nurse up for possible lawsuit. Documentation is depended upon as evidence of nursing assessment and diagnosis, the plan of nursing care, along with its implementation and evaluation of patient responses. Nurses' notes with few explanations, little description of key findings, or no mention of periodic patient checks could be construed as negligence by a court on the frequently shared nursing adage that "if it is not documented, it was not done." High-quality documentation is also timely, contemporaneous, and sequential as well as legible/readable particularly in terms of the resolution related to qualities of the electronic health record (EHR) as it is displayed on the screens of various devices (ANA, 2010b).

Constant monitoring and assessment of a patient's condition is an important responsibility of nursing practice. It is not appropriate to simply follow unit protocol or a physician's order to assess and obtain vital signs. When the patient's condition warrants more frequent assessment and monitoring, it is the nurse who decides to increase that frequency. This is most important as changes in the health status of a patient can be gradual or sudden and nurses are usually the first to take note of these and act (Croke, 2003).

Failure to use equipment in a responsible manner hinges on the nurse being aware of the safety features, capabilities, and limitations of any equipment they use. Nurses should not modify equipment from the specifications of the manufacturers' usage recommendations. Additionally, nurses need to be aware of an agency's policies regarding their use of certain equipment as well as their nurse practice act and guidelines. Nurses may not be permitted, for example, to insert a small-bore gastric tube using a stylet or reposition a Swan-Ganz catheter. These tasks may be beyond their purview.

Finally, nurses may fail to delegate nursing tasks appropriately. One of the most complex nursing skills is delegation. Delegation requires sophisticated clinical judgment and final accountability for patient care. Effective delegation is based on one's state nurse practice act and an understanding of the concepts of responsibility, authority, and accountability. Nurses delegate care to other RNs, licensed practical/vocational nurses, and unlicensed personnel. When delegating tasks to others, nurses must consider the five rights of delegation: (1) right task, (2) right circumstances, (3) right person, (4) right communication, and (5) right supervision/evaluation.

In 2006, the ANA and the National Council of State Boards of Nursing (NCSBN) issued a joint statement on delegation. This joint statement is very helpful to advanced nurses as it offers principles to follow for delegation and includes overarching principles, nurse-related principles, and organization-related principles. Most importantly, a decision tree for delegation to nursing assistive personnel is provided. In early 2015, the NCSBN convened two panels of experts representing education, research, and practice. The goal was to develop national guidelines based on current research and literature to facilitate and standardize the nursing delegation process. These guidelines provide direction for employers, nurse leaders, staff nurses, and care delegates by building on the earlier works of ANA and NCSBN (NCSBN, 2016).

Medical Malpractice Insurance

The most common question nurses have is whether they should carry medical malpractice insurance. Many nurses depend on the insurance carried by the employing institution. The danger in doing so is that they usually do not know whether they are named individually in the institution's insurance policy and for what amount. The policy may not fully cover the expenses incurred. Unfortunately, if the judgment against the nurse is more than the available on-the-job insurance coverage, the nurse must pay from savings, liens on certain properties, possible wage garnishment, or future inheritance (Collins, 2002). The nurse also may not have followed agency policy or protocol or acted within his or her scope of practice. In these instances, the institution may decide not to cover the nurse. An institution's medical malpractice insurance usually provides an attorney; however, this attorney represents the hospital. This is usually not an issue except the nurse needs to understand that this attorney has the hospital's best interest at the forefront (Pohlman, 2015).

Professional liability insurance typically pays for a defense attorney and any settlement or judgment against the nurse, up to the policy limits. Depending on the policy, the added benefit is that this will often cover licensure defense if the nurse is reported to the board of nursing. Few employer policies offer this benefit and it covers attorney fees and expenses when the nurse faces an investigation or disciplinary charges by the licensing board. When nurses have private malpractice insurance, the company provides an attorney to represent their individual interests. Some policies even allow nurses to choose their own attorneys. When covered by both their own and an employer's policies, the two insurance companies coordinate representation, benefits, and allocation of claim costs and any indemnity or settlement payments (Oliver, 2016).

How to Proceed if Sued

A nurse who is being sued will receive a summons sent via a courier service representing the plaintiff's attorney and directly placed in hand while at work or at home. Immediately after receiving the summons, the nurse should contact the liability insurance company. If the nurse is still employed at the institution where the incident occurred, notification should be made to that institution. Once these notifications are made, the nurse will be contacted by the law firm representing the institution and/or the attorney providing representation as determined by the liability insurance company. Nurses not having medical malpractice insurance should hire their own attorney (Larson & Elliott, 2009).

The attorneys defending the nurse may ask that the nurse complete written documentation regarding the event and names of any witnesses that he or she recalls. If the nurse kept private notes from the time of the event detailing the incident, these notes are considered discoverable and the nurse will most likely be required to hand them over to the defense attorney. It is important to know that such notes can be used against the nurse. Finally, it is extremely important that the nurse not discuss the case with anyone except his or her attorney (Reising, 2007).

Steps of a Malpractice Case

Once the nurse has been served with a summons and met with the attorney, a deposition is arranged. A deposition is taken under oath in the form of a question-and-answer session called an *interrogatory*. The interrogatory is led by the opposing attorney. This session is recorded by a court reporter, transcribed, and kept confidential. Any information given during the deposition is admissible during a trial (Larson & Elliott, 2009). Questions that the nurse can expect to answer include current address, credentials, current place of employment, any past employment, education, certifications, and possibly information about the unit in which the incident occurred and the staff working during that time. Specific questions involving policies and procedures, agency orientation, inservices, or continuing education that focus on the issue at hand may be asked. The nurse should prepare by reviewing the medical records involved in the case and practicing a line of questioning with his or her attorney.

Once *discovery* is completed and all data have been gathered, both the plaintiff and defendant attorneys determine the next steps of the lawsuit. Some states require mediation as a next step, others do not. The defendant's attorney may settle with the plaintiff for monetary payment, referred to as damages, thus avoiding trial. The decision to settle a case is a business one made between the attorneys and does not involve the defendant. The defendant should remember that a settlement is by no means an admission of guilt (Larson & Elliott, 2009).

If the case results in a trial, the nurse's attorney will prepare the nurse to take the stand. While a deposition can be stress provoking, a trial can be even more so as it involves jurors, a judge, and the complainant. At the deposition, the nurse sits with the representing attorney at a table with other attorneys asking questions. If the nurse has been sued as an individual, daily trial attendance is required. The jury is continuously observing the nurse and the nurse must act accordingly, including attention to professional dress and behavior. The nurse will be cautioned not to speak with anyone who may be a juror. The attorney should take the nurse to the court room ahead of time to become familiar with the setting (Butler & Lostritto, 2015). Whenever a claim filed against a nurse is settled or receives a trial judgment, it is best that the nurse shares this information with any future employers rather than have them obtain the information from the National Practitioner Data Bank (Resnick & Guarino, 2001).

Impact of a Malpractice Suit

One of the least discussed issues regarding a malpractice suit is the psychological impact that it can have for the defendant. Termed *medical malpractice stress syndrome*, this response includes psychological and physical symptoms. Psychological symptoms can include feelings of guilt, anxiety, depression, poor self-image, and anger. Isolation sets in especially since the nurse has been told not to speak to anyone regarding the case. A feeling of shame is particular to the sued individual in the medical field and is cited in several research studies on medical errors. Larson and Elliot (2010) state that the emotional stages of malpractice follow a common theme and are dynamic with the defendant moving back and forth on a continuum. Physical complaints often manifest as gastrointestinal disturbances, headaches, and fatigue (Ryll, 2015).

Coping strategies for adequately dealing with this stress syndrome include seeking out a psychologist or therapist. As opposed to a spouse or other confidant, discussions with the licensed professional, such as a counselor, are protected by client-provider privilege. Taking an active role in the malpractice case by keeping up to date with the progress of the case can help to ease anxiety and help the nurse to feel more in control of the situation. Participating in regular physical activities, sports, or other leisure activities also helps alleviate the stress experience (Larson & Elliott, 2010).

Preventing Malpractice Lawsuits

Nurses can protect themselves from malpractice lawsuits by doing the following: (1) refuse assignments and tasks that cannot be performed safely, (2) delegate safely, (3) obtain clear orders, (4) provide a safe patient and work environment, (5) follow agency policies and procedures, (6) administer medications safely, (7) provide accurate and complete documentation, and (8) establish good nurse-patient relationships.

Much has been written in the nursing literature about the lack of information provided to nurses on legal issues. Pappas, Clutter, and Maggi (2007) describe a legal seminar for undergraduate nursing students with seven key areas: (1) emancipation of a minor, (2) hospital lawsuits, (3) nurse malpractice and the attorney, (4) liability of nurse managers, (5) physician's orders, (6) nursing charting and technology, and (7) end-of-life authorizations. The program was evaluated as successful by the faculty and students. The goal was to help graduate nurses think more critically and provide optimum nursing care. Having been exposed to current legal information in the seminar, it was thought that students would have a deeper insight into identifying the accurate legal issue pertaining to complicated patient care situations. These strategies can be further enhanced through the use of case scenarios, role play, and simulation.

Reaching the practicing nurse has long been a problem; however, Nellis and George (2012) explored the use of a self-paced educational module. They investigated knowledge acquisition about medical malpractice and litigation and assessed learner satisfaction with the self-paced module as an alternative to traditional educational models. The program assessment survey indicated that the educational module provided content in a format that was valuable to the participants. More importantly, after the use of the module, participant total mean knowledge scores showed a statistically significant increase from pre- to posttest. Educating nursing students and practicing nurses is one way to potentially reduce malpractice events while supporting the nursing profession.

▶ Role of the Nurse Expert

The nurse, practicing in an advanced role with a graduate degree and nationally recognized credentials, may be called upon by a law firm to render an expert opinion in a malpractice case. Nurse *experts* are those who have special education or experience about a professional matter in a case and are permitted to give their opinions regarding the matter. Nurse experts assist the judge and jury in understanding scientific evidence and standards of care (Grant, 2018a). An advanced nurse does not need to be certified as a legal nurse consultant or take courses in this area to render such opinions. Attorneys seek out nurse experts based on their area of clinical practice, degree of experience, and level and area of education. Basic requirements include the following: (1) licensed to practice as a RN, (2) registered to practice nursing in the state in which the incident occurred (preferable but not required), (3) credentials that are equal to or beyond those of the nurses involved in the case, and (4) no professional or private relationship with anyone involved with the case (Helm, 2003), and (5) certification in the practice area of nursing related to the case is preferred.

There is a difference between a witness and an expert witness. As a general rule, a *lay* witness (also called *fact* witness), as opposed to an *expert* witness, usually testifies as to facts and does not provide opinion. A jury, however, normally does not have extensive scientific knowledge pertaining to nursing issues. Because nursing activities commonly involve the exercise of professional judgment and the application of advanced knowledge, how the nurse deviated from the standard of care is often difficult for a jury to decide. An expert witness, therefore, is often used to assist the jury by offering an opinion as to whether the nurse committed malpractice. Specifically, expert testimony will be required to show the nursing standard of care, how the nurse deviated from or breached that standard, and how the nurse's breach in care caused the patient's harm.

Initial Legal Contact

An attorney initially contacts the nurse expert to present a brief summary of the main facts of the case in an attempt to learn if the nurse expert can support a particular side of the case. This is termed *finding* for the defense or the plaintiff named in the complaint. The advanced nurse must first learn if the law firm is representing the defendant or the plaintiff. The *plaintiff* is the party initiating a lawsuit and demanding damages, performance, and/or court determination of rights. The *defendant* is the party who denies or defends against a legal claim brought against them. In many instances there is more than one plaintiff or defendant. Advanced nurses must be very clear in communications with the attorney to specify that this is a preliminary opinion and a more informed one will be provided after review of pertinent medical records involved with the case. It is very important that the advanced nurse's opinion be objectively based on the aspects of the case and pertinent nursing standard of care. Only recently have courts recognized nurses as the appropriate health professional for offering expert opinion on nursing standards of care. Previously, this expert opinion could be offered by physicians.

Many state nurse practice acts now define nursing in broad and independent terms that do not depend on physicians or other HCPs. Additionally, the Illinois Supreme Court reviewed the evolving recognition of nurses' unique practice and concluded that a physician was not qualified to testify as to a nursing standard of care because he was not a nurse (*Sullivan v. Edward Hospital* 806 N.E.2d 645, 653-61 [Ill. 2004]). While this decision was specific to the Illinois statutory and judicial context, it is fairly characterized as "judicial recognition [of] nurses' long-time assertion that nursing is an independent profession with a unique body of knowledge" (Cohen, Rosen, & Barbacci, 2008, p. 5). In 2006, the American Association of Legal Nurse Consultants (AALNC) published a position paper stating, "Nurses are uniquely prepared to perform a critical review and analysis of clinical nursing care and administrative nursing practice to provide the foundation for testifying on nursing negligence issues" (p. 1).

TABLE 10-4 Fee Schedule	
Charge Description	**Fee**
Clinical Evaluation, Research, Review of Patient/Client-Related Materials, Record Chronology, Case History, Telephone Time, Report Preparation	$150/hour
Preparation for Trial/Deposition	$250/hour
Deposition (for Trial or *de bene esse*)	$250/hour [2 hour Retainer Fee required]
Trial Testimony	$2,000 per day $1,000 per ½ day [$500 Retainer Fee required]
Travel Expenses (Personal Travel by Car to Courtroom, Deposition Site, or Evaluation Location)	$50/hour; $0.50 mile if driving
Lodging and Meal Expenses	Reimbursed at Actual Cost

Following the preliminary discussion, the attorney will usually request a current curriculum vitae (CV) and fee schedule. The CV serves as documentation of the advanced nurse's clinical expertise, experience, and education. Include any publications and research as these may further support content and practice expertise. Before being retained by the attorney, the CV and fee schedule will be shared with other involved parties (e.g., malpractice insurance provider for the defendant) for prior approval. The fee schedule includes review of client-related materials, development of chronology of events, research conducted, clinical analysis, and report preparation (**TABLE 10-4**). Additional fees for conference calls, preparation for trial or deposition, as well as actual trial and travel expenses are to be included. Some experts have difficulty collecting payment in a timely manner, so it is acceptable to request partial payment ahead of time in the form of a *retainer*. The fees charged may be different from those provided in Table 10-4 as they should be based on the advanced nurse's specialty area, level of education, and experience. In this situation, it is best to contact others within the relevant professional network for input.

Avoiding Conflict of Interest

A nurse expert should not be involved with a case if it involves a current or previous employer. If the expert work involves an institution from recent past experience, then the attorney involved in the case would need to be notified and permission obtained from the institution. Nurses and other HCPs are often mobile in their positions. Nurse experts may face situations in which they are asked to be involved in a case in which they know the defendant(s) or plaintiff(s). In such circumstances, they must recuse themselves. Nurse experts should avoid involvement with cases in other organizations within the same corporate umbrella in which they work. It is always important for nurse experts to provide unbiased and nonprejudiced opinions, and for this reason they should also consider personal beliefs that may taint a case (Creel & Robinson, 2010).

▶ Expert Review and Analysis

Record Keeping

The nurse expert should first review the complaint. The *complaint* is the initial document a plaintiff files with the clerk of court to begin a lawsuit. The complaint outlines the facts of the case, what the defendant(s) did wrong, and what the plaintiff is seeking in damages (typically the plaintiff seeks some sort of monetary compensation). The advanced nurse will also need to review additional documents, including medical records; agency policies and procedures; and depositions of HCPs, the patient, family members, and other pertinent individuals.

All records are delivered to experts either via mail or electronically. Most firms are moving toward electronic records with a passcode given for review and download. Keep a copy of downloaded records on a password-protected computer as well as a password-protected travel drive. These records are to be safeguarded until notice is received that the case has come to a resolution. A locked cabinet in a home office is a good place to keep paper records related to the case as well as travel drives. Electronic records are then deleted, and paper records are taken to a professional shredder whereby a receipt for payment is saved as proof that the records were safely destroyed. Paper records are never to be shredded at home or thrown into personal trash. It is important to recognize that all legal documents are confidential and in the case of medical records, the Health Insurance Portability and Accountability Act (HIPPA) legislation applies. The HIPAA 1996 provides data privacy and security provisions for safeguarding medical information (USDHHS, 2017). Furthermore, the nurse expert is not to discuss the case with anyone other than the attorneys involved with the case.

A case may be active for several years and so a system for record keeping needs to be set up ahead of time. As records are received, log these into the spreadsheet and save by case name and date received. This spreadsheet will also be useful when tracking conference calls with attorneys, invoices sent, and payment received. The log can be created in a Word document as a table or spreadsheet, depending on preference (**TABLE 10-5**).

Standards of Care

The nurse expert reviews the records to answer the following question: Did the nurse(s) in the case act as a nurse similarly trained in the same or similar circumstances would have acted? To answer this question, the expert nurse looks to the standards of care that nurses should follow. Standards of care are used as the basis for proving a breach of duty (Aiken & Warlick, 2010). It is very important that the reviewed standard of care be contemporaneous with the incident. Standards that have been enacted several years after the date of the incident do little to inform the analysis. Sources for the standards of care can be found in three main areas: legal and regulation sources, accreditation organizations, and authoritative sources (**TABLE 10-6**).

TABLE 10-5 Case Log*

Law Firm Case	Date In	Date Out	Conference Call #1 Date/Time	Conference Call #2 Date/Time	Invoice #1 Date Sent Date Paid	Invoice #2 Date Sent Date Paid	Date Resolved
Firm A Smith							
Firm A Dennis							
Firm B Doe							
Firm B Everly							
Firm C Morris							
Firm C Nance							

*Note: The table does not contain real information.

TABLE 10-6 Sources for Nursing Standards of Care*

Source	Website
Agency for Healthcare Research and Quality (AHRQ) Clinical Guidelines and Recommendations	https://www.ahrq.gov/professionals /clinicians-providers/guidelines -recommendations/index.html
American Association of Critical-Care Nurses (AACN) Scope and Standards for Acute and Critical Care Nursing Practice; AACN Scope and Standards for Acute Care Clinical Nurse Specialist Practice; AACN Scope and Standards for Acute Care Nurse Practitioner; AACN Tele-ICU Nursing Practice Guidelines	https://www.aacn.org/store /books/130300/aacn-scope-and-standards -for-acute-and-critical-care-nursing -practice; https://www.aacn.org/store/books /128110/aacn-scope-and-standards -for-acute-care-clinical-nurse-specialist -practice; https://www.aacn.org/store/books /128102/aacn-scope-and-standards -for-acute-care-nurse-practitioner -practice-2017; https://www.aacn.org/store/books/128115 /aacn-teleicu-nursing-practice-guidelines
American Association of Critical-Care Nurses Certification Corporation Certification for: Critical Care Nurse (Adult, Neonatal, Pediatric, Progressive Care, Cardiac Medicine); Cardiac Surgery; Acute Care NP; Acute Care CNS; Acute Care Neonatal CNS; Acute Care Pediatric CNS	https://www.aacn.org/certification /get-certified
American Association of Nurse Anesthetists (AANA) Scope of Nurse Anesthesia Practice; Standards for Nurse Anesthesia Practice	https://www.aana.com/practice
American Academy of Nurse Practitioners (AANP) Certification: Adult-Gerontology NP, Family NP, Emergency NP	http://www.aanpcert.org/
American Association of Nurse Practitioners (AANP) Scope of Practice; AANP Standards of Practice	https://www.aanp.org/images/documents
American College of Nurse Midwives Scope and Standards of Practice	http://www.midwife.org/index.asp?bid =59&cat=2&button=Search

Source	Website
American Heart Association (AHA) Guidelines for CPR; Advanced Cardiac Life Support	http://cpr.heart.org/AHAECC/CPRAndECC /ResuscitationScience/Guidelines /UCM_473201_Guidelines.jsp
American Midwifery Certification Board	http://www.amcbmidwife.org/
American Nurses Association (ANA) Code of Ethics for Nurses with Interpretive Statements	http://nursesbooks.org/Main-Menu/Ethics /Code-of-Ethics.aspx
American Nurses Association (ANA) Scope and Standards of Practice	http://nursesbooks.org/Main-Menu /Standards/Nursing-Scope-and-Standards -3rd-Ed.aspx
American Nurses Association (ANA) Scope and Standards of Practice (Multiple Specialties)	http://www.stopre.nursebooks.org /Main-Menu/Standards/
American Nurses Credentialing Center (ANCC) Certification: Adult-Gerontology Acute NP, Adult-Gerontology Primary NP, Family NP, Pediatric Primary NP, Psychiatric-Mental Health NP	http://www.nursecredentialing.org /Certification
American Psychiatric Nurses Association Scope and Standards of Practice	https://www.apna.org/i4a/pages/index .cfm?pageid=3342
Board of Certification for Emergency Nursing (CEN, BCEN)	http://www.bcencertifications.org/Get -Certified/CEN.aspx
Centers for Disease Control and Prevention (CDC) Guidelines	https://www.cdc.gov/infectioncontrol /guidelines/index.html
Emergency Nurses Association (ENA)	https://www.ena.org/
Joint Commission Standards	https://www.jointcommission.org /standards_information/standards.aspx;
Infusion Nurses Society; Infusion Therapy Standards of Practice	https://www.ins1.org/Store/ProductDetails .aspx?productId=113266
National Board of Certification and Recertification of Nurse Anesthetists (NBCRNA)	https://www.nbcrna.com/

(continues)

TABLE 10-6 Sources for Nursing Standards of Care*	*(continued)*
Source	**Website**
National Council of State Boards of Nursing (NCSBN) (This site is particularly useful for information on licensure compact states, delegation, substance abuse, use of social media.)	https://www.ncsbn.org/boards.htm
National League for Nursing Certification for Nurse Educators	http://www.nln.org/professional -development-programs /Certification-for-Nurse-Educators
National League for Nursing Scope of Practice for Academic Nurse Educators	http://www.nln.org/advocacy -public-policy/issues/scope-of-practice
Nurse Practice Acts, Rules & Regulations for Each State (see NCSBN)	https://www.ncsbn.org/nurse-practice-act .htm
Oncology Nursing Certification Board	https://www.oncc.org/
Oncology Nursing Society (ONS) Statement on the Scope and Standards of Oncology Nursing Practice: Generalist and Advanced Practice	https://www.ons.org/store/books /statement-scope-and-standards-oncology -nursing-practice-generalist-and -advanced-practice

*This listing of resources is not comprehensive and serves to provide select examples.

Legal and regulatory sources consist of the NCSBN and the nurse practice act applicable to the state in which the incident occurred. The nurse expert needs to be aware of the fact that other laws and regulations may impact practice, and other boards may play a role. Examples of these sorts of situations include (1) nurse midwives that may be regulated by a specific board of midwifery or public health, (2) nurse anesthetists with a scope of practice that may not be evident in the nurse practice act in all states, and (3) clinical nurse specialists without consistent title recognition across nurse practices. Given the variance in the inclusion of advanced practice regulations in nurse practice acts, it is vital that the nurse expert know where to access this information. This can be complicated by the fact that interpretation of specific acts, not evident conclusively in the nurse practice act, is provided by the regulatory body in the form of an opinion (ANA, 2017).

Specialty organizations provide documents such as position statements along with scope and standards of practice that can be helpful in defining the parameters of professional practice (**TABLE 10-7**). Certification organizations seek to protect the public by ensuring that certified individuals have met predetermined criteria for safety in practice. These organizations have standards that an individual must meet

TABLE 10-7 Select Specialty Organizations	
Name of Specialty Organizations	**Home Page Web Address**
American Academy of Nurse Practitioners	https://www.aanp.org/
American Association of Nurse Anesthetists	https://www.aana.com/
American Association of Critical Care Nurses	https://www.aacn.org/
Oncology Nursing Society	https://www.ons.org/
National Association of Pediatric Nurse Practitioners	https://www.napnap.org/
American Psychiatric Nurses Association	https://www.apna.org/i4a/pages /index.cfm?pageid=1
Academy of Medical Surgical Nurses	https://www.amsn.org/
National Association of Orthopedic Nurses	http://www.orthonurse.org/

to obtain and maintain certification (**TABLE 10-8**). All advanced nurses, particularly those serving as expert nurses, need to be familiar with the work products of relevant specialty organizations. It is also important to recognize nurse credentials and the eligibility requirements needed to sit for such an examination and to maintain the earned credential.

Some states have incorporated the Code of Ethics into their nurse practice acts. The District of Columbia amended their act in 2014 to read: "A [registered/practical] nurse shall adhere to the standards set forth in the 'Code of Ethics for Nurses' as published by the ANA, as they may be amended or republished from time to time" (Stokes, 2015, p. 6). As licensed professionals, nurses have a relationship with the state BONs that regulate nursing practice and protect the public by ensuring that the standards of nursing practice are met and that nurses are competent to practice. "Nurses must always comply with and adhere to state nurse practice acts [NPAs], regulations, standards of care, and ANA's Code of Ethics for Nurses with Interpretive Statements" (ANA, 2015, p. 15). The code is used as a resource by nurse regulators as they consider cases related to violations of the nurse practice act.

Accreditation organizations have established guidelines for the operation of hospitals and health care facilities with the goal of maintaining patient safety. For many years, TJC was the only accrediting body for hospitals and health care agencies in the United States. Since 2008, two other organizations in addition to TJC are available to offer accreditation to health care organizations: the American Osteopathic Association (AOA) and Det Norske Veritas Healthcare's National Integrated Accreditation

TABLE 10-8 Nursing Certification Organizations

Name of Certification Organization	Home Page Web Address
American Nurses Credentialing Center	http://www.nursecredentialing.org/
American Academy of Nurse Practitioners Certification Board	https://www.aanpcert.org/
American Midwifery Certification Board	http://www.amcbmidwife.org/
National Board on Certification and Recertification of Nurse Anesthetists	https://www.nbcrna.com/
Pediatric Nursing Certification Board	https://www.pncb.org/
Oncology Nursing Certification Corporation	https://www.oncc.org/
Board of Certification for Emergency Nurses	https://www.bcencertifications.org/Home.aspx
American Association of Critical-Care Nurses Certification Corporation	https://www.aacn.org/certification?tab=First-Time%20Certification
National League for Nurses Certification for Nurse Educators	http://www.nln.org/professional-development-programs/Certification-for-Nurse-Educators

for Healthcare Organizations (DNV HC NIAHO®). These three organizations have standards used in surveying agencies and are excellent resources to nurse experts.

Authoritative sources consist of scientific literature and institutional resources. When looking for scientific literature, advanced nurses should consider peer-reviewed journal articles and current textbooks, representative of care provided at the time of the incident. An example of the scientific literature that an advanced nurse might review for a case involving a patient error in critical care related to silencing an ECG monitor may be the following: (1) AACN Alarm Management Practice Alert (https://www.aacn.org/clinical-resources/practice-alerts/alarm-management); (2) AACN Accurate Dysrhythmia Monitoring in Adults Practice Alert (https://www.aacn.org/clinical-resources/practice-alerts/dysrhythmia-monitoring); (3) AACN Scope and Standards for Acute and Critical Care Nursing Practice (https://www.aacn.org/store/books/130300/aacn-scope-and-standards-for-acute-and-critical-care-nursing-practice); (4) *AACN Core Curriculum for High Acuity, Progressive, and Critical Care Nursing* (7th ed.) (https://www.aacn.org/store/books/128700/aacn-core-curriculum-for-high-acuity-progressive-and-critical-care-nursing-7th-ed); (5) current critical care textbook;

and (6) ECG monitoring textbook. Most experts have available textbooks pertaining to their specialty; if not, the advanced nurse can rent them online for a fee that is much less than the purchase cost. Ancillary organizations may also have standards that apply to the case. In this particular example, the *Update to Practice Standards for Electrocardiographic Monitoring in Hospital Settings: A Scientific Statement from the American Heart Association* (Sandau et al., 2017) would be an excellent choice for review and consideration.

Again, all scientific literature obtained must address the clinical practice at the time of the incident. References can be sent to the attorney with whom the nurse expert is working along with photocopies of the original sources. These references help to support the expert nurse's written report and testimony.

The involved health care facility is a source of important policy and procedures, standards and guidelines. The nurse expert is responsible for reviewing these documents and addressing their currency and consistency with the standard of care. A *policy* is an institutional expectation for employees and reflects the philosophy of the organization. A *procedure* is a step-by-step description of what to do in a given situation. Examples of procedures include suctioning of a tracheostomy, medication administration, and measurement of cardiac output. A nurse's failure to adhere to a policy or procedure can be seen as a deviation from the standard of care by the plaintiff. Compliance with procedures, however, is viewed by the defense as adherence to the standard of care. How nurses follow policies and procedures are critical to the outcome of a legal case (Grant, 2018b).

Reviewing the Records

Nurse experts need to conduct a systematic review of the collected records. In doing so, it is important that they address only the care provided by the nurse. While the expert may have an opinion on the care provided by other professionals, they cannot speak to the nonnursing standard of care. Begin the review with the complaint followed by an exhaustive analysis of the medical records. Nurse experts can place "sticky" tabs on records as labels for quick review. They are advised not to write any notes on these documents as they are *discoverable*, meaning their notes are able to be requested by an opposing party through a legal process such as a subpoena. All notes should be written on paper separate from the records and kept in a safe place. Since notes are also discoverable, do not include opinions or thoughts that may be damaging to the case.

It is helpful if the nurse expert develops a chronology or timeline of events pertinent to the case. These can be useful in establishing whether any gaps exist for which additional information is needed (Murphy, 2005). Chronologies can be written as a table or timeline. The end product needs to be helpful for rendering an opinion as to the actions of the nurses involved in a malpractice case. The most important details to include are the event, date, time, and brief description of the event. Timelines can be created using a document or PowerPoint in landscape view and inserting lines, arrows, and shapes as needed. Similarly, free software for the development of timelines is available through Timegraphics (https://time.graphics/), Office Timeline (https://www.officetimeline.com/), Preceden (https://www.preceden.com/), and Smartdraw (https://www.smartdraw.com/). A sample timeline created using Smartdraw can be found in **FIGURE 10-1**.

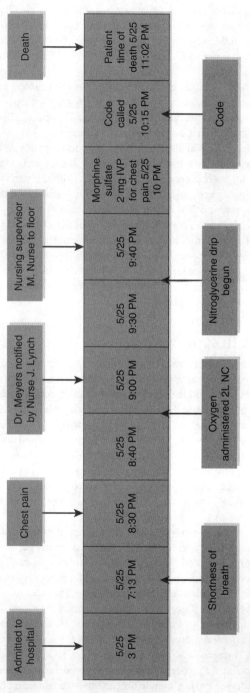

FIGURE 10-1 Timeline of Events.

FIGURE 10-2 Example of Bates Numbering

Medical records usually contain a unique identification number on each page called a Bates number (also known as Bates stamp or Bates code) (**FIGURE 10-2**). Bates numbering is done by scanning or manual production and is used as an organizational method to label and identify legal documents. This method allows for easy reference and retrieval. The nurse expert may want to include the Bates number when referring to particular events in the chronology (Jones, 2008). Bates numbering may also be applied using some versions of Adobe Acrobat.

The nurse expert reviews the records and investigates any areas of concern regarding the nursing care provided, including breaches of standards of care, inaccurate record keeping by the nurses involved, and other issues. The expert should include the names of specific HCPs in the developing chronology as well as any pertinent data such as vital signs, medications, complaints, assessment, and plan of care. It is important to label the chronology as attorney-client privileged material. The chronology should be for in-house use only and not available to anyone other than the attorneys on the case for the firm with whom the nurse expert is working.

Nurse experts also review the deposition transcripts of the involved providers and the fact witnesses (those having knowledge of the events but not named as defendants). *Depositions* are a witness's sworn out-of-court testimony (Legal Information Institute, n.d.). They are used to gather information as part of the discovery process, and may be used at trial. They provide an opportunity for the lawyers to learn, in advance, what the other party and witnesses will say at trial. Depositions are usually taken in an attorney's law office. When reviewing depositions, the nurse expert looks for explanations of events that may differ among the defendants. Depositions may reveal fuller descriptions of nursing practices which may not match with what should be done. As the deposition is reviewed, the nurse expert needs to determine whether opinions about the case have been expanded or altered by the information in the deposition.

Most states permit expert witness depositions except for New York and Pennsylvania, whereby these are only conducted in special instances. Thus, the nurse expert will prepare for either an expert testimony in a pretrial deposition or the development of a written report regarding their opinions. The plaintiff expert witness's deposition or written report is typically completed before the defense expert's report. When reviewing the opposing nurse expert, investigate the background of the nurse expert. The CV is helpful in this regard. Examine any publications or research the opposing expert has conducted, if it applies to the case. Interestingly, one of the primary ways that jurors decide which expert to trust is a comparison of their qualifications (Demorest & Whiteman, 2004). Probe the opposing expert's testimony/report with a critical eye, looking for any weaknesses in facts or supporting evidence.

▶ The Written Report

When providing a written report, the nurse expert summarizes developed opinions along with the facts of the case. There are six key elements that should be included in the report: (1) description of expert's qualifications to render an opinion, (2) list of information reviewed in formulating opinion, (3) summary of the facts of the case, (4) standard of care pertaining to the HCPs, (5) expert's opinion, and (6) conclusion (Myers & Boutier, 2011). Writing this report can seem to be a daunting task as examples of these are usually not found in the literature (**EXEMPLAR 10-1**).

The initial paragraph of the report should begin with a statement about the expert's specialty, place and length of employment, length of time in specialty and nursing in general, along with education and certifications. This helps to establish the advanced nurse as the expert in the context of the legal case. Next, the nurse expert lists the materials that have been reviewed for report preparation. A brief summary of the facts of the case is included to establish that the expert is familiar with the records, testimony, and other materials provided. The nurse expert can later highlight certain facts in support of his or her position regarding the appropriateness of the care provided. In this part of the report, the expert identifies the care that should have been provided the patient in the case and supports this with the relevant standards of care.

The summary sets the stage for the next section of the report in which the nurse expert renders an opinion as to causation. *Causation* makes the crucial link between

---

 EXEMPLAR 10-1 Sample Nurse Expert Report Format

January 10, 2018
Martha Smith, MSN, RN, CCRN
800 World Place
Spring Hill, PA 19100

Ms. Hortense Bragg, Esq.
1313 Mockingbird Lane
Mockingbird Heights, PA 14330
Re: Delores Dee v. St. Elsewhere Hospital CASE NUMBER

Dear Ms. Bragg: [Use business letter format. Available via Web search]

[Introductory comments:

- Thank you for the opportunity.
- Acknowledge expertise.
- Review credentials, including certifications and academic degrees.
- May provide relevant work history. Keep this information brief.]

[(1) Acknowledge the relevant medical records that have been reviewed and the associated dates.

(2) Following this sentence or two, list the additional records that have been reviewed. For example:

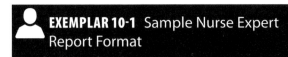

EXEMPLAR 10-1 Sample Nurse Expert Report Format *(continued)*

"I have reviewed the records for the care of Ms. Dee. Specific attention was paid to those aspects of care provided the plaintiff on May 21, 2015 to May 23, 2017. Additionally, I have examined the following in preparation of this report:

- Complaint Delores Dee v. St. Elsewhere Hospital, et al.
- Medical Records from St. Elsewhere Hospital (5/21/2017 to 5/23/2017)
- Medical Records from Mountville Family Practice
- Medical Records from Friendly Family Practice
- Medical Records from Meister Orthopedic Group
- Deposition of Anna Hunt, MD
- Deposition of Amy Welsh, RN
- Plaintiff's Expert Witness, Harriett Falcone, MS, RN"]

[Provide a statement that acknowledges that the provided opinion is offered with a reasonable degree of professional certainty. Make clear that the opinion is based on the provided materials. Include that the opinion has been considered within the context of acceptable and relevant professional nursing standards. If there are specific standards of nursing care, provide this information.]

[Provide succinctly detailed case information. Avoid jargon. Avoid abbreviations unless they have been identified earlier in the summary. Details should be chronological. Make certain that details are consistent. For example, when addressing the right side of the body, ensure that the right side is consistently included and is, in fact, the correct side.]

[Respond to the plaintiff's expert summary. What is the expert missing? Why is the expert incorrect? Keep this evaluation professional and based on facts, including professional standards of care, policies and procedures, and other evidence-based information.]

[Summary statements. Keep this brief and clearly stated. Incorporate professional, peer-reviewed (ideally) references if such are available, to support conclusions.]
Sincerely,

[Signature block. A proper signature should be inserted. Do not include handwritten credentials.]
Full name, credentials

[Once the document is signed and completed, save it in Word form for personal records. Save it in portable text format (PDF), locked to editing, and submit this version electronically to the attorney using delivery and read receipts. If sent via postal mail, send certified with signature required.]

a person or agency's behavior and harm to another individual. These opinions should be offered within a "reasonable probability" (greater than 51% certainty) and that phrase should appear in the report (Myers & Boutier, 2011). The final area of the report is a conclusion or summation of what has been written. Include the fact that the expert reserves the right to alter or amend the opinion if additional information were to become available. The written report is usually reviewed by legal counsel before being officially submitted.

▶ Expert Testimony

Should a deposition be required, it takes place in a less formal atmosphere than a courtroom, but it is still sworn testimony. In certain circumstances, the deposition may be conducted via telephone conference, Web conference, or video recording, if the expert lives in a distant state. A court reporter is available to transcribe the testimony given during the deposition. Opposing counsel uses this opportunity to learn about the nurse expert's opinions, the basis for these opinions, and a sense of the expert's credibility. Therefore, it is very important that the nurse expert fully prepare for the deposition.

The nurse expert should be prepared for the deposition by the attorney with whom he or she is working. The attorney should describe the deposition process and all that it entails. It is helpful if information about the opposing attorney's style is shared with the nurse expert. Important aspects of the case such as the facts, opinion, and the basis for that opinion will be discussed. This includes any supporting standards of care.

It is important to know which documents the nurse expert can bring to the testimony. The deposition notice outlines documents and materials that must be brought by the expert, but care must be given not to include attorney work product. Written or oral materials prepared by or for an attorney, in the course of legal representation, are considered *attorney work product* and are undiscoverable by opposing counsel unless presented at the deposition.

The nurse expert must be ready to support opposition to the opposing nurse expert's opinion. Some attorneys will conduct a mock cross examination so that the expert can anticipate some of the questions that may be asked. This activity helps the attorney and expert in understanding areas needing more preparation (Taggart, 2012).

Basic guidelines for nurses when providing testimony include the following: (1) dress professionally; (2) arrive on time; (3) turn off cell phone and pager; (4) avoid eating, drinking, or chewing gum; (5) sit up in a straight manner; (6) speak in a courteous manner, avoiding the use of slang; and (7) remain calm during questioning. The nurse expert should be well rested for the day of testimony. If the testimony is prolonged, he or she should request a break. A brief time away can aid in replenishing fluids and getting a small snack. This also provides an opportunity to clear one's thoughts and refocus attention (McAuliffe, 2007; Smalls, 2013).

The expert is to listen very carefully to all questions and take time when answering. Only the question posed should be answered and ask for clarification as needed. Questions may range from short yes/no questions to open-ended questions, compound questions, and leading questions. The expert should be careful with open-ended questions that the answer does not include more than needed. Giving lengthy answers to questions and elaborating too much, instead of just answering simply with the facts, can lead to an endless line of questioning.

The nurse expert should be objective, credible and firm in stated convictions without appearing inflexible. It is advantageous to be alert to situations that offer a good time to teach the jury. The expert describes complex nursing and medical tasks and explains medical jargon and abbreviations. On the other hand, opposing counsel may ask questions with the intent to provoke the nurse expert into an emotional response. An emotional response can come back to cause problems. Opposing counsel will note which questions are provoking or causing a hesitant or angry response. Once on the stand at trial, this could affect whether a jury believes the nurse expert (Combs, 2015; Grandjean, Ward, McMullen, & Howie, 2008; Zorn, 2015).

▶ Negotiations and Settlement

Less than 10% of malpractice cases proceed to trial (Boehler, 2007). The overwhelming majority settle out of court. But, of the medical malpractice cases that do go to trial, most result in verdicts for the defense, because insurance companies settle most of the cases they feel they are likely to lose. As a general rule, there are no serious discussions of settlement in medical malpractice cases until after the plaintiff's experts have been deposed. Settlement is not an admission of guilt. It is purely a business decision between attorneys and is based on money. If an agreement between the two parties is unable to be reached, the case will move to a jury trial (Larson & Elliott, 2009).

Occasionally, when negotiations toward settlement are unsuccessful, the parties will agree to participate in either mediation or arbitration. *Mediation*, also called alternative dispute resolution (ADR), is negotiation facilitated by a neutral third-party mediator and its most important characteristic is that it is nonbinding. If either party decides to break off negotiations, they may do so at any time and all content is, by law, confidential. If a case cannot be settled through mediation, the parties then consider whether arbitration, rather than jury trial, would be the best alternative in prosecuting the case to its conclusion. Arbitrators can be selected for their medical background or experience in medical negligence cases. Such an arbitrator will likely understand the issues, both legal and medical, better than a lay jury would. Often in arbitrations, expert reports, rather than live expert testimony, are used to prosecute or defend the action. Both of these techniques offer a solution that is less costly financially and psychologically to the parties involved (Bal, 2009).

▶ Going to Trial

When the involved parties are not able to reach a settlement, the case is set for trial. Arrangements are made for expert witnesses to testify at trial, either in person or by deposition. Pretrial meetings are held with the expert witness so that one knows exactly what to expect. Trial testimony practices are similar to those for depositions. A credible, professional, composed expert witness is likely to have a positive impact on the jury, portraying themselves as a truthful and caring provider (Zimmerman, 2008).

The day of trial can be tiring and may take longer than anticipated. Food and water are not permitted in the court room, so it is beneficial to bring hard candy or mints. Nurse experts should be prepared to wait. The testimony of others may take longer than anticipated or the attorneys may decide to delay the expert's testimony until later in the trial. The role of the nurse expert is to present the facts, the evidence, and the opinion as to the practice of the nurses involved in the case. Responses should be factual and if an answer is not known, it is appropriate to say so. The expert should be mindful that testimony is being given under oath and so all statements must be truthful. Giving an untruthful answer can cause the expert to lose credibility with the jurors and judge and set them up for a charge of perjury and being sued for negligence (Smalls, 2013).

When testifying, it is best to maintain direct eye contact with both the judge and the questioning attorney. When explaining nursing standards, some attorneys prefer that the nurse expert look directly at the jury. In this way, the expert is teaching the jury about an area in which they lack knowledge and need a firm understanding. Simple language that is devoid of medical slang is best so the juror, who is most likely a layperson, can more easily comprehend the information being conveyed.

Even an experienced nurse expert can leave a courtroom feeling uncertain about his or her testimony, and unsuccessful, defeated, and unsatisfied with the experience due to verbal attacks by the opposing attorney. Debriefing following testimony can be a welcome resource at this time. In some instances, the lawyer with whom the nurse expert is working will offer this. Most likely, however, the expert will need to seek out a trusted confidante or counselor (Murray, 2005).

The nurse expert will want to send invoices for completed work commensurate with the agreed upon fee schedule. A W-9 form must also be sent along as the nurse expert will be paid as an independent contractor. When law firms and malpractice insurance companies pay an independent contractor $600 or more over the course of a tax year, they are required to report these payments to the Internal Revenue Service (IRS) on an information return called form 1099-MISC. Law firms and insurance companies use the name, address, and social security number of from the W-9 to complete form 1099-MISC (Patterson, 2006). Since a case can span over several years, invoices can be sent periodically, as files for review are sent to the nurse expert. The final invoice is sent when the notice is received that a case has settled or a trial has ended. Invoices are sent to the attorney with whom the expert has been working. They in turn may send the invoice to the malpractice insurance company representing the defendant as appropriate. Therefore, it is best to allow 6 to 8 weeks for payment.

Begin the invoice by thanking the firm for providing the opportunity to contribute as a nurse expert. Additional information includes the nurse expert's contact information, the case name and file number assigned by the law firm, and dates covered by the review. Most law firms prefer detail such as the records reviewed, date and length of a conference call and individual spoken with, as well as meetings with counsel, time spent, and fee charged. Detailed records of time spent on a case are also helpful should a dispute arise over billable hours (Patterson, 2006). An invoice example is provided in **EXEMPLAR 10-2**.

Calculations can be simplified by billing in 15-minute increments of time. It is suggested that the nurse expert develop a system to track time spent while reviewing records as this is accomplished. Unless the costs are substantial, it is recommended that the nurse expert not bill for costs such as photocopying, parking fees, tolls, and postage for mailing reports or the cost for faxing. It is best to save the receipts as a business expense on taxes (Patterson, 2006). A second and third invoice can be sent if payment is not received in a timely manner. Once a second invoice has not been paid after several weeks, it may be best to have a phone conversation with the attorney, send an email reminder, and/or fax the invoice and W-9 form. Communication is the best way to avoid problems with prompt payment.

A question asked by many nurse experts is whether malpractice insurance, other than that held by the agency in which they work, is needed. Certainly, when a nurse is acting as an expert in a legal matter, it is a good idea to carry malpractice insurance. Traditionally, expert witnesses were considered immune from lawsuit for the testimony they provided in court, even if a mistake was made in providing that testimony. Such testimony was considered common law doctrine upheld by the Supreme Court in *Briscoe v. LaHue*, 460 U.S. (1983), in which the Court ruled that fact witnesses in criminal proceedings were immune from suit for the declarations they made in court. Over time, this idea was broadened through other court decisions to cover expert witness testimony. In recent years, however, several states now allow attorneys to sue their expert witnesses (Hatcher, 2017). While this is a rare occurrence, it is best to carry malpractice insurance.

EXEMPLAR 10-2 Invoice

Dee v. St. Elsewhere Hospital
NO. 2017-14230
Dates Reviewed: Feb-July 2017

Martha Smith
800 World Place
Spring Hill, PA 19100
678-739-4444

November 6, 2017
Mr. Adam Bragg, Esq.
1313 Mockingbird Lane
Mockingbird Heights, PA 14330

Dear Mr. Bragg:
Thank you for submitting to me the Dee v. St. Elsewhere Hospital records for review.
This is the invoice for the final review.

Description	Time (hours)	Fee ($)
Conference Call with Mr. Bragg (July 14, 2017)	1	150.00
Review of Case for Conference Call	2	300.00
Complaint Delores Dee v. St. Elsewhere Hospital, et al.	½	75.00
Medical Records from St. Elsewhere Hospital (5/21/2017 to 5/23/2017)	3	450.00
Medical Records from Mountville Family Practice	½	75.00
Medical Records from Friendly Family Practice	½	75.00
Medical Records from Meister Orthopedic Group	½	75.00
Deposition of Anna Hunt MD	2	300.00
Deposition of Margaret Fan MD	1	150.00
Deposition of Amy Welsh RN	1	150.00
Deposition of Gregory Dee	¼	37.50
Deposition of Linda Dee	¼	37.50
Plaintiff's Expert Witness, Harriett Falcone MS, RN, CLNC	1	150.00
Research conducted for Attorney	2	300.00
Preparation of Expert Report	2	300.00
Total	**17.5**	**2,625.00**

Sincerely,
Martha Smith
Martha Smith, MSN, RN, CCRN
Legal Nurse Consultant

▶ Conclusion

Advanced nurses may be interested in pursuing opportunities to engage as nurse experts, providing that they have the expertise required of a particular case. Other nurses may not be interested in such experiences; however, all advanced nurses need a basic understanding of the mechanisms and expectations underlying the litigation process, particularly related to malpractice and negligence lawsuits. As advocates and leaders, advanced role nurses have an obligation to enlighten and educate colleagues about malpractice beyond suggestions for safe patient care and thorough documentation. These include familiarizing nurses with legal terms, the process of malpractice, and the stress and emotions that accompany the entire process.

References

Adelman, R., & Allen, J. (2014). Reducing the risk of litigation. *Geriatric Nursing, 35*, 80–81.

Agency for Healthcare Research and Quality. (2017, December). AHRQ quality and safety review system. Improved patient safety monitoring. Retrieved January 4, 2018, from https://www.ahrq.gov/professionals/quality-patient-safety/qsrs/index.html

Aiken, T. D., & Warlick, D. T. (2010). The law, standards of care, and liability issues. In A. M. Peterson, & L. Kopishke (Eds.). *Legal nurse consulting principles and practices* (3rd ed., pp. 9–10). Boca Raton, FL: CRC Press.

American Association of Legal Nurse Consultants. (2006). Position statement providing expert nursing testimony regarding nursing negligence. Retrieved from http://www.aalnc.org/page/position-statements.

American Nurses Association. (2010a). Position statement. Just culture. Retrieved January 5, 2018, from http://nursingworld.org/psjustculture.

American Nurses Association. (2010b). ANA's principles for nursing documentation. Silver Springs, MD: Author. Retrieved June 6, 2018, from https://www.nursingworld.org/~4af4f2/globalassets/docs/ana/ethics/principles-of-nursing-documentation.pdf

American Nurses Association. (2015). *Code of ethics for nurses with interpretive statements.* Silver Springs, MD: Author.

American Nurses Association. (2017). State law and regulation. Retrieved from http://www.nursingworld.org/statelawandregulation.

American Nurses Association and National Council of State Boards of Nursing. (2006). Joint statement on delegation. Retrieved from https://www.ncsbn.org/Delegation_joint_statement_NCSBN-ANA.pdf.

Baker, G. R. (2004). Commentary. Harvard Medical practice study. *BMJ Quality & Safety, 13*, 151–152. Retrieved January 3, 2018, from http://qualitysafety.bmj.com/content/13/2/151.

Bal, B. S. (2009). An introduction to medical malpractice in the United States. *Clinical Orthopaedics and Related Research, 467*, 339–347. doi:10.1007/s11999-008-0636-2

Boehler, R. (2007). Malpractice stress and coping: The role of the physician executive. *The Physician Executive, 33*(4), 84–86.

Brady, J. (2016). New system aims to improve patient safety monitoring. Retrieved January 3, 2018, from https://www.ahrq.gov/news/blog/ahrqviews/new-system-aims-to-improve-patient-safety-monitoring.html.

Brennan, T. A., Leape, L. L., Laird, N. M., Hebert, L., Localio, A. R., Lawthers, A. R., . . . Hiatt, H. H. (2004). Incidence of adverse events and negligence in hospitalized patients: Results of the Harvard Medical Practice Study. *Quality Safety Health Care, 13*, 145–152.

Butler, K. A., & Lostritto, M. D. (2015). Malpractice 101: Strategies for defending your practice. *Journal of Radiology Nursing, 34*, 13–24. doi:10.1016/j.jradnu.2014.12.006

Clarke, C., & Mantle, R. (2016). Using risk management to promote person-centred dementia care. *Nursing Standard, 30*, 41–46.

Cohen, M., Rosen, L. F., & Barbacci, M. (2008). Past, present, and future: The evolution of the nurse expert witness. *Journal of Legal Nurse Consulting, 19*(4), 3–8.

Collins, S. E. (2002). Nursing malpractice insurance: Individual insurance policy purchase. *The Florida Nurse, 50*(1), 14–15.

Combs, L. (2015). Nurse experts: Are you prepared for cross-examination? *Journal of Legal Nurse Consulting, 26*(3), 31–33.

Creel, E. L., & Robinson, J. C. (2010). Ethics in independent nurse consulting: Strategies for avoiding ethical quicksand. *Nursing Ethics, 17*(6) 769–776. doi:10.1177/0969733010379179

Croke, E. M. (2003). Nurses, negligence, and malpractice. *American Journal of Nursing, 103*(9), 54–64.

Davis, R., Briggs, M., Arora, S., Moss, R., & Schwappach, D. (2014). Predictors of health care professionals' attitudes towards involvement in safety-relevant behaviours. *Journal of Evaluation in Clinical Practice, 20,* 12–19. doi:10.1111/jep.12073

Demorest, L. E. & Whiteman, N. S. (2004). Voir dire of expert witnesses: Tactical considerations when challenging qualifications. *Medical Malpractice Law and Strategy, 21*(4), 1, 3, 6.

Edwards, M. T. (2017). An organizational framework for patient safety. *American Journal of Medical Quality, 32,* 148–155. doi:10.1177/1062860616632295

Eldridge, N. (2016). Software developers meeting—AHRQ common formats. AHRQ Patient Safety Surveillance for Adverse Events. Retrieved January 4, 2018, from https://www.psoppc.org/psoppc_web/DLMS/downloadDocument?groupId=626&pageNa me=for%20developers%20and%20vendors.

Etchegaray, J. M., Gallagher, T. H., Bell, S. K., Sage, W. M., & Thomas, E. J. (2017). *Advances in patient safety and medical liability. Error disclosure training and organizational culture.* Rockville, MD: Agency for Healthcare Research and Quality. Retrieved from http://www.ahrq.gov/professionals/quality-patient-safety/patient-safety- resources/resources/liability/advances-in-patient-safety-medical-liability/etchegaray.html.

Fowler, M. D. M. (2015). *Guide to the code of ethics for nurses with interpretive statements* (2nd ed.). Silver Spring, MD: Nursesbooks.org. The publishing program of the American Nurses Association.

Grandjean, C., Ward, R., McMullen, P., & Howie, W. (2008). Surviving the deposition blues: Instructions for Advance Practice Nurses in preparing for and participating in a deposition. *Journal for Nurse Practitioners,* November/December, 754–759. doi:10.1016/j.nurpra.2008.08.023

Grant, P. D. (2018a). Anatomy of civil and criminal trials. In D. Ballard and P. DiMeo (Eds.), *Law for nurse leaders* (2nd ed., pp. 72). New York, NY: Springer Publishing.

Grant, P. D. (2018b). Nursing malpractice/negligence and liability. In D. Ballard and P. DiMeo (Eds.), *Law for nurse leaders* (2nd ed., pp. 59–60). New York, NY: Springer Publishing.

Groves, P. S., Finfgeld-Connett, D., & Wakefield, B. J. (2014). It's always something: Hospital nurses managing risk. *Clinical Nursing Research, 23,* 296–313. doi: 10.1177/1054773812468755

Harrison, R., Walton, M., Manias, E., Smith-Merry, J., Kelly, P., Iedema, R., & Robinson, L. (2015). The missing evidence: A systematic review of patients' experiences of adverse events in health care. *International Journal for Quality in Health Care, 27,* 424–442.

Hatcher, T. (2017, February 7). Can an expert witness be sued? [web log]. Retrieved from https://www.theexpertinstitute.com/can-expert-witness-sued/.

Helm, A. (2003). *Nursing malpractice: Sidestepping legal minefields.* Philadelphia, PA: Lippincott Williams & Wilkins.

Hunt, D. R., Verzier, N., Abend, S. L., Lyder, C., Jaser, L. J., Safer, N., & Davern, P. (n.d.). Fundamentals of Medicare patient safety surveillance: Intent, relevance, and transparency. Retrieved January 3, 2018, from http://www.ahrq.gov/downloads/pub/advances/vol2/Hunt.pdf.

Institute for Healthcare Improvement. (2009). *IHI global trigger tool for measuring adverse events* (2nd ed.). IHI Innovation Series white paper. Cambridge, MA: IHI. Retrieved January 3, 2018, from http://www.ihi.org/resources/Pages/Tools/IHIGlobalTriggerToolforMeasuringAEs.aspx.

Institute for Healthcare Improvement. (2018). *IHI global trigger tool for measuring adverse events.* Retrieved January 4, 2018, from http://www.ihi.org/resources/Pages/Tools/IHIGlobalTriggerToolfor MeasuringAEs.aspx.

Jackson, D., & Wilson, S. (2016). Editorial: Harm-free care or harm-free environments: Expanding our definitions and understandings of safety in health care. *Journal of Clinical Nursing, 25,* 3081–3083.

Jacoby, S. R., & Scruth, E. A. (2017). Negligence and the nurse: The value of the code of ethics for nurses. *Clinical Nurse Specialist, 31*(4), 183–185. doi:10.1097/NUR.0000000000000301

Jones, M. P. (2008). Strategies for an effective medical chronology. *Journal of Legal Nurse Consulting, 19*(3), 7–11.

Kohn, L. T., Corrigan, J., & Donaldson, M. S. (2000). *To err is human: Building a safer health system.* Washington, DC: National Academy Press.

Larson, K., & Elliott, R. (2009). Understanding malpractice: A guide for nephrology nurses. *Nephrology Nursing Journal, 36*(4), 375–378.

Larson, K., & Elliott, R. (2010). The emotional impact of malpractice. *Nephrology Nursing Journal, 37*(2), 153–156.

Legal Information Institute. (n.d.). *Deposition.* Wex Legal Dictionary. Retrieved from https://www .law.cornell.edu/wex/deposition.

Martin, J., Benjamin, E. M., Craver, C., Kroch, E. A., Nelson, E. C., & Bankowitz, R. (2016). Measuring adverse events in hospitalized patients: An administrative method for measuring harm. *Journal of Patient Safety, 12*, 125–131.

Mathes, M., & Reifsnyder, J. (2014). *Nurse's law: Legal questions & answers for the practicing nurse.* Indianapolis, IN: Sigma Theta Tau International.

McAuliffe, D. M. (2007). Practice pointers for deposition preparation. *Journal of Nursing Law, 11*(2), 80–83.

Mollon, D. (2014). Feeling safe during an inpatient hospitalization: A concept analysis. *Journal of Advanced Nursing, 70*, 1727–1737. doi:10.1111/jan.12348

Mortaro, A., Moretti, F., Pascu, D., Tessari, L., Tardivo, S., Pancheri, S., . . . Naessens, J. M. (2017). Adverse events detection through global trigger tool methodology: Results from a 5-year study in an Italian hospital and opportunities to improve interrater reliability. *Journal of Patient Safety.* doi:10.1097/PTS.0000000000000381. [Epub ahead of print].

Murphy, E. K. (2005). The expert nurse witness. *Association of Operating Room Nurses Journal, 82*(5), 853–856.

Murray, R. B. (2005). The subpoena and day in court: Guidelines for nurses. *Journal of Psychosocial Nursing, 43*(3), 38–44.

Myers, T. D., & Boutier, B. P. (2011). Preparing a nursing negligence expert report in six paragraphs. *Journal of Legal Nurse Consulting, 22*(2), 13–15.

National Council of State Boards of Nursing. (2016). National guidelines for nursing delegation. *Journal of Nursing Regulation, 7*(1), 5–14.

Nellis, D. L., & George, L. (2012). Preliminary exploration of the use of a medical malpractice self-study module. *The Journal of Continuing Education in Nursing, 43*(5), 225–229. doi:10.3928/00220124-20111115-03

Oliver, R. (2016, February 17). Should nurses consider medical malpractice insurance, too? Minority Nurse. [Web log]. Retrieved from http://minoritynurse.com/should-nurses-consider-medical-malpractice -insurance-too/.

Olson, L. L., & Stokes, F. (2016). The ANA code of ethics for nurses with interpretive statements: Resource for nursing regulation. *Journal of Nursing Regulation, 7*(2), 9–20.

Pappas, I. E., Clutter, L. B., & Maggi, E. (2007). Current legal changes: Innovative legal seminar for nursing students. *Journal of Nursing Law, 11*(4), 197–209.

Parry, G., Cline, A., & Goldmann, D. (2012). Deciphering harm measurement. *JAMA, 307*, 2155–2156.

Patterson, P. (2006). Billing and collections. In P. W. Iyer, J. Aken, & K. W. Condon (Eds.), *Business principles for legal nurse consultants.* Boca Raton, FL: CRC Press.

Pittet, D., Panesar, S. S., Wilson, K., Longtin, Y., Morris, R., Allan, V., . . . Cleary, K. (2011). Involving the patient to ask about hospital hand hygiene: A National Patient Safety Agency feasibility study. *Journal of Hospital Infection, 77*, 299–303.

Pohlman, K. J. (2015). Why you need your own malpractice insurance. *American Nurse Today, 10*(11), 28–30. Retrieved from https://www.americannursetoday.com/need-malpractice-insurance/.

PSNet. (2017). Patient safety primer. Adverse events, near misses, and errors. Retrieved January 5, 2018, from https://psnet.ahrq.gov/primers/primer/34/adverse-events-near- misses-and-errors.

Reising, D. L. (2007). Protecting yourself from malpractice claims. *American Nurse Today, 2*(2). Retrieved from https://www.americannursetoday.com/protecting-yourself-from-malpractice-claims/.

Relias, formerly AHC Media. (2016). More nurses, hospitalists being sued for malpractice, studies say. Retrieved from https://www.ahcmedia.com/articles/137567-more-nurses- hospitalists-being-sued-for-malpractice -studies-say.

Resnick, B., & Guarino, K. (2001). Professional practice what to do if you are sued. *Journal of the American Academy of Nurse Practitioners, 13*(3), 99–100.

Ryll, N. A. (2015). Living through litigation: Malpractice stress syndrome. *Journal of Nursing Radiology, 34*, 35–38. doi:10.1016/j.jradnu.2014.11.007

Sandau, K. E., Funk, M., Auerbach, A., Barsness, G. W., Blum, K., Cvach, M., . . . Wang, P. J., on behalf of the American Heart Association Council on Cardiovascular and Stroke Nursing, Council on Clinical Cardiology, and Council on Cardiovascular Disease in the Young. (2017). Update to practice standards for electrocardiographic monitoring in hospital settings: A scientific statement from the American Heart Association. *Circulation, 136*, e273–e344. doi:10.1161/CIR.0000000000000527

Serembus, J. F., Wolf, Z. R., & Youngblood, N. (2001). Consequences of fatal medication errors for health care providers: A secondary analysis study. *MEDSURG Nursing, 10*, 193– 201.

Smalls, H. T. (2013). So you want to be an expert witness. *Neonatal Network, 32*(2), 125–126. doi:10.1891/0730-0832.32.2.125

Stokes, F. (2015). Code of ethics for nurses. *District of Columbia Nurse: Regulation, Education, Practice, 12*(2), 6. Retrieved from https://doh.dc.gov/sites/default/files/dc/sites/doh/release_content /attachments/DCNurse_43.pdf.

Sullivan v. Edward Hosp., No. 95409, 2004 WL 228956 (Ill. Feb 5, 2004) Amicus brief submitted to Illinois Supreme Court – Karen Butler, Esq. American Association of Nurse Attorneys. Retrieved from http://www.illinoiscourts.gov/opinions/supremecourt/2004/february/opinions/html/95409.htm.

Taggart, M. D. (2012). How to prepare for and manage the depositions of expert witnesses. *Los Angeles Lawyer*, July-August, 20–25.

U.S. Department of Health and Human Services. (n.d.). *National practitioner data bank medical malpractice payment reports (MMPR) and adverse action reports (AAR)*. Retrieved from https:// www.npdb.hrsa.gov/resources/npdbstats/npdbStatistics.jsp#contentTop.

U.S. Department of Health and Human Services. (2017). *HIPPA for professionals*. Retrieved from https://www.hhs.gov/hipaa/for-professionals/index.html.

Walsh, K. E., Harik, P., Mazor, K. M., Perfetto, D., Anatchkova, M., Biggins, C., . . . Tjia, J. (2017). Measuring harm in health care. Optimizing adverse event review. *Medical Care, 55*, 436–441.

Winning, A., M., Merandi, J. M., Lewe, D., Stepney, L. M. C., Liao, N. N., Fortney, C. A., & Gerhardt, C. A. (2018). The emotional impact of errors or adverse events on healthcare providers in the NICU: The protective role of coworker support. *Journal of Advanced Nursing, 74*, 172–180. doi:10.1111/jan.13403

Wolf, Z. R., Serembus, J. F., Smetzer, J., Cohen, H., & Cohen, M. (2000). Responses and concerns of healthcare providers to medication errors. *Clinical Nurse Specialist, 14*, 278–290.

Zimmerman, P. G. (2008). Providing expert witness testimony: Lessons learned. *Journal of Legal Nurse Consulting, 19*(2), 15–17.

Zorn, E. (2015). Serving as a nurse expert witness: A virtual roundtable discussion. *Journal of Legal Nurse Consulting, 26*(3), 41–44.

Index

Note: Page numbers followed by *b, f,* or *t* indicate material in boxes, figures, or tables, respectively.

C

E

N

Q

QSEN (Quality and Safety Education for
Nurses), 289–290, 291*b*
QSRS (Quality and Safety Review System), 346
Quality and Safety Education for Nurses
(QSEN), 289–290, 291*b*
Quality and Safety Review System (QSRS), 346
quality improvement, 318–335
lean thinking, 326–335, 334*f*, 335*f*
measurement for improvement/
measurement for research, 319, 319*t*
plan-do-check act (PDCA). *See* plan-do-
check act (PDCA/PDSA)
Six Sigma, 324–326, 324*f*, 326*t*, 330–331
Quick Start Guide, 232–233, 232*f*

R

rapid cycle improvement model (RCIM),
327–328
Rapid Estimate of Adult Literacy in Medicine
(REALM), 243
RCA (root cause analysis), 248, 332–333
RCA² (Root Cause Analysis and Actions), 332
RCIM (rapid cycle improvement model),
327–328
readability tools, 240–242
REALM (Rapid Estimate of Adult Literacy in
Medicine), 243
records. *See also* reports
electronic, 78
electronic health record (EHR), 335–336
expert review and analysis, 362, 363*t*
reviewing, 369, 370*f*, 371
timeline, 369, 370*f*
references included on résumé, 29–30
reflection, 2–11
discussion opportunity, 63–65
relationships, 11
self-care practices, 3–10
reflective activity, 13
reflective practice, 11–13
regulations
variability in practice requirements, 17
workplace violence, 146–147, 151–152
relationships
performance management, 76–77
self-care practices, 11
staff and students, 259
student-preceptor, 92
reliability of competencies, 250–251
religious views on environmentalism, 185
remote video monitoring, 125

reports. *See also* records
budget variance reporting, 127
To Err Is Human report, 271
outcome report card, 303–304
Quality Reports*, 306
voluntary incident reporting, 348
workplace violence, 153, 163–164
written, 372–373
resources
*Children's Environmental Health:
Online Resources for Healthcare
Providers*, 207
community, 330
consumption reduction, 190–191
distribution, 184
error disclosure, 350*t*
health literacy, 222–234
health literacy Web resources, 222*t*–223*t*
Medical Society Consortium on Climate
and Health, 209
outcomes, 310–312
workplace violence, 172–173
results standards, 83
résumé
constructing, 25–26
credentials, 26–27, 26*t*
critique, 28
curriculum vitae vs., 22, 22*t*
designing, 25–28
discussion boards and forums, 33–34
disseminating, 28–29
education information, 27
electronic, 29
electronic expertise, 34–35
experiences/employment, 27
LISTSERV, 32–33, 33*b*
organizational involvement, 31–32
professional association leadership,
30–31, 31*b*
references, 29–30
retainer, 361
revenue budget, 115–116
risk, liability, 353
risk oversimplification, 280
Robert's Rules of Order, 55
Root Cause Analysis and Actions
(RCA²), 332
root cause analysis (RCA), 248, 332–333

S

safety
concerns, 132
culture of safety, 345